Survival Strategies for Nurses in Managed Care

Visit our website at **www.mosby.com**

SURVIVAL STRATEGIES FOR NURSES IN MANAGED CARE

TONI G. CESTA, PhD, RN, FAAN
Director of Case Management
Saint Vincent Catholic Medical Centers of New York
Manhattan Region
New York, New York;
Principal, Case Managers Solutions, LLC
Tucson, Arizona

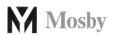 Mosby

An Imprint of Elsevier Science

St. Louis   London   Philadelphia   Sydney   Toronto

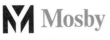

Mosby

An Imprint of Elsevier Science

Vice President, Publishing Director: Sally Schrefer
Acquisitions Editor: Yvonne Alexopoulos
Senior Developmental Editor: Melissa K. Boyle
Project Manager: Patricia Tannian
Production Editor: Steve Hetager
Book Design Manager: Gail Morey Hudson
Cover Design: E. Rohne Rudder

Mosby, Inc.
An Imprint of Elsevier Science
11830 Westline Industrial Drive
St. Louis, Missouri 63146

Printed in the United States of America

Library of Congress Cataloging-in-Publication Data

Survival strategies for nurses in managed care / [edited by] Toni G. Cesta.
   p. ; cm.
  Includes bibliographical references and index.
  ISBN 0-323-01397-X
    1. Managed care plans (Medical care) 2. Nursing. 3. Nursing—Effect of managed care
on. I. Cesta, Toni G.
  [DNLM: 1. Managed Care Programs—Nurses' Instruction. 2. Nursing. 3. Case
Management. 4. Nurse's Role. W 130.1 S963 2002]
  RA413 .S87 2002
  610.73—dc21
                                                                    2002019264

02 03 04 05 06 TG/FF 9 8 7 6 5 4 3 2 1

Contributors

Eileen Barton, RN, MA
Manager, Case Management
Saint Vincent Catholic Medical
    Centers of New York
Manhattan Region
New York, New York

Elizabeth A. Bonetti, RN, MA, MS
Director, Patient Care Management
The Brooklyn Hospital Center
Brooklyn, New York

Sandra Schmidt Bunkers, RN, PhD, FAAN
Associate Professor and Chair of Nursing
Department of Nursing, Augustana College
Sioux Falls, South Dakota

Connie Burgess, MS, RN
Partner, Health Inter Connexions
Sioux Falls, South Dakota

Patricia A. Chin, RN, DNSc
Associate Professor, School of Nursing
California State University–Los Angeles
Los Angeles, California

Christine Coughlin, RN, EdD
Chief Nurse Executive
Vice President, Clinical Services
Montefiore Medical Center
Bronx, New York

Margaret Davino, JD, RN
Vice President and General Counsel
St. Joseph's Hospital and Medical Center
Paterson, New Jersey

**Deborah V. DiBenedetto, RN, BSN, MBA,
    COHN-S/CM, ABDA**
President, DVDiBenedetto & Associates, Ltd.
Yonkers, New York;
Executive Vice President, CMGT, Inc.
Scottsdale, Arizona;
President, American Association of
    Occupational Health Nurses
Atlanta, Georgia

Susan M. Erickson, RN, MPH
Case Management Industry Advisor
3M Health Information Systems Consulting
    Services
Atlanta, Georgia

Elizabeth Corso Falter, RN, CNAA, BC
Falter & Associates, Inc.
Tucson, Arizona

William A. Falter, MA
Falter & Associates, Inc.
Tucson, Arizona

Laurie J. Frahm, RN, BSN, MSN
Case Management Training Consultant
    Health Partners
Minneapolis, Minnesota

Ruth A. Hanson, MS, RN
Internal Consultant, MeritCare Health System
Fargo, North Dakota

Linda Hertz, RN, CNS
Nurse Case Manager—Behavioral Health
Immanuel–St. Joseph's Hospital
Mayo Health System
Mankato, Minnesota

Lauren Hoffmann, BS, MA
Medical Writer
Atlanta, Georgia

Mary Krentzman, MS, RN
Community Case Manager
Hartford Physician Hospital Organization
Hartford Hospital
Hartford, Connecticut

Laura A. Kukowski, BSN, RN
Critical Care Nurse
New York Presbyterian Hospital
New York, New York

Gerri S. Lamb, PhD, RN, FAAN
Associate Dean for Clinical & Community
    Services
University of Arizona
College of Nursing
Tucson, Arizona

Sandra B. Lewenson, EdD, RN, FAAN
Professor and Associate Dean for
    Academic Affairs
Lienhard School of Nursing, Pace University
Pleasantville, New York

Francesca Losito, RN, MPA
Director of Hospital Relations
Visiting Nurse Service of New York
New York, New York

Diana J. Mason, PhD, RN, FAAN
Editor-in-Chief
American Journal of Nursing
Lippincott Williams & Wilkins
New York, New York

Ellen R. Mitchell, RNC, MA
RN Case Manager
Department of Case Management
Saint Vincent Catholic Medical Centers
    of New York
Manhattan Region
New York, New York

Laurel Nadler, MPA
Manager, Ambulatory Managed Care Operations
Saint Vincent Catholic Medical Centers
    of New York
Manhattan Region
New York, New York

Jeffrey P. O'Donnell, MS, RN, FNP
Lecturer and Family Nurse Practitioner
Lienhard School of Nursing, Pace University
Pleasantville, New York

Judith L. Papenhausen, PhD, RN
Chairperson and Professor
Department of Nursing
California State University–Los Angeles
Los Angeles, California

Barbara A. Ryan, RN, BS, JD
Partner
Aaronson, Rappaport, Feinstein & Deutsch, LLP
New York, New York

Tina H. Sernick, BSN, JD
Associate
Aaronson, Rappaport, Feinstein & Deutsch, LLP
New York, New York

Lawrence F. Strassner, RN, MS
Manager, Healthcare Consulting
Cap Gemini Ernst & Young, LLC
New York, New York;
Associate Faculty
School of Hygiene and Public Health
Department of Health Policy and Management
Johns Hopkins University
Baltimore, Maryland

Hussein A. Tahan, MS, DNSc(c), RN, CNA
Director of Nursing, Cardiac Specialties
Columbia Presbyterian Medical Center
New York, New York

Carol Taylor, CSFN, RN, MSN, PhD
Director, Center for Clinical Bioethics;
Assistant Professor, Nursing
Georgetown University
Washington, DC

Donna Zazworsky, MS, RN, CCM
Principal, Case Manager Solutions, LLC;
Director of Home Health and Outreach
St. Elizabeth of Hungary Clinic;
Adjunct Clinical Assistant Professor
College of Nursing, University of Arizona;
Tucson, Arizona

Lisa M. Zerull, MSN, RN
Program Director, Valley Health System
Winchester, Virginia;
Case Management Consultant
Future Health Care
Chapel Hill, North Carolina

Reviewers

Sherry L. Aliotta, RN, BSN, CCM
CEO, S.A. Squared, Inc.
Farmington Hills, Michigan

Michal Boyd, RN, MSN, MS, ND, C-ANP
Professor
University of Colorado Health Sciences Center
Denver, Colorado;
Adult Nurse Practitioner
Boulder Internal Medicine
Boulder, Colorado

Michelle M. Boylan, DM(c), MA, BSN, RN
Vice President, Quality Management
  Community Healthcare, Inc.
Wausau Hospital, Wausau, Wisconsin;
Adjunct Faculty, University of Phoenix;
Adjunct Faculty, National American University
Colorado Springs, Colorado

Joyce Brett, MS, RN, CCM, CRRN, CDMS
Team Manager, Zurich Services
Schaumburg, Illinois

Connie Commander, RN, CCM, ABDA
Director of Medical Management
Methodist Care Health Plan
Houston, Texas

Connie Gardner, BA, RN, CCM
Vice President of New Business Development
Careguide
Northbrook, Illinois
National Treasurer
Case Management Society of America
Little Rock, Arkansas

Betty Guleserian, RN, MS, CCM, CDMS, CRC
Case Manager
Proficient Case Management, LLC
Carol Stream, Illinois

Judy A. Harris, BSN, MS, MSN
Advanced Registered Nurse Practitioner, Nurse
  Practitioner Certified
Seniors First HealthCare
Tallahassee, Florida

Alison Johnson, BSN, MBA
Healthcare Management Consultant
Milliman & Robertson, Inc.
Minneapolis, Minnesota

Dee McGonigle, PhD, RNC, LCCE, FACCE
President
Educational Advancement Associates (EAA)
Kittanning, Pennsylvania;
Associate Professor of Nursing and Information
  Sciences & Technology (IST)
Pennsylvania State University
University Park, Pennsylvania;
Editor, Online Journal of Nursing Informatics
Kittanning, Pennsylvania;
Member
Tri-State Healthcare Informatics Professionals
Pittsburgh, Pennsylvania

Tommie L. Norris, RN, DNS(c)
Assistant Professor
Loewenberg School of Nursing
University of Memphis
Memphis, Tennessee

Patricia Orchard, BSN, Med, MSHA
Assistant Vice President
Case Management Virtua Health
Voorhees, New Jersey

To

my family and friends.

Thank you. I love you.

Flowers

Flowers come in all different colors,
All shapes and sizes too.
Why the flowers come that way,
We really have no clue.
But, if you stop to think about it,
They're much like me and you.

Zara Cesta Fishkin, age 10
2001

Foreword

In the years ahead, managed care will be considered one of the most profound influences on the American healthcare system. Started as a social experiment, it has emerged as the focal point for debate over basic values and rights in healthcare. Managed care is the lightning rod around which we are evaluating our most deeply held beliefs about patient rights, choice, access to healthcare, and accountability for quality and cost-effectiveness. No sector of the American public or the healthcare system has been immune from the controversy. With consumers at the core, all stakeholders, including employers, health plan administrators, legislators, and healthcare professionals, have been deeply touched and changed by their experiences with managed care.

Although some analysts are now predicting the demise of managed care, most observers suggest that we are now witnessing a critical transition point in its history. Soon, we may see important shifts in some of the most basic structures of healthcare and managed care. If the forecasters are correct, consumers are waiting in the wings to take center stage—a state of affairs that has been central to nursing belief and practice for over a century. It is likely that all players on the healthcare scene will continue to experience major changes in what they currently are doing and what they can expect to be doing in the decades ahead. This, in great part, is the legacy of managed care as we have known it.

The publication of *Survival Strategies for Nurses in Managed Care* could not be timed better. We are approaching a critical mass of voices calling for revolutionary changes in healthcare. It is absolutely essential that nurses fully understand and appreciate managed care in the context of its history, its opportunities, and its pitfalls to influence the shape of a new healthcare system. Make no mistake about this: the experience and lessons of managed care *will* dominate thinking and decision making for the future. We must survive together to translate what we have learned into creating the system we want for the future.

It is essential that we bring together critical analysis of managed care with our passions for equitable access, choice, and quality in order to sit at the table with the policymakers, the CEOs of Fortune 500 companies, the leaders of the healthcare industry, and others who are likely to drive the coming changes. Numerous surveys have shown that the American public trusts nurses, perhaps more than any other profession, to make the right decisions for the right reasons. This book and the wisdom shared by its authors provide us with tools that are essential for the rigorous work ahead.

The chapters of this book document the history and experiences of nurses and nursing practice in managed care. Managed care has been a source of tremendous opportunities to design, implement, and evaluate new and innovative nursing programs. It has taught us important and frequently difficult lessons about incentives and payment structures that can nurture or destroy promising programs. It has opened doors for contracts for advanced practice nurses and new practice models that reward some of our most cherished contributions, including health promotion, disease prevention, chronic illness management, and care coordination. It has closed other doors. My own experiences in designing and leading nursing programs in managed care, including one of four national Community Nursing Organization demonstrations, have been among the most exhilarating, frustrating, and fulfilling of my 30 years in nursing.

This book offers testimony to the skill and competence of nurses in analyzing and refining managed care in ways that are consistent with the mission of nursing and the will of the American public. In their roles as administrators of managed care plans, chief hospital executives, acute care and community nurses, faculty, case managers, and nurse practitioners, our colleagues have demonstrated that nurses, whether on the front lines or behind the scenes, have contributed in many significant ways to the evolution of managed care.

As all good books do, *Survival Strategies for Nurses in Managed Care* leaves us wanting more. We want to turn the last page and be transported into the future to see how our healthcare system will fare in the years ahead. I for one would like to be assured that the healthcare system that I am likely to use in the next 20 or 30 years, along with my aging cohort of baby boomers, will match my vision for caring and quality. No such luck. We will all need to take these lessons of survival to heart and use them—with all of the strategy and passion we can muster—to create our future together.

Gerri S. Lamb, PhD, RN, FAAN

Preface

Healthcare continues to change at lightning speed. Nursing in the twenty-first century continues to evolve in response to the challenges posed by never-ending change. Clearly, one of the most dramatic paradigm shifts affecting nursing and nurses has been the rapid and pervasive growth of managed care in the United States. Although you may not yet be directly affected by these changes, you are probably affected in a myriad of indirect ways. You may have experienced changes in your healthcare insurance, downsizing at the organization where you work, increasing demands by your patients, systems stretched to their maximum capacity, or fewer resources with which to care for your patients.

Whether you have been affected directly or indirectly, you have most certainly been affected. When Mosby asked me to edit this book, I began to think of all the ways in which nurses might be influenced by managed care or might themselves have an influence on managed care. I tried to select chapter topics that would cover a broad range of issues related to managed care today as well as in the future. The selected chapter topics span from the business side of managed care, including Wall Street and resource management, to patients as consumers, and quality and outcomes. They include personal experiences, case studies, and vignettes. They also include practical information related to managed care, its inner workings, and its effects on the healthcare industry.

Among the many challenges that the nursing profession will face over the next 10 years will be the need to address managed care as it relates to the ways in which we educate our nurses, including both new nurses and nurses seeking advanced practice degrees. Additional challenges will include defining new strategies for educating our patients and responding to their fears and concerns. Finally, nurses will need to find their place in our emerging healthcare delivery systems. How we define our roles across the continuum of care, in our managed care organizations, in our educational settings, and in our professional organizations will be critical to our effectiveness in helping to shape healthcare over the next two decades.

So much of what has been written on managed care has been written by physicians and business people; nurses deal with the implications of a managed care world every day. It is important that our voices be heard and that we begin to define the elements of healthcare delivery from a nursing perspective. To sit back and let this turmoil of change occur around us would be a huge mistake. To allow others to define our response to managed care would also be a mistake. Therefore this book attempts to bring nursing's voice to the forefront and to allow nurses an opportunity to read the experiences and struggles of their peers. After all, nursing's experience is a unique one. Therefore our reactions and responses should also be unique.

The brave authors who contributed chapters to this book did so with a vision. That vision was to address a specific issue directly affected by managed care and to pro-vide information and experiences that might help other nurses as they struggle with similar issues. This approach is a unique approach to the literature on managed care. It will hopefully set the stage for many more nurses to share their ideas, experiences, and suggestions for future change.

Toni G. Cesta, PhD, RN, FAAN

Contents

Detailed Contents

Introduction to Managed Care

Nursing's Voice and Presence in Today's Managed Healthcare Environment

Hussein A. Tahan

KEY LESSONS IN THIS CHAPTER

- The increase in managed care's popularity has led to new and nontraditional roles for nurses.
- The dominant driving force for change in the roles assumed by nurses in a managed care environment is financially based.
- Demand management is a technique used by managed care organizations to reduce member demand for healthcare services and ultimately contain costs.
- Even if managed care were to disappear, cost-effectiveness and quality of care would continue to remain a priority in healthcare management and delivery.
- The survival of nurses in tomorrow's managed care/healthcare market will depend on their knowledge, skills, competencies, and openness to new roles.

Managed care has rapidly dominated healthcare delivery, financing, and reimbursement structures in the United States. Although its roots go back to the early part of the twentieth century, it did not gain wide acceptance and popularity until the 1990s. Today it is very unlikely that a healthcare organization does not deal on some level with managed care organizations (MCOs). This popularity has led healthcare and nursing executives to implement new methods and strategies to deliver cost-effective and high-quality care, resulting in new and nontraditional roles for nurses. These strategies have enhanced the status of the nursing profession and increased the visibility and voice of nurses, specifically in the strategic decisions made to address the demands and needs of managed patient care delivery systems. Moreover, today nursing is often represented at the managed care contracts negotiating table, where nurse executives collaborate with the chief operating, chief financial, and chief managed care officers in their organizations in the evaluation and negotiation of prospective managed care contracts. It also is not unusual to witness the rejection of a contract because of nursing care delivery issues or demands that are considered outrageous or unrealistic. This chapter focuses on the contributions of nurses to the delivery of healthcare services in the current managed care environment.

OVERVIEW OF MANAGED CARE

Healthcare consumers, payers, providers, and others have exchanged the term *managed care* as if it were a simple and most desirable way of delivering healthcare services. In fact, it is a complex phenomenon that means different things to different people. Some think that managed care is any type of health insurance with utilization review components. Others view it as capitation; still others equate managed care with integrated delivery systems, where services are provided across the full continuum of care (Tindall et al, 2000). Although these thoughts may not be unusual to managed care practices, the intensity of the managed care services provided and the types of reimbursement methods applied varies widely. Moreover, the involvement of nursing in these environments differs based on the degree and complexity of the managed services offered to the consumers or demanded by the payers. Nurses play crucial roles in the success or failure of the efforts their organizations exert to meet the demands of managed care. The intensity of their roles and the scope of their services usually depend on the stage of managed care (i.e., the level of managed care penetration) that describes their healthcare organization and geographical region. Figure 1-1 presents some examples of these roles and describes the scope of services provided by nurses based on the five stages of managed care markets defined by Tindall et al (2000).

The efforts exerted to control the escalating healthcare costs in the 1990s brought about unprecedented new roles and a new voice for nurses. The environment of managed care has changed where and how nurses practice (Kersbergen, 2000). For example, nurses are found today in roles in which decisions are made to authorize or deny healthcare services or in independent practice, such as owners of independent case management companies, where they are responsible and accountable for total patient care, including rehabilitative services.

The term *managed care* has become a generic label but still lacks a clear or standardized definition. The many definitions described in the literature are dependent on the structure of the care delivery model and the reimbursement strategies employed. Although it lacks a universally accepted definition, managed care may be described simply as a system of healthcare delivery that aims to manage the cost and quality of healthcare services and to enhance access to these services. The most desirable system is one that demonstrates an effective balance between access, cost, and quality. Attaining such a balance is not easy, however, and it demands the cooperation and collaboration of the payers, providers, and consumers of healthcare.

Managed care attempts to create an "organized system where care that is medically necessary is delivered by properly trained and educated healthcare professionals, in appropriate locations and facilities, and under practice guidelines that are likely to produce the best results for patients" (Knight, 1998, p 21). Managed care is both a type of health insurance and a type of healthcare delivery system, that is, it focuses on both delivery and reimbursement of healthcare services. It is a health insurance in that MCOs contract with purchasers

Least
Managed
Care

Stage % Managed	Characteristics of Environment	Role of Nurse/ Practice Environment

Stage I
5%-10%
	Unstructured framework
	• Little managed care/indemnity
	  insurance dominance
	• Hospitals and physicians
	  function independently with little
	  or no affiliations
	• Overuse of inpatient care
	• Mostly FFS
	• Hospitals are revenue centers
		• Nurses are primarily hospital-based
		• Patient care is fragmented and
		  duplicative
		• No pressure to discharge patients
		  from hospitals
		• More services are considered more
		  revenue
		• Competition is based on technology

Stage II
10%-30%
	Loose alliances
	• Primarily discounted FFS and
	  per diem
	• Limited capitation
	• Some consolidation of hospitals
	• Some affiliations of hospitals
	  and physicians
	• Focus on cost of care
	• Hospitals no longer revenue
	  centers; excess beds
	• Purchasers have more power
		• Use of nurses as case managers
		  begins
		• Focus on elimination of delays and
		  duplication of care processes
		• Streamlining provision of services
		• Focus on cost-effectiveness begins
		• Pressure to reduce length of
		  hospital stay and number of beds
		• Increased interest in providing care in
		  settings other than hospital,
		  particularly in home

Stage III
30%-50%
	Consolidation
	• Strong managed care
	  penetration
	• More capitation
	• HMOs, PPOs, and medical
	  groups begin to consolidate
	• Increased presence of primary
	  care practices
	• Hospital beds continue to
	  decline
	• Coordinated continuum of care
	  services
	• Specialty medical groups begin
	  to form
		• Integrative approach to care begins
		• Nurses in case management roles:
		  payer-based and provider-based
		• Continuum of care approach to
		  patient care management
		• Smaller hospitals
		• Nurses focus on reimbursement
		  issues: authorization of services,
		  denials, and appeals
		• Competition is based on price

Stage IV
50%-80%
	Competing systems
	• Minimal FFS
	• Mostly capitation
	• Employer coalitions compete to
	  control market
	• Large providers and insurers
	  align together
	• Physician networks grow larger
		• Integrated approach to care delivery
		  is the norm
		• Discharge planning, utilization
		  review, and clinical care
		  management are integrated in role
		  of nurse case managers
		• Continuum of care focus for patient
		  care management regardless of

Figure 1-1   The five stages of managed care and the role of the nurse.

Continued

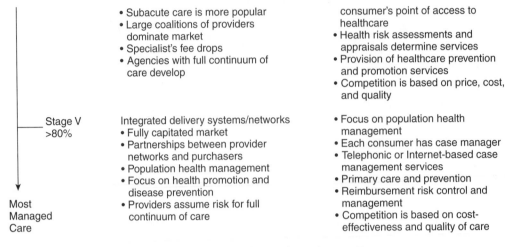

- Subacute care is more popular
- Large coalitions of providers dominate market
- Specialist's fee drops
- Agencies with full continuum of care develop

consumer's point of access to healthcare
- Health risk assessments and appraisals determine services
- Provision of healthcare prevention and promotion services
- Competition is based on price, cost, and quality

Stage V
>80%

Integrated delivery systems/networks
- Fully capitated market
- Partnerships between provider networks and purchasers
- Population health management
- Focus on health promotion and disease prevention
- Providers assume risk for full continuum of care

- Focus on population health management
- Each consumer has case manager
- Telephonic or Internet-based case management services
- Primary care and prevention
- Reimbursement risk control and management
- Competition is based on cost-effectiveness and quality of care

Most
Managed
Care

Figure 1-1, cont'd For legend see p. 5.

(e.g., individuals, employers, unions) to provide comprehensive health insurance in return for a certain fee called a *premium*. It is a healthcare delivery system because a contractual agreement or arrangement is made between the purchaser and the MCO to provide certain agreed-upon healthcare services and between the MCO and the healthcare services provider in return for a specific reimbursement schedule. The health plan or policy (insurance policy) the purchaser chooses determines the services provided. Healthcare professionals usually provide the services stipulated in the policy in return for a certain fixed fee (i.e., reimbursement) schedule such as a capitated rate. How managed care services are provided to purchasers is discussed in Chapter 3.

MCOs are more complex today than ever before. They are organized in a variety of ways, depending on the managed care services or products they provide and the reimbursement methods they apply. They are owned by managed care firms, physician groups and associations, hospital associations, physician-hospital organizations, private investors, commercial health insurers, integrated delivery systems or networks, or other organizations. MCOs are either for-profit or not-for-profit and provide services to consumers on a local, state, regional, or national level (Knight, 1998). The wider their geographical coverage, the more complex are their structure and processes. They may offer comprehensive healthcare services or specific medical services such as mental health, dental, or vision care. The variety of services provided by an MCO is indicative of its complexity and intensity. Usually the services provided are defined and clarified in the health policy or plan purchased by a consumer or employer.

Attempting to define the different types of MCOs is not an easy task, considering today's dynamic healthcare environment. Nevertheless, distinctions can be made regarding the degree of cost, utilization of services, and quality control exerted by the MCO. Kongstvedt (2001) describes MCOs based on a continuum of managed care intensity (i.e., from least to most managed). Examples of the different types of MCOs and managed care practices are presented in Figure 1-2. Depending on the degree to which the care is provided as "managed

Least
Managed

Type of Organization	Characteristics	Reimbursement Methods
Indemnity plan with fee for service (FFS)	Complete freedom of choice to consumers	FFS
Managed indemnity plan	Free choice and FFS; however, insurer exercises some degree of control over utilization of services.	Discounted fees, managed FFS
Preferred provider organization (PPO)	Provides medical care to individuals at negotiated fee. Usually insurer accepts financial risk.	Negotiated/10%-30% discounted FFS
Point-of-service plan (POS)	Members are required to choose primary care provider (PCP). Staying within network of providers is not mandatory.	100% reimbursement if staying within network. As low as 70% if outside network
Independent practice association (IPA)	Insurer contracts directly with provider groups who have agreed to bear some financial risk for performance.	Capitation or FFS with financial incentives
Health maintenance organization (HMO)	Prepaid organization that provides services to members at preset fee. Services provided by either staff or independent group of providers.	Capitation/per-member-per-month (PMPM) rate
Open panel HMO	Members are required to select PCP who functions as gatekeeper. Referral to specialist by PCP is not mandatory.	PMPM, copayment is higher for self-referral
Network IPA	Multispecialty provider group in contract with HMO on exclusive basis	Capitation; network IPA may reimburse its providers on either capitation or FFS basis
Closed panel HMO	Members are required to select PCP who functions as gatekeeper. Referral to specialist by PCP is mandatory.	PMPM; all coverage via PCP referral only

Most
Managed

Figure 1-2   Continuum of managed healthcare organizations.

care," nurses play various roles. For example, in the most managed environment, nurses assume the gatekeeper role (e.g., MCO-based case manager, payer-based case manager). As case managers, they are involved in authorizing or denying healthcare services, utilization review, telephonic triage and case management activities, enrollee risk assessment and health appraisal, and health education and promotion.

According to Tindall et al (2000), MCOs are characterized by the following:

1. Sharing of risk among patients, payers, and providers
2. Limitation on provider choice (i.e., preauthorization of services)
3. Limitations on consumer choice (i.e., consumer's ability to access provider's services within or outside the network)
4. Accessibility to services (i.e., the need for referral by a primary care provider to a specialty care provider)
5. Control over utilization of services (i.e., prospective, concurrent, or retrospective review of utilization of services)
6. Contracts for best prices (i.e., negotiation with prospective providers and agencies until desired prices are met)
7. Use of information technology to manage the value and delivery of quality and cost-effective healthcare services
8. Conduct of health risk assessment and appraisal of enrollee
9. Provision of preventive healthcare services (e.g., patient and family education services, telephone triage services).

In all these aspects of managed care, nurses play important roles. They facilitate communication between the payer, provider, and consumer; act as gatekeepers; evaluate the quality of the services provided and their related costs; control the use of unnecessary resources and services through utilization review and authorization of services; and ensure the provision of preventive health services. These roles are achieved through business management processes (e.g., communication, collaboration, cooperation, negotiation) and are primarily driven by the goals of cost containment and cost-effectiveness, improved access to care, and quality care and outcomes.

MANAGED CARE ENROLLMENT

Managed care now exists in virtually every region of the United States, including both rural and urban areas. Nevertheless, the number of people enrolled in managed care plans varies from one city, state, or region to another. Some are still at the unstructured or loose alliances stage, whereas others are already at the utmost stage (i.e., integrated delivery networks). Arizona and California are considered stage V managed care penetration. Managed care enrollment has reached greater popularity in 2000, according to a survey conducted and reported by the Utilization Review Accreditation Commission (URAC) (Greenberg, 2000). The survey, conducted in the spring of 2000, showed that preferred provider organizations (PPOs) were the nation's most popular healthcare delivery system. Over 98 million Americans were enrolled in PPOs, compared with 81 million in health maintenance organizations (HMOs) and 18 million in indemnity plans with fee-for-service (FFS). Experts estimate that managed care enrollment will continue to rise and that people insured by their employers will receive healthcare services almost exclusively through managed care plans.

Managed care has also reached the Medicare and Medicaid populations. Although not yet very popular, managed Medicare programs were expected to enroll 11.8 million Americans in the year 2000 compared with 7.3 million enrolled in 1998 (Tindall et al, 2000). Nevertheless, 17,756,603 Medicaid beneficiaries are enrolled in managed Medicaid programs as of June 1999, that is, 55.59% of the total Medicaid population (HCFA, 2000). The percentage of enrollees in Medicaid managed care programs varies from state to state. Box 1-1 summarizes the distribution of enrollees according to their state of residence. The increased numbers of Medicaid managed care enrollment called for new roles for nurses, such as those associated with case management and risk reduction programs. Nurses in these programs assume a responsible, accountable, autonomous, and intimate relationship with Medicaid managed care recipients. Nurses in these programs are responsible for either actual provision or supervision of the following services:

1. Delivery of patient-centered care
2. Health risk assessment and appraisal
3. Health risk behavior modification, counseling, and management
4. Provision of care management and telephonic case management services
5. Guarantee of enrollee's ongoing medical follow-up
6. Encouragement of enrollee to keep appointments with healthcare providers
7. Encouragement of enrollee to identify a primary care provider and adhere to his or her medical services
8. Provision of patient and family education regarding healthcare benefits, medical services, disease processes, medication usage, and so on

---

BOX 1-1

Distribution of Medicaid Managed Care Enrollee by State (June 30, 1999)

100%	Michigan, Montana, Tennessee
90%-99%	Arizona, Colorado, Washington
80%-89%	Iowa, North Carolina, Oregon, Utah
70%-79%	Alabama, Connecticut, Delaware, Georgia, Hawaii, New Mexico, Pennsylvania, Puerto Rico, South Dakota
60%-69%	District of Columbia, Florida, Indiana, Kentucky, Maryland, Massachusetts, Minnesota, Rhode Island, Virginia
50%-59%	Arkansas, California, Kansas, New Jersey, North Dakota, Oklahoma, Vermont
40%-49%	Mississippi, West Virginia, Wisconsin
30%-39%	Idaho, Missouri, Nevada
20%-29%	New York, Ohio
10%-19%	Illinois, Maine, Texas
1%-9%	Louisiana, New Hampshire, South Carolina
0%	Alaska, Wyoming

9. Brokerage of community services
10. Financial management and counseling
11. Psychosocial support and counseling
12. Arrangement of transport services to and from healthcare providers and agencies
13. Provision of rehabilitative services
14. Consumer advocacy

ATTRIBUTES AND CHARACTERISTICS OF MANAGED CARE SERVICES

In an effort to clarify the confusion surrounding the term *managed care,* Kersbergen (2000) developed the concept *managed care* and identified its attributes, characteristics, and consequences. She based her conclusions on a critical review and analysis of the multidisciplinary literature on managed care, observations of practicing case managers, and interviews with managers and administrators involved in managed care. The results of this analysis are presented in Tables 1-1 and 1-2, and examples of the roles assumed by nurses

TABLE 1-1
Predominant Attributes and Defining Characteristics of Managed Care

Attribute	Defining Characteristics	Role of the Nurse
Business framework	Discounted or capitated contracts Preauthorization for care Prospective, concurrent, or retro-spective reviews	Contract negotiation Utilization review and management Cost-effectiveness analysis and reporting
Organization of delivery of healthcare services	Integrated healthcare systems MCOs: HMO, PPO, POS	Case/care management Payer-based case management Advocacy
Control of services and resource utilization	Standardized practice patterns Gatekeepers	Practice guidelines/clinical pathways development and use Facilitation/coordination/brokerage of healthcare services Variance/delays management
Incentives to control costs	Provider/consumer assumes part of financial risk of care Limited provider and consumer choices	Risk stratification of population Care/case management based on identified risk Gatekeeper
Decisions based on business parameters	Allocation or denial of service decisions made by nonhealthcare providers (third-party payers) Shift from altruistic healthcare model to business framework	Payer-based case management Utilization review and management Cost-effectiveness analysis

Modified from Kersbergen AL: *Nurs Health Care Perspect* 21(2):81-83, 2000. This copyrighted material is used with the permission of the National League for Nursing.
HMO, Health maintenance organization; *MCO,* managed care organization; *POS,* point-of-service plan; *PPO,* preferred provider organization.

are shared based on Kersbergen's thoughts regarding the effects of managed care on nursing practice. The popularity of managed care has resulted in an added focus for nursing. There now exists, in addition to the patient-driven nursing model of care delivery, a business framework in which reimbursement methods and processes play an integral role in healthcare delivery. Nurses, more than ever before, are now found functioning in payer-based healthcare organizations where they are responsible for authorizing or denying healthcare services. Even in provider-based organizations, they assume nontraditional

TABLE 1-2
Predominant Consequences of the Concept of Managed Care

Consequences	Defining Characteristics	Role of the Nurse
Changing base of power	Payers are dictating clinical decision making through incentives Payers have power over consumers' choice of providers Payers are the "customers" of healthcare providers and organizations	Authorization and certification of healthcare services Case management and variance/delay management Cost control
Ethical dilemmas	Concerns about jeopardizing quality of care Concerns about access to appropriate care Concerns about disrupting therapeutic relationships	Quality improvement/management Consumer satisfaction Brokerage of healthcare services Advocacy for consumers, providers, payers
Conflicts	Intrapersonal conflicts: providers torn between personal and professional values and coping with practice guidelines and decisions imposed by managed care entities Interpersonal conflicts between provider-payer-patient/consumer regarding values, perceived healthcare needs, and parameters of care allowed by payers Group conflicts over market economics and community values and healthcare needs Professional conflicts within and among disciplines regarding scope of practice, emerging roles, and professional values versus economic values of managed care Financial conflicts resulting from perceived need to provide care beyond contracted dollar amounts, resulting in potential loss of income for provider/organization	Practice guidelines/clinical pathways Managed care contract negotiation Patient and family education, specifically regarding health insurance plan's benefits Advocacy for consumers, providers, payers Balancing cost, quality, and access to healthcare services Adherence to standards of regulatory agencies such as NCQA and URAC Leadership of multidisciplinary healthcare teams (informal leader and gatekeeper) Cost-effectiveness analysis and reporting

Modified from Kersbergen AL: *Nurs Health Care Perspect* 21(2):81-83, 2000. This copyrighted material is used with the permission of the National League for Nursing.
NCQA, National Committee for Quality Assurance; *URAC*, Utilization Review Accreditation Commission.

roles, such as case management, resource utilization management, quality management, or reimbursement denials and appeals management.

Based on the predominant attributes, characteristics, and consequences found in the literature, Kersbergen was able to define managed care as a "business framework for organizing the delivery of healthcare services while controlling service and resource utilization through incentives to control cost and decision making based on business parameters" (Kersbergen, 2000, p 82). Five characteristics that clearly describe the impact of managed care on healthcare delivery and the roles played by nurses are highlighted in this definition. These characteristics are discussed as follows:

1. *Business framework.* This framework aims at the reimbursement methods of managed care and the shift in power from the provider or consumer to the payer. The business model is driven by the bottom line: the cost of healthcare services. Nurses have assumed an important role in controlling cost, such as that of a payer- or provider-based case manager.

2. *Organization of the delivery of healthcare services.* This is related to the surge of new healthcare organizations, which are both payer- and provider-based. Examples of payer-based organizations are HMOs and PPOs. Examples of provider-based organizations are integrated delivery systems and physician-hospital organizations. Nurses in these new organizations play a more visible role and are responsible for deciding whether healthcare services should be authorized and what degree or amount should be reimbursed.

3. *Control of services and resource utilization.* This highlights the trend of requiring authorizations of services before delivering care. Controlling services is driven by the need to reduce escalating healthcare costs. Control tries to prevent the delivery of unnecessary or duplicate services. The nurse's role in this regard is that of a gatekeeper. For example, from a payer-based organization's perspective, nurses are involved in authorizing or denying services. From a provider-based organization's perspective, however, they ensure appropriate reimbursement (reduce or limit reimbursement denial rate) for the healthcare services provided and prevent delays in the provision of care. Nurses are also found to manage practice guidelines and clinical pathways programs. They oversee the development, implementation, and evaluation of such programs that are implemented as proactive approaches to effective care delivery, quality, and outcomes.

4. *Incentives to control costs.* This entails shifting the financial risk from the payer to the provider of healthcare services. Controlling costs is another aspect of the impact of the business model on healthcare. Providers who are able to demonstrate cost-effective and quality practices and desirable portfolios are rewarded with financial incentives by MCOs. This characteristic brought about a new role for nurses—that of a managed care reviewer—in provider-based organizations. These nurses are constantly negotiating services and reimbursement with the payer-based case manager. They exchange information regarding the necessity of services to be provided and obtain timely authorizations for these services.

5. *Decisions based on business parameters.* This highly important characteristic acts as the theme that threads through all the other characteristics of managed care services. Business strategies and parameters have become integral factors to the success of healthcare organizations. Cost, quality, and access to care are the driving forces of change in the delivery of healthcare services. Nurses play an important role in ensuring the delivery of cost-effective and quality care. In their roles as gatekeepers of healthcare delivery, they communicate with the payers, providers, and consumers of healthcare. Therefore they are in the best position to ensure that the decisions made align with the business parameters determined by the organization and to prevent undesired effects. Examples of nurses' roles that focus on keeping in line with business parameters are prevention of delays or duplication in the delivery of healthcare services, integration of services, and negotiation with consumers of healthcare organizations or MCOs regarding care delivery.

NURSING'S ROLE IN MANAGED CARE: DRIVERS OF CHANGE

The dominant driving force for change in the roles assumed by nurses in a managed care environment is financially based. Experts contribute the escalating healthcare costs to many reasons, including the following:
1. Fragmentation and duplication of services
2. Hospitals as the predominant setting for care provision
3. Availability of provider-focused delivery systems/models rather than patient-focused
4. A healthcare environment that is too complex for consumers to understand or navigate
5. Healthcare plans/policies and reimbursement methods that are too complex for consumers to understand, which makes them unable to differentiate between covered and not-covered services based on their benefits/entitlements
6. Lack of knowledge and understanding of the administrative processes required by the MCOs, such as preauthorization of services, claims management, denials and appeals management, and reimbursement

These reasons and others have lead healthcare executives to develop new roles for nurses. The case manager's role has been the most visible one. Case managers today are available in any setting across the healthcare continuum and in both provider- and payer-based organizations. It is no surprise that the main focus of case management programs is financial tightening. Case managers are the professionals best equipped to make synergistic decisions that address both the financial and clinical demands of care delivery. They are able to reduce cost and expenditure without compromising the quality of care. For example, case managers can decrease duplication of services by coordinating care delivery with the payers/insurers, providers, employers, and consumers and assuring that appropriate and timely information is communicated to all parties. Another example is disease management programs, in which case managers conduct health risk assessments and appraisals of enrollees and use the results to proactively determine the level of case management services needed. The case management services provided range from least to most intensive and usually must correlate with the risk groups (low, moderate, and high risk) identified as a result of the assessments.

Quality is another driving force for change in the role of nurses. Quality of care is an evaluative variable taken into consideration by MCOs when deciding whether to renew or terminate a managed care contract with a provider or agency. As the managed care market reaches stages IV or V, the provision of "accountable care" becomes more desirable. Although the primary driver of the movement toward managed care is financial, clearly clinical benefits result from this move. By making healthcare providers accountable for the outcomes of the services they deliver, they are pressured to focus on quality and to implement strategies that enhance the quality of care. One important outcome of this trend is the focus on the continuum of care that has been operationally organized through the development of integrated delivery systems (Geary and Smeltzer, 1997). Healthcare providers realized that meeting the health needs of their consumers across the continuum of care assures quality outcomes. As a result, physicians and hospitals have been working together through established partnerships toward the same goals: quality of care and cost-effectiveness. Quality of care can be improved only after these partnerships are established and differences are put aside.

The increased focus on the continuum of care has improved the status of case management and also has led to the development and implementation of disease management programs. Whereas case management programs focus on managing care of the individual patient, disease management programs focus on managing care of an entire patient population (i.e., aggregate patient populations, such as persons with heart failure, diabetes, or asthma). Such chronic illnesses, if not managed well, result in increased cost of care that is (in most cases) preventable. The bottom line of both programs is quality. These changes resulted in expanded and more powerful roles for case managers. With a managed care market at stages IV or V, case managers had to shift their focus from episode-based care to continuum-based care. This shift assures that patients' health conditions are managed more effectively and that acute care episodes, which traditionally are more costly, are kept to a minimum—only when necessary. Such focus of case managers results in improved quality of care and outcomes and allows them to be a more visible force in healthcare delivery.

Case managers in disease management programs have expert knowledge specific to a particular disease. Their practice is similar to those in case management programs in that they focus on the continuum of care. To improve quality of care and patient care outcomes, disease management programs aim to understand a disease population by examining and analyzing the information obtained from the population in an aggregate fashion and on an ongoing basis. Over time, case managers and disease management program administrators are able to identify subtle changes in the outcomes of the care provided and are able to attribute these outcomes to specific interventions. These programs allow providers to evaluate the short- and long-term benefits of specific interventions and treatment protocols over a period of time and across the continuum of care. By understanding a disease population, care providers and case managers can then determine which treatment modalities contribute to the most desired outcomes. In addition, these programs allow providers to identify areas for potential improvements. Ultimately, the goal is to continuously improve the quality of care and outcomes. Case managers have been able to capitalize on the knowledge gained from disease management programs to develop clinical practice guidelines and clinical pathways as prospective tools for the care and management of specific chronic and costly diseases.

Another factor that contributes to quality is the collaborative nature of today's case management programs. Although case managers were first popular in acute care, today they are found in every care setting across the continuum. The case managers of the different settings collaborate to assure that patients receive care in the most appropriate environment and that continuity of care is maintained. Collaboration has also extended to MCOs. The payer- and provider-based case managers are in constant communication to ensure that patients receive the best quality care possible and in the most appropriate setting, control overutilization of resources, discuss treatment options, and negotiate the approval of community-based services. These collaborative efforts are considered indispensable and necessary for maintaining cost-effective and quality care and outcomes for all, including the providers, payers, purchasers, and consumers.

CONSEQUENCES OF MANAGED CARE ON NURSING: CASE MANAGEMENT

As managed care intensified, the need to decrease hospital-based care grew stronger. This need was a direct result of the cost reduction strategies of MCOs and the costly state of hospital-based services. MCOs had pressured acute care institutions to decrease their length of stay by discharging patients as rapidly as possible and by attempting to deliver care in other, less costly settings such as the community or home. By decreasing the use of costly hospital care, MCOs were able to lower their average cost per enrollee and therefore decrease the premiums paid by employers and purchasers. Organizations that decreased costs had a more competitive advantage over others and were more able to secure cost-effective managed care contracts (Buerhaus, 1994). Acute care institutions employed case management programs and case managers to address the demand for hospital length of stay reduction and the restrictions on resource utilization imposed by MCOs. They also relied on case managers for their managed care contract negotiations.

Case Managers and Acute Care

Care integration has always been a primary role for case managers in acute care settings. Case managers bring an understanding of the healthcare continuum and the importance of providing care in settings other than acute care to the interdisciplinary care teams. They help the teams meet the cost control efforts imposed by MCOs, such as constraints on utilization of services and preauthorized services. Case managers do not restrict access to services but instead encourage consumers to use services that promote healthy lifestyles, enhance functional abilities, and monitor chronic illnesses so that chronically ill enrollees are managed outside the hospital setting and their need for acute care or hospitalization is reduced.

Not all healthcare professionals have appropriate knowledge of managed care operations and reimbursement, availability of community resources, and standards of regulatory bodies such as the Joint Commission on Accreditation of Healthcare Organizations (JCAHO), the National Committee for Quality Assurance (NCQA), and the American Accreditation Healthcare Commission/Utilization Review Accreditation Commission (URAC). The presence of case managers on interdisciplinary healthcare teams allows for better outcomes, such as cost-effectiveness, quality care, low reimbursement denial rates, and compliance with the standards of regulatory bodies. Today the role of case managers mainly focuses on the integration of clinical care management, resource utilization and managed care reviews, psychosocial counseling, and transitional planning to a different level of care. Case management models with this integrative nature tend to be based on a continuum of care and have been proven to be most effective and more desired by MCOs. The proliferation of such a continuum-of-care case management approach is viewed as an enhancement of the old models that were present either predominantly in acute care settings or only in MCOs. The continuum-of-care approach to case management brought case managers more political influence in their roles and made them more respectable and appreciated members of interdisciplinary healthcare teams.

Case Managers and Managed Care Contracts

For nursing and healthcare executives, case managers constitute a group of most desired participants in the managed care contract negotiation process, due in part to their knowledge, involvement, and understanding of the day-to-day activities and dealings with MCOs. Contract negotiations usually arise to generate new business, to prevent the erosion of existing market shares (Rehberg, 1996), or to save a preexisting contract from dissolving. These functions are true for both the payers and providers of healthcare services. Traditionally the presence of clinicians such as nurses was minimal. As managed care penetration approaches stages IV and V, however, risk contracts and reimbursement at a capitated rate are becoming the norm, and the presence of clinicians is becoming mandatory. Therefore in today's healthcare market, more nurses, especially nurse case managers, participate in managed care contract negotiations. Their presence at the negotiation table contributes the following benefits:

1. Understanding of the level of overutilization or inappropriate use of services
2. Knowledge of the impact the managed care contract may have on clinical care
3. Intimate familiarity with the daily life of the case manager and the desires of consumers
4. Practical insight regarding the administrative and clinical issues that may be encountered by the providers and the case management department
5. Knowledge of how best to provide care for the contracted population
6. Understanding of the reimbursement practices, the process of claims management, denials and appeals management, and issues of noncoverage
7. Knowledge of the processes of authorizing services, choosing referral providers, and gaining access to community-based resources
8. Familiarity with the process of evaluating resource utilization, quality of care provided, and consumer satisfaction with care
9. Knowledge of necessary information technology that can be used to track the care of the contracted population

10. Ability to foresee the impact of the contract language
11. Knowledge of the current healthcare organization's structure, systems, processes of care, staffing patterns, and use of technology and whether these resources are able to support the potential managed care contract

Administrators of case management programs are best suited to participate in the managed care contract negotiation process, since they are the link between the payers, the providers, and the consumers. Like case managers, their involvement in all aspects of patient care management (e.g., clinical, financial, administrative, evaluative) makes them essential to the effectiveness of the negotiating team, which may include the chief medical, financial, marketing, and managed care officers. By demonstrating the effectiveness of case management programs, administrators of these programs can bring the benefits of case management to the contract discussion table and perhaps negotiate some compensation for these services. It is not unusual for an MCO to compensate providers a fixed amount per-member-per-month (PMPM) or on a per-admission basis for case management services (Rehberg, 1996).

NURSES AND DEMAND MANAGEMENT PROGRAMS

MCOs use demand management to reduce members' demand for healthcare services and ultimately contain costs. The goals of demand management programs are many. They help members maintain healthy lifestyles. They also are designed to encourage the appropriate use of healthcare services and to help members make better-informed health decisions. In addition, they provide members with information about their health condition, their disease and the disease process, use of medications, how to monitor symptoms to avoid complications and deterioration of condition, the importance of seeking treatment early, and how to self-treat minor ailments (Knight, 1998; Kongsvedt, 2001). These programs are usually run by nurses, particularly the payer-based case managers. Demand management programs created a new opportunity for nurses to function in a health promotion and prevention role with a main focus on wellness. Some of the services provided by nurses in these programs include triage call centers and hotlines, health education classes and newsletters, outreach programs such as health risk assessment and appraisal, and health education using electronic media.

Demand management differs from case management in that it takes place before actual care is provided. It is preventive rather than treatment-oriented and is provided in a virtual medium either over the telephone or through the Internet. Moreover, unlike case management, it is provided to all enrollees regardless of health condition. Payer-based case managers are available telephonically to consumers to answer their questions, provide advice, and triage the need for services to the appropriate level of care and setting to reduce unnecessary use of resources. Nurses who provide these services use automated protocols for providing appropriate advice or referring the consumer to the appropriate care setting. To make effective decisions, they also have access to consumers' files that contain their medical histories, medication use, and information regarding previous encounters with healthcare providers.

The increased popularity of integrated delivery systems and networks has resulted in a surge of demand management programs that are administered by providers rather than by payer-based organizations. Because providers are pressured to reduce the cost of healthcare and the inappropriate use of resources, demand management programs are a desired strategy. They are seen as advantageous because of their special focus on health promotion and prevention and telephone triage activities, which in some cases may delay the need for acute care. These programs also improve consumer satisfaction with care and enhance their perception of access to care. Moreover, they contribute to better outcomes by helping consumers become more involved in the management of their own care.

NURSES AND MANAGED CARE ACCREDITATION

Nurses can play important roles in helping MCOs attain accreditation and guiding healthcare providers in selecting accredited organizations. Accreditation of MCOs has gained increased importance and credibility over the past decade. Consumers of managed healthcare services are more aware of the necessity of accreditation before they choose a health plan. Healthcare providers and agencies interested in becoming members of managed care panels of providers are more inclined to pursue participation in MCOs that demonstrate accreditation status and good standing.

Despite this popularity and trend, accreditation remains voluntary. Nevertheless, the market demands accreditation, as evidenced by the desire of leading businesses and corporations for accreditation before they purchase managed care services for their employees. The public has demonstrated similar demands as well. Three agencies now accredit MCOs: NCQA, URAC, and JCAHO. The accreditation standards of these agencies are similar; however, the main focus of each varies somewhat.

Nurses' role in the accreditation process is essential for the success of the survey. Nurses have demonstrated competence and success in preparing organizations for accreditation and guiding them through the process. They are effective in leading the teams charged with planning and preparing for the survey process. In addition, nurses are given the authority to manage quality and performance programs, prepare reports to be shared with the surveyors, train and educate staff about accreditation procedures, and implement strategic changes to attain compliance with the accreditation standards. Some of the functions assumed by nurses regarding accreditation are as follows:

1. Management of quality improvement programs
2. Provision of demand management services to ensure the availability of health promotion and disease prevention services
3. Telephonic case management and triage services
4. Consumer education regarding healthcare services and plan benefits
5. Provision of health assessments and appraisals services such as risk assessment, cholesterol, hypertension, and cancer screening, child immunizations, and flu shots for the elderly
6. Claims processing and appeals management

7. Authorization and reauthorization of services
8. Utilization review and management
9. Training and education of providers and MCO staff
10. Ensuring accessibility of consumers to healthcare services

NURSES AND THE ADVOCACY ROLE

Advocacy is an important and essential role for nurses, particularly case managers. Case managers function as "coordinators of care, catalysts, problem solvers, facilitators, impartial advocates, and educators" (Mullahy, 2001, p 250). Case managers act on behalf of patients and their families in ensuring that they receive the necessary treatments and interventions and that the care they receive is ethical, legal, and valuable. In addition, they have a responsibility to maintain a balance between the competing forces and priorities of healthcare consumers, employers, insurers and payers, providers, and regulatory systems and agents.

Case managers and nurses in general have demonstrated an effective advocacy role for those who are impaired and unable to advocate for themselves. Nurses are in the ideal and most desired position to work the healthcare system within and outside the walls of their organization to ensure that their patients' needs are met and that their care is safe, necessary, and effective. Effective patient advocates are required to have a wide knowledge and understanding of the dynamics of the healthcare system and reimbursement. Due to their education, training, and background, nurses and case managers are best positioned to provide this role. They make well-educated decision-makers whom patients and their families can rely on and benefit from.

The advocacy role of case managers is evident in the following functions:

1. Contacting the medical staff and other members of the healthcare team to discuss the patient's needs, required services, and progress
2. Arranging for services required after discharge such as community resources, home care, and durable medical equipment
3. Instituting interventions that prevent complications and deterioration in the patient's medical condition
4. Obtaining payer authorizations for services on behalf of the patient and family
5. Obtaining information regarding living wills, healthcare proxies, and do-not-resuscitate status
6. Working with team members to achieve goals and representing patients by sharing information obtained from patients and families
7. Advising patients of the available treatment options and medically appropriate alternatives and ensuring that their interests are identified and supported
8. Encouraging patients and their families to advocate for themselves and to participate in decision making regarding care and lifestyle changes
9. Educating and counseling patients regarding the disease process and health benefits
10. Negotiating with representatives of MCOs or health insurance plans for out-of-network services and coverage

11. Helping patients sort through bills and finances and prioritizing payments
12. Visiting patients' place of employment and negotiating return-to-work plans
13. Assisting patients and families in understanding the need for healthcare services to obtain informed consents and reach informed decisions

NURSING EDUCATION AND MANAGED CARE

As more nurses find themselves employed in an MCO or managed care setting, adequate preparation of nurses for such roles and the unique demands of such an environment have begun, but more still needs to be addressed. Today's graduating nurses are somewhat exposed to managed care systems; however, they are not appropriately prepared to effectively function in an MCO or managed care environment. Basic knowledge of managed care systems has been incorporated into the graduate and undergraduate nursing curricula, but it has been implemented only in a limited number of nursing schools. Nursing case management curricula have been more successful in producing case managers who are knowledgeable and well qualified to assume such roles successfully.

Case management programs have demonstrated that the use of nurses in the case manager role contributes to better and more desired outcomes. Therefore nursing faculty must not continue to exhibit their cautious attitude toward the desire to change nursing curricula. They must be encouraged to incorporate nursing case management and managed care content into their curricula. Such content will only produce nurses who are better prepared to meet the demands of the real world.

THE FUTURE OF NURSES IN MANAGED CARE

Even if MCOs disappear, cost-effectiveness, cost containment, and quality of care will remain priorities in healthcare delivery and management. The business framework of healthcare where economic decision making takes place also will grow more complex. Therefore what nurses have learned and achieved in the current managed care market will be a prerequisite for their continued survival in the future. Nurses will remain the most desired force for healthcare delivery. They will remain the best positioned to facilitate care and educate patients and their families toward health and wellness. In addition, they will continue to act as consumer advocates, especially for those who are uninsured or who may not know how to navigate the complex healthcare system.

The survival of nurses in tomorrow's managed care/healthcare market will depend on their knowledge, skills, competencies, and openness to new roles. To ensure their place in tomorrow's world, they must pay close attention to the following issues of future healthcare delivery and practices:

1. Understand the intricacies of the healthcare reimbursement systems (private and governmental) so that they are able to build cost-effective clinical care programs.
2. Maintain an acceptable level of knowledge, skills, and competence in the fiscal management of healthcare delivery. Nurses will be held directly responsible for market

shares, profit margins and losses, and risk contracts and will be required to answer to these issues.

3. Identify, implement, and manage the use of appropriate technologies, especially those that are Internet-based. Such technologies will become the number-one desired method of communication between payers, providers, and consumers of healthcare services, and nurses must know how to manage them. They must also be able to assist consumers in the use of such technologies.

4. Understand the different healthcare regulations that govern different regions or states. This information will become more important as the Internet allows providers to provide healthcare services (especially wellness services) across state lines.

5. Practice in collaborative team settings as the complexity of the delivery of healthcare services continues to increase and becomes more reliant on the interdependence of the various disciplines and their combined contribution rather than on the contribution of individual disciplines. Healthcare providers will be held accountable and responsible for team-based outcomes instead of individual outcomes. This collaborative practice will be necessary for both the clinical and managerial aspects of healthcare delivery.

6. Focus on the continuum of care regardless of where the consumer accesses services. This focus raises the importance of the provider's accountability for outcomes across the continuum of care and not for a single setting or episode of care.

The future will provide nurses with new roles. As the consumer becomes more sophisticated in the use of information technologies, so will nurses. For example, consumers will self-manage their health records. They will house them on the Internet so that they are accessed easily by providers anywhere in the nation. As consumers are required to access demand management services through the Internet, case managers will be able to access and review patients' health records before giving any advice. They also will be able to document the Internet-based communication and assessment and the advice given in the record afterwards. Such service will be provided regardless of the proximity of the provider to the consumer. This universal health record will become more popular as consumers' interest in self-management of healthcare needs increases. Consumers will call on nurses to help them establish their own health records, and nurses will function as consultants for such services. For a small fee, consumers will be able to get their health records set up on the Internet by nurses. Nurses will play an important role in these services because of their healthcare knowledge, background, and educational preparation. They will assist consumers in storing their health-related information in a way that makes it easy to access and locate any piece of information by payers and providers.

Another future role of nurses is that of the nurse practitioner (NP) as a primary care provider. Although their presence in today's managed care market is limited, NPs will be a powerful force and will assume primary care roles similar to those of physicians. Consumers will have the option to choose a NP or a physician from their MCO's directory or panel of providers. NPs will be listed independently rather than under a collaborating physician practice. The services NPs provide will be best suited for both demand management and acute care or disease-based services. They will continue to provide competition for physician practices. Such competition will only result in further reductions in the cost of healthcare and will force the "survival of the fittest," that is, the "accountable" providers who are able to provide supportive evidence of cost-effective and quality outcomes practice.

Nurses as managers of practice guidelines and clinical pathway programs will also continue to exist, but these programs will shift their focus from an episode of care or a single care setting to the care continuum. They also will become truly interdisciplinary, that is, reflective of the team's goals and desired outcomes instead of those of individual disciplines. Nurses in such programs will continue to coordinate these efforts, however, and will play a more formal rather than an informal leadership role. The guidelines will combine the efforts of the interdisciplinary collaborative team in meeting the needs of the consumer across the continuum of care. These guidelines also will be developed in collaboration with the consumer and the payer. In addition, to meet the continuum-based healthcare needs of consumers, the guidelines will also be developed in collaboration with providers from different sites or even different organizations. Such collaborative practices will be essential for the survival of healthcare organizations. They will allow continuity of care as the consumer navigates the healthcare system, possibly seeing different providers yet experiencing a seamless approach to care delivery.

REFERENCES

Buerhaus P: Economics of managed competition and consequences to nurses. Part II, *Nurs Econ* 12(2):75-80, 106, 1994.

Geary RC, Smeltzer HC: Case management: past, present, future—the drivers for change, *J Nurs Care Qual* 12(1): 9-19, 1997.

Greenberg L: *The state of PPO performance measurement: case study report*, 2000, Utilization Review Accreditation Commission.

Healthcare Financing Administration: *National summary of Medicaid managed care programs and enrollment*, 2000, The Administration, Available online: http://www.hcfa.gov/medicaid/trends99.htm, accessed on 3/20/01.

Kersbergen A: Managed care shifts healthcare from an altruistic model to a business framework, *Nurs Health Care Perspect* 21(2):81-83, 2000.

Knight W: *Managed care: what it is and how it works*, Gaithersburg, Md, 1998, Aspen.

Kongstvedt P: *Essentials of managed healthcare*, Gaithersburg, Md, 2001, Aspen.

Mullahy C: Case management and managed care. In Kongstvedt P: *Essentials of managed healthcare*, Gaithersburg, Md, 2001, Aspen.

Rehberg C: Managed care contracts: a guide for clinical case managers, *Nurs Case Manag* 1(1):11-17, 1996.

Tindall W, Williams W, Helmer L, et al: *Paving the way to managed care medicine*, 2000, Available online: http://acmcm.org/cme/Pathway_Course_1.htm, accessed on 3/20/2001.

Historical Perspectives on Managed Care

Sandra B. Lewenson

KEY LESSONS IN THIS CHAPTER

- Little has been documented in the literature concerning nursing's responses or contributions to the development of managed care in the United States.
- Public health nursing at the beginning of the twentieth century provides us with examples of early nursing models in a managed care environment.
- Nurses have been present and have witnessed the changes in healthcare that created the managed care environment of today.
- Nurses, as case managers, assist in operationalizing cost-effective, outcome-driven, and process-oriented care.
- To survive in a managed care environment, nurses must continue to identify and measure their contributions to the healthcare team.

Managed care organizations and their associated business language have become a familiar part of the healthcare marketplace since the 1970s. Given the need to control the high costs of healthcare and still provide better access, managed care organizations have spread throughout various regions of the United States between the 1970s and 1990s. Knight notes that managed care aims to provide an appropriate mix of healthcare providers and care to a given population. In addition to providing care, these same organizations provide health insurance to consumers (Knight, 1998).

Cohen and Cesta define managed care as a "system that provides the generalized structure and focus for managing the use, cost, quality, and effectiveness of healthcare services" (Cohen and Cesta, 1997, p 32). Viewed as an umbrella, managed care encompasses many healthcare cost containment measures, one of which is nursing case management. Case management considers quality of care, efficiency of care, and cost-effectiveness of care (Cohen and Cesta, 1997). Bower (1992) notes an interrelationship among the cost, processes, and outcomes of care. Nursing case managers address these variables within the managed care environment.

Nursing has traditionally assumed the responsibility for the management of healthcare for individuals, families, and communities. Conti notes that insurance companies historically had sought the expertise of nurses in the management of "catastrophic cases because of their knowledge and understanding of medical and nursing practice" (Conti, 1996, p 13). Since the opening of nurse training schools in 1873, nurses have played a major role in improving healthcare outcomes of patients. The extent to which nurses have had a role in ensuring the cost and outcomes of their care, however, has been largely unexplored (Conti, 1996).

Managed care is seen as a late-twentieth-century phenomenon; however, its roots predate the Health Maintenance Organization Act of 1973 (Knight, 1998). The literature about managed care rarely identifies nursing's participation in its evolution, suggesting that nursing had little influence in its development. What little has been written about the history of managed care has all but omitted nursing's responses or contributions to the development of this evolving healthcare system. This omission from our collective understanding of nursing's influence or lack of influence prevents nursing from understanding its necessary role in participating in decision-making opportunities at the proverbial "table." As managed care systems become larger and perhaps more controlling of healthcare in the United States, nursing must recognize its history and bring it to the bargaining table. Thus as we look at the evolution of managed care, we look for specific examples of nursing's contribution to this history.

Hamilton's research on Lillian Wald's leadership in the managed care experiment with the Metropolitan Life Insurance Company in 1909 exemplifies one of nursing's direct links to the evolution of managed care (Hamilton, 1988a, 1988b). Hamilton analyzes the public health nurses' ambivalence about the conflict they experienced balancing their nursing care with cost containment measures. A second example of bringing cost and care together is found in one of the many studies of nursing commissioned during the twentieth century. In 1940, the National League of Nursing Education (NLNE) and the American Hospital Association published a study, "Administrative Cost Analysis for Nursing Service and Nursing Education" (Pfefferkorn and Rovetta, 1940). Blanche Pfefferkorn, Director of Studies for the NLNE, in collaboration with Charles Rovetta, an MBA from the University of Chicago, studied the effect of applying accounting principles to nursing service and education. Both the study of managed care and the cost analysis provide some historical insight into nursing's response to providing care within a cost containment model.

HISTORICAL OVERVIEW OF NURSING

Knight identifies the use of a managed care approach dating back to the mid-1800s. According to Knight, railroad and mining companies offered prepaid healthcare plans in the hopes of attracting and retaining the immigrant labor force. In the form of benevolent societies, these companies engaged local physicians, built hospitals and clinics, and provided hospital beds for their workers and families (Knight, 1998). The Mayo Clinic, founded in the 1880s, was one of the earliest prepaid medical group practices. The idea of prepaid groups did not become firmly established until the 1920s and 1930s, when industrial development of the lumber, railroad, and construction industries demanded this type of healthcare benefit for its employees (Knight, 1998). The founding of the organization Kaiser Permanente in the 1930s was attributed to a Southern Californian physician, Sidney Garfield, who convinced Henry J. Kaiser and his son of the value of paying him directly for the care of the construction workers on their sites. From this first agreement, Garfield was asked to provide healthcare at other construction sites run by Kaiser. In San Francisco, the plan expanded to include the public, as well as Kaiser's employees, and a healthcare facility was built to serve the prepaid members of the new plan. In 1945, another prepaid plan was started by 400 families who contributed $100 apiece to start a medical clinic. The group became the Group Health of Puget Sound in Seattle and faced a legal battle from the local medical association, who opposed the cooperative plan. In this instance, Knight noted that the prepaid group won the right to establish a prepaid plan (Knight, 1998). Knight outlines a number of other examples in which prepaid plans were formed throughout the 1920s, 1930s, and 1940s (Knight, 1998).

Knight does not refer to the role nursing may have played in providing healthcare to these workers (Knight, 1998). This omission may be understandable given the history of nursing in the United States. The modern nursing movement did not begin until 1873, with the opening of Nightingale training schools. Before 1873, few training opportunities for nurses existed except through an apprenticeship model. There may have been nurses involved in the early attempts at managed care in the mid-1800s; however, they were most likely to be either volunteer or untrained nurses. To understand nursing's participation in the evolution of managed care, one must understand the emergence of the nursing profession in the United States and how these early professionals participated in shaping twentieth-century healthcare.

THE MODERN NURSING MOVEMENT

Florence Nightingale became a heroine of epic proportions after her successful use of nurses to improve the conditions found in military hospitals during the Crimean War between 1854 and 1856. The implementation of her ideas about improving the sanitary conditions of hospitals and later, her views on opening nurse training schools and using trained nurses in practice dramatically improved patient mortality rates. This significant outcome contributed to the rapid spread of her ideas to other parts of the world. Nightingale's nurse training program at the St. Thomas Hospital in London, England in 1860 became a model for the nursing schools that opened in the late nineteenth and early twentieth centuries. Nightingale insisted that nurses teach nursing and that nurses needed a formal training period to learn the art of nursing (Lewenson, 1996).

Training Schools for Nurses

After the American Civil War ended in 1865, the opening of three Nightingale-influenced training schools in 1873 marked the beginning of the modern nursing movement in the United States. Although a few unsuccessful attempts had been made at establishing training schools for nurses in the United States before this time, the three schools that opened in 1873 became successful examples of Nightingale's ideas. These schools were the Bellevue Training School for Nurses at Bellevue Hospital in New York City, the Connecticut Training School for Nurses at the New Haven Hospital in New Haven, Connecticut, and the Boston Training School of Nurses at Massachusetts General Hospital in Boston, Massachusetts (Dock and Stewart, 1931; Roberts, 1954; Bullough, Bullough, and Stanton, 1990; Lewenson, 1996). The training schools at Bellevue, New Haven Hospital, and Massachusetts General provided some of the earliest opportunities for women to receive a nursing education and the opportunity for professional employment. Before these schools opened, women nursed their families at home or volunteered during wartime to nurse the soldiers. Nursing was considered women's work, an extension of their role as mother and daughter. Nightingale advocated that women control the newly opened nurse training schools and that nursing education be in the hands of nurses. This revolutionary notion influenced the development of what became known throughout the world as the modern nursing movement (Reverby, 1987; Lewenson, 1996).

The new nursing schools provided an opportunity for women to become economically self-sufficient. During the nineteenth and early twentieth centuries, upper- and middle-class women were expected to marry, live at home, and care for their families. Women were financially dependent and were not expected to work outside the home. Few options existed for women outside of this arrangement. Nurse training, described by North in 1882 as "A New Profession for Women," provided an avenue of independence and a viable alternative to marriage (North, 1882). Women learned the art of nursing while caring for patients. Hospitals used these student nurses as a source of revenue for the hospital. The students cared for the patients and provided a healthier hospital environment that promoted healing. This dramatic change in the care of the sick prompted the proliferation of nursing schools in the United States (Burgess, 1928; Fitzpatrick, 1983). More nursing schools opened and educated greater numbers of nurses to manage the care of the sick than did medical schools (Table 2-1).

TABLE 2-1
Medical and Nursing Schools and Graduates: 1880-1926

Year	Medical Schools	Nursing Schools	Medical Graduates	Nursing Graduates
1880	100	15	3241	157
1890	133	35	4454	471
1900	160	432	5214	3456
1910	131	1129	4440	8140
1920	85	1775	3047	14,980
1926	79	2155	3962	17,522

From Burgess MA: *Nurses, patients, and pocketbooks,* Report of a study of the economics of nursing conducted by the Committee on the Grading of Nursing Schools, New York, 1928, Committee on the Grading of Nursing Schools.

Professional Nursing Organizations

Trained nurses, the term used for nurses who were educated in the new schools, found that once trained, they were no longer employed by the hospital. Hospitals found it cheaper to use the students as nurses and rarely hired their own graduates (Roberts, 1954; Fitzpatrick, 1983; Lewenson, 1996). After graduation, trained nurses found work as private duty nurses or visiting nurses in the newly emerging field of public health nursing. As private duty nurses and visiting nurses, these trained professionals managed the care of their patients.

To control their practice, nurses organized the Nurses Associated Alumnae of the United States and Canada (Associated Alumnae) in 1896, which became the American Nurses Association (ANA) in 1911. The ANA focused on the concerns of the working graduate nurse. To protect both the public and the trained nurse from someone without training who called herself a nurse, the ANA advocated the passage of nurse registration laws. The first nurse registration laws passed in 1903 in North Carolina, New Jersey, and New York. This important nursing legislation served to protect the public from untrained nurses, as well as protect the livelihood of trained nurses (Roberts, 1954; Lewenson, 1996).

Before establishing the ANA, nursing educators at the newly opened training schools recognized that to control practice, they had to control the education of nurses. These early pioneers founded the American Society of Superintendents of Training Schools (Superintendents Society), forerunner of the NLNE in 1912 and the National League for Nursing (NLN) in 1952. The Superintendents Society had organized 3 years before the Associated Alumnae and was interested in raising the standards of education and practice. The leaders of the Superintendents Society organized and supported the development of the Associate Alumnae, and many of the leaders were active in both organizations. Women such as Isabel Hampton Robb, Lavinia Dock, and Linda Richards supported the advancement of the nursing profession and sought recognition for their professional worth and contributions to healthcare in the United States (Roberts, 1954).

The National Association of Colored Graduate Nurses (NACGN), established in 1908, was organized for the same reasons as the Superintendents Society and the Associated Alumnae. Standards of practice and control of nursing education constituted a good part of the activities of this third national organization. The overriding reason for NACGN's existence, however, was related to the need to address the racism experienced by many African-American nurses. The NACGN was formed to provide a professional organization for African-American nurses that responded to their experiences of racism (Hine, 1989; Carnegie, 1991; Lewenson, 1996).

Public Health Nursing

By 1912, increasing interest in public health supported the rapid growth of public health nursing. Visiting nurse services opened in many cities throughout the United States, offering home care to families in the community. In 1890, almost 20 years after the opening of nurse training schools in the United States, 21 visiting nurse organizations existed. Gardner, an early public health nursing leader, explained that "these organizations had no connection with one another, and no common standard of efficiency, either in practical work or in the educational requirements for the nurse" (Gardner, 1933, p 19). A need to set public health nursing care standards prompted the formation of the National Organization of Public Health Nurses (NOPHN) in 1912 (Gardner, 1933; Fitzpatrick, 1975). The purpose of this new professional organization was to increase interest and responsibility in public health nursing, to establish ethical and technical standards of care, to facilitate the joint efforts of those interested in public health in the community, and to establish a central clearinghouse for information about public health nursing (Fitzpatrick, 1975).

Public health nursing at the beginning of the twentieth century provides early nursing models in a managed care environment. Even before Wald's work with the Metropolitan Life Insurance Company in 1909, public health nurses worked in settings that provided care for groups of people as part of the employees' benefits. One of the earliest accounts of the use of a public health nurse in industry can be traced to the Vermont Marble Company. In 1895 this company, under the leadership of its owner Fletcher Proctor, employed a trained nurse to provide healthcare to its employees. The John Wanamaker Department Store in 1897 and the National Cash Register Company in 1902 both provided healthcare for their employees (Gardner, 1933; Fitzpatrick, 1975).

Industrial nurses were trained nurses who provided a range of public health nursing services, as well as care of the sick, in the home to employees of a particular company. Gardner described how companies used and paid for industrial nursing:

The entire responsibility may be borne by the employer who furnishes the funds and controls policy; the employees themselves may assume this responsibility through group association in a single plan or through a labor union; or responsibility may be shared by the employer and the employees each contributing a part of the cost, and each having a voice in the administration (Gardner, 1933, p 362).

The rationale behind these various arrangements needs further study; however, the arrangements seem to relate to control of healthcare costs for a group of people, similar to the goals of managed care companies in the 1990s. Public health nurses, through their work in visiting nurse services, health departments, industry, and schools, provided communities with links to the healthcare system. Wald reflected how the public health nurses at the Henry Street Settlement improved the health of the community:

Doubtless among the outstanding phenomena within the memory of the living are the vast sums and the vast educational programs that have been poured out in efforts to care for the sick, to prevent illness, and to popularize the subject of health (Wald, 1934, p 70).

The public health nurses at Henry Street joined with others interested in improving the health and welfare of the immigrant poor in New York City. They argued for child labor laws, school nurses, and playgrounds for children. Nevertheless, although these nurses advocated social, political, and economic changes for the families they served, as women, they did not yet have the right to vote. Keeping this in mind, the contributions that nurses made before they won suffrage in 1920 were extraordinary. Under Wald's visionary leadership, the nurses at Henry Street joined with the Metropolitan Life Insurance Company in 1909 to create an experiment that lasted almost 50 years and led to the creation of the Metropolitan

Visiting Nurse Service (MVNS). This activity exemplifies nursing's historical involvement with the management of care of an aggregate.

THE METROPOLITAN VISITING NURSE SERVICE

In the early 1900s, the Metropolitan Life Insurance Company sold insurance policies to the families who had recently immigrated to the United States. Men and women bought policies that would assure a family's existence during a period of loss. The leadership of the Metropolitan Life Insurance Company faced fierce competition in the marketplace. To address this competition, the company targeted low-income immigrant families living in the crowded cities and sold them low-cost industrial life insurance policies. With the cost so low and the promised security so high, families bought insurance for each member of the household (Hamilton, 1988a, 1988b). Simultaneously, urban reformers advocated the adoption of public health reform measures. The newly emerging profession of nursing, already engaged in the health of the public, provided nursing services to overpopulated communities in cities throughout the United States.

By 1893, Wald had established the Henry Street Settlement. It was one of the first settlement houses in the country to provide nursing care in the community. Wald and her friend, Mary Brewster, both 1891 graduates of the New York Training School for Nurses, started the Henry Street Settlement with support from socially responsible philanthropists and like-minded trained nurses who had graduated from the newly opened training schools. A sliding scale for payment allowed all families to pay something for their care. This practice, Wald felt, removed the stigma of "charity" and "handout," which families who received care often experienced (Wald, 1915).

Wald wrote that "in the year 1909 the Metropolitan Life Insurance Company undertook the nursing of its industrial policy holders—an important event in the annals of visiting nursing" (Wald, 1915, p 63). Hamilton (1988a) likened the joining of these two diverse forces as the confrontation between faith and finance. Haley Fiske, vice president of the Metropolitan Life Insurance Company, believed in the redeeming social benefits of owning industrial life insurance policies. In response to muckrakers' attacks on the honesty of the insurance industry, Fiske spoke in defense of his company and touted the benefits of its policies to the owners. At one meeting where Fiske spoke, Dr. Lee Frankel challenged Fiske to provide healthcare to policyholders. Wald heard of Frankel's ideas and convinced him and the Metropolitan Life Insurance Company that use of public health nurses would benefit the company. Nurses, she noted, decreased mortality rates and provided health education to families. Policyholders, with little access to healthcare, could receive needed nursing care in the home (Hamilton, 1988a, 1988b).

The Metropolitan Life Insurance Company and the nurses of the Henry Street Settlement established the MVNS, which lasted from 1909 until 1953 (Hamilton, 1988a, 1988b). What had begun as a 3-month experiment lasted 43 years. In keeping with the separate philosophy of each group and to benefit policyholders, health education and nursing home care visits merged with business acumen. The statistics gathered by nurses and prepared by statisticians supported the rationale of providing healthcare for "improving" health. Hamilton (1988b) noted that during the 43-year history of the MVNS, nurses defended their ability to provide quality nursing care in the home, whereas businessmen argued for cost containment and cost consciousness.

This tension continues in the 1990s, since the ethics of managed care and nursing sometimes conflict (Wurzbach, 1998). Cost versus quality was an issue that created the schism between the two groups that eventually, along with other significant factors, led to the demise of the MVNS. Hamilton (1988b) explained how nursing care became too costly for the Metropolitan Life Insurance Company. The demographics and environment had changed significantly since it first sold industrial insurance to the urban, immigrant poor on the Lower East Side of New York.

During its prime, the MVNS became a national entity in which visiting nurses were contracted by the company to provide home care and health education to Metropolitan Life's policyholders in cities throughout the United States. Usually the contract was made with existing Visiting Nurse Services, but when one did not exist, the company started its own service. Nurses were paid a yearly salary of $1200 and reported over 4 million visits in 7000 cities throughout the United States (Hamilton, 1988b). Expanding business and providing access to healthcare services were the two central reasons for the Metropolitan Life Insurance Company to develop the MVNS. Frankel spoke at the first annual meeting of the National Organization of Public Health Nurses in 1913. At that meeting, only 4 years after the MVNS began, he spoke in a talk titled, "Visiting Nursing—A Business—How it is to be Conducted," about the need for public health nurses to incorporate business practices in their agencies (Fitzpatrick, 1975).

The conflict that nurses experienced between their ideas about quality and the need to be cost-efficient and accountable, however, contributed to the closing of the MVNS and the loss of nursing positions. Other contributing factors that led to the end of the MVNS included a change in the demographics of policyholders and the introduction of Social Security in 1935, which provided healthcare options for American workers, as well as other health insurance companies. Insurance companies such as Blue Cross offered newer ways for people to obtain affordable healthcare. In addition, the positive outcomes from the early public health campaign created a healthier population and the need for fewer public health nursing visits. An increase in immunizations and childbirth hospital deliveries and a decrease in infant mortality contributed to the decrease in public health nursing services by the Metropolitan Life Insurance Company policyholders (Hamilton, 1988a, 1988b).

The MVNS closed in 1953. Although a number of factors influenced the decline of the MVNS, Hamilton (1988a, 1988b) believed that the nurses' lack of understanding of the relationship between the care they delivered and economic influences on care was a major factor.

. . . when early nursing leaders resisted involvement with finances, they created a situation in which patient policy decisions were made for them. Nurses, believing that patient needs determine policy, did not fully comprehend that, from a business perspective, finances would be included in policy formation (Hamilton, 1988a, p 127).

COST ANALYSIS STUDY

Pfefferkorn and Rovetta opened the report of the Joint Committee on the Cost of Nursing Service and Nursing Education (Joint Committee) study with the words, "the subject of nursing costs is not new" (Pfefferkorn and Rovetta, 1940, p 3). Whether it was new or not, nurses' understanding of finance and the application of its principles in determining care was a dilemma that has haunted the profession throughout the twentieth century. As a result of the apprenticeship training nurses received during the first half of the twentieth century, the cost of care was directly linked to the cost of education. Pfefferkorn and Rovetta (1940) examined the cost of using nursing students to provide nursing service as opposed to using a graduate staff. More importantly, they wanted to develop procedures for measuring and comparing the outcomes of one hospital with another. Tools and accounting formulas were designed to help administrators collect the data on staffing and census at a particular hospital. Pfefferkorn and Rovetta wrote that to determine the appropriate cost procedure, "it is essential to know the conditions under which costs are being measured and the purpose for which the particular costs are being used" (Pfefferkorn and Rovetta, 1940, p 10).

Results of the analysis of Pfefferkorn and Rovetta (1940) revealed that graduate nurses were cheaper and better than student nurses for direct patient care. Graduate nurses spent fewer hours than student nurses on similar tasks. Moreover, their report revealed an interesting discussion on how to link cost with outcomes and with financial matters in general. The term *budget*, they said, did not become widely used in the United States until the 1920s. Separate administrative budgets, to be determined by nursing cost data, were needed in hospitals that provided patient care and nursing education. Budgets based on collected nursing cost data enabled administrators to set policy, compare the costs of one institution with another, and give an "account of how funds of the institution have been used and the value the institution has received in return" (Pfefferkorn and Rovetta, 1940, p 189).

The issue of cost containment and nursing services provided in hospitals was important to hospitals, nursing organizations, government agencies, private foundations, nursing schools, and other interested stakeholders. These groups often collaborated and sponsored studies such as that of the Joint Committee. In addition, they studied the status of nursing and the relationship between nursing and cost, education, value, and roles. Earlier studies pointed nursing leaders in the direction of raising nursing education to a baccalaureate level and in later studies, to an advanced graduate level for some of the newer roles in nursing.

CONTEMPORARY PERSPECTIVES ON MANAGED CARE

How some of the previous examples related nursing's contribution to the history of managed care may be a bit of a stretch, but the case can be made that nursing has always cared for patients and at times has been concerned about the cost of that care. Historical examples inform the conversation but by no means tell the whole story of nursing's role or contribution to the development of managed care. Nurses have been present and have witnessed the changes in healthcare that created the managed care environment in the 1990s. Their contributions can be found in their roles as case managers, educators, and practitioners.

Changes in Healthcare After World War II

By the 1960s, the U.S. healthcare system had adjusted to the social, political, and economic changes since the mid-twentieth century. World War II had brought great changes that dramatically altered the way healthcare was delivered. Changes in the management of illness, the building of more hospitals, the use of advanced technology in care, the rise of critical care units, and a general belief that science would cure the ills of society framed the thinking of the second half of the twentieth century (Fairman and Lynaugh, 1998). Nursing had undergone scrutiny by several mid-twentieth-century studies, such as Brown's *Nursing for the Future* (1948), which called for broad planning for collegiate education in nursing. Brown urged nursing to collect data to make the decisions needed to meet the demands of the future. She wrote that "no group of persons, however well informed about nursing education in the particular state, has enough basic data for construction of a blueprint" (Brown, 1948, p 180). In addition, with the need for more and better-prepared nurses, Brown challenged nursing to recruit from a broader cross-section of American culture, regardless of "sex, marital status, economic background, or ethnic, racial and religious origins" (Brown, 1948, p 197).

After World War II, interest in rebuilding American communities to accommodate growing families encouraged women to leave the job market and return home. More nurses were needed to fill the vacancies created by the increasing number of hospitals built as a result of the Hospital Survey and Reconstruction Act (Hill-Burton Act). The increase in employer-provided private health insurance, scientific and technological advances, and economic prosperity created public demand for the "best healthcare money could buy" (Lynaugh and Brush, 1996, p 22). This demand for care created an even greater demand for more and better-prepared nurses.

Lynaugh and Brush noted that post-World War II hospitals were seen as a place to restore health, mirroring the rest of society's return to "peace and prosperity" (Lynaugh and Brush, 1996, p 23). As hospitals grew in structure and stature, nurses who could work within the increasingly complex environments were needed. Lynaugh and Brush (1996) noted that although the need increased for more specialized nursing care, the education and status of nursing did not accompany that change. Hospitals were interested in making money. Nurses could not and did not articulate their worth, nor did they define themselves as a monopoly requiring the appropriate economic reward. As a result, nurses were underpaid and often were replaced through the use of less expensive staffing patterns (Lynaugh and Brush, 1996).

The demand for nurses supported the need for better preparation and more educational resources to produce the desired professional (Petry and Vreeland, 1952). Nursing organizations recognized this need and struggled to improve the quality and standards of nursing education. The early 1950s saw a restructuring of the professional nursing organizations. The first four organizations that formed at the beginning of the twentieth century—the ANA, the NLNE, the NACGN, and the NOPHN—had been joined by several other specialty organizations. Groups representing collegiate education, industrial nursing, religious institutions, and the like had assumed the responsibility of setting and maintaining standards for these specialties. A consolidation of many of these organizations into the ANA and the NLN created two powerful nursing groups. In this period of restructuring, the newly formed NLN accepted the responsibility of being designated the sole accrediting body for nursing education. To meet the demand for more and better-prepared nurses, accreditation became an increasingly important activity of the NLN. In addition to the need for better nurses, there was a need for better nursing schools and better-prepared faculty.

Changes Since the 1960s

Medicaid and Medicare legislation established in the 1960s created a dramatic change in the provision of healthcare. This new federal legislation exerted pressure on hospitals to provide increasingly specialized care to more people. The concomitant increase in costs that accompanied this change precipitated a redefinition of the professional practices of nurses and physicians (Lynaugh and Brush, 1996). In an effort to match the education of nurses to the more complex care required, in 1965 the ANA supported the controversial platform of baccalaureate entry into practice. In the 2000s this goal has not been realized; however, the nursing profession has spent over 35 years discussing the merits of such a stand. While nursing debated this issue, advanced degrees in nursing became more prevalent. Federal money to support nursing education contributed to the increasing number of nurses who returned to school. The nurse practitioner movement began in the 1960s and provided the healthcare system with a much needed primary care provider. Additionally, other advanced practice nurses such as clinical specialists and nurse clinicians began to provide advanced nursing care both in the hospital and in the community (Lynaugh and Brush, 1996).

The 1970s and Beyond: Managed Care and Nursing Case Management

Managed care was an outgrowth of the need to control costs and provide access to care in a reasonable manner; it was a perceived vehicle to contain such costs. The late 1960s and early 1970s saw society's discontent with an expensive fee-for-service (FFS) system and an increasing suspicion of physicians and hospitals (Knight, 1998). The women's movement raised women's consciousness of their health and their bodies. The once sought-after traditional health insurance policies from the 1930s, 1940s, and 1950s served as a barrier between the consumer and the service provider by the 1970s, and insurance companies paid an ever-increasing healthcare bill. The structure of hospitals in the 1970s promoted and supported the increase in such costs, so much so that Jennings and Jennings noted, "more insurance begets more expensive care, and more expensive care begets more insurance" (Jennings and Jennings, 1977, p 1155).

In 1973 Congress passed the HMO Act, creating a new way of providing healthcare for the American people. In the early 1970s, health maintenance organizations (HMOs) sought federal certification, which enabled providers to receive federal grants and awards and also gave them creditability with consumers. HMOs expanded throughout the country, more successfully in some regions, such as the West, than in others. Concern for the high cost of FFS led to even larger numbers of HMOs; newer versions of this managed care plan that allowed greater flexibility emerged in the 1980s (Knight, 1998).

Eventually the need to demonstrate tangible outcomes from receiving care in the out-of-control healthcare environment had became evident (Corder, Phoon, and Barter, 1996). Consumers, insurance companies, managed care companies, and healthcare professionals needed data that would support cost containment measures while ensuring level of quality. Each group had a different stake in the collected data and the delivered outcomes. The increasing costs of insurance benefits prompted business in the 1980s to control the spiraling cost of employee benefits. Employers began to share the cost of insurance with their employees by requiring deductibles, nominal copayments, or partial premium payments. This shift in cost did not sufficiently decrease the high cost of healthcare for the employer, and other solutions had to be found (Corder, Phoon, and Barter, 1996).

The demand for managed care to control healthcare costs became omnipresent in the 1990s. Employers, who since the 1950s had assumed most of the cost, now challenged insurance companies, hospitals, and physicians to provide less expensive healthcare benefits for their employees. The younger and older populations, both unemployed, also needed an affordable avenue to purchase healthcare. The cost of insurance for unemployed persons was so high that alternatives to this form of payment were essential. Consumers' discomfort with the earlier HMO models led to adaptations and the rise of other forms, such as the point-of-service plan (POS) and the preferred provider organization (PPO). The POS gave consumers some flexibility in choosing their healthcare provider; the PPO gave the purchaser of healthcare services a wide array of networks from which to select medical care. Additional services such as case management and utilization review needed to be purchased separately (Bower, 1992).

CASE MANAGERS

Nurses historically have managed the care of individuals, families, and communities. Nightingale's direction to nurses that they "ought to signify the proper use of fresh air, light, warmth, cleanliness, quiet, and the proper selection and administration of diet" (Nightingale, 1858/1969, p 8) pointed to the responsibility nurses were given to control the patients' environment. From Nightingale's early advice to the ANA's updated social policy statement in 1995, nursing has defined itself by the management of care.

The ANA's Social Policy Statement defined nursing's role as the:

attention to the full range of human experiences and responses to health and illness without restriction to a problem-focused orientation; integration of objective data with knowledge gained from an understanding of the patient or group's subjective experience; application of scientific knowledge to the processes of diagnosis and treatment; and provision of a caring relationship that facilitates health and healing (ANA, 1995, p 6).

Nurse case managers operate within this recent definition of nursing. The principles underlying case management—cost containment, outcome-driven care, and process-oriented care—frame the work that nurses do. Whereas managed care refers to the measures used by the purchasers of healthcare to "influence aggregate utilization levels of various types of services in order to maintain quality and control cost" (Bower, 1992, p 2), case management has become one of the strategies used by MCOs to provide care to individuals, families, and communities while balancing the cost, outcomes, and processes.

MEASURING THE VALUE OF NURSING

Before 1903 when the first nursing registration laws were passed, any woman could call herself a nurse. Through professional organizations, nurses sought control of practice and education. They did so among conflicting ideas about the roles of women and nurses and changing expectations of practice and education. Nurses and nursing have been there for patients and communities, yet their contributions are rarely acknowledged or understood. The value of nursing to the healthcare system has been difficult to measure. Outcomes for the care provided have been sought throughout the twentieth century. For nurses and nursing to survive in this managed care environment, their worth must be measured. Like the earlier experiment at the Henry Street Settlement, nurses need to understand the language of business and translate it into the language of care. Similarly, like the earlier hospital studies, nurses need to know the cost of their services and to inform others of these costs, as well as the benefits accrued through the use of nursing services. Costs, outcomes, and the way care is provided are so essential to nursing's survival that nurses need to assume responsibility and knowledge and become major players in healthcare. Knowing this, however, nurses and nursing need to recognize the "nursism" that surrounds the perception of their work, education, and role. Overcoming nursing's lack of recognition at the "table" will require visionary leadership, new ways to educate the profession and public, and greater visibility of nursing's work. Nurses need to be multilingual—to understand the language of care and frame it in a way that others can understand, as well as to understand the language of others. They also need their history to inform their work and to inform others.

REFERENCES

American Nurses Association: *Nursing's social policy statement*, Washington, DC, 1995, American Nurses Publishing.

Bower KA: *Case management by nurses*, Kansas City, Mo, 1992, American Nurses Association.

Brown EL: *Nursing for the future*, A report prepared for the National Nursing Council, New York, 1948, Russell Sage Foundation.

Bullough V, Bullough B, Stanton MP, editors: *Florence Nightingale and her era: a collection of new scholarship*, New York, 1990, Garland.

Burgess MA: *Nurses, patients, and pocketbooks*, Report of a study of the economics of nursing conducted by the Committee on the Grading of Nursing Schools, New York, 1928, Committee on the Grading of Nursing Schools.

Carnegie ME: *The path we tread: blacks in nursing 1854-1990*, New York, 1991, National League for Nursing.

Cohen EL, Cesta T: *Nursing case management: from concept to evaluation*, ed 2, St Louis, Mo, 1997, Mosby.

Conti RM: Nursing case manager roles: implications for practice and education, *Nurs Admin Q* 2(1):67-81, 1996.

Corder KT, Phoon J, Barter M: Managed care: employers' influence on the healthcare system, *Nurs Econ* 14(4): 213-218, 1996.

Dock LL, Stewart IM: *A short history of nursing from the earliest times to the present day*, New York, 1931, GP Putnam's Sons.

Fairman J, Lynaugh J: *Critical care nursing: a history*, Philadelphia, 1998, University of Pennsylvania Press.

Fitzpatrick ML: *The national organization for public health nursing: 1912-1952*, New York, 1975, National League for Nursing.

Fitzpatrick ML: *Prologue to professionalism: a history of nursing*, Bowie, Md, 1983, Brady Communications.

Gardner MS: *Public health nursing,* ed 2, New York, 1933, Macmillan.

Hamilton D: Faith and finance, *Image J Nurs Sch* 20(3): 124-127, 1988a.

Hamilton D: Clinical excellence, but too high a cost: the Metropolitan Life Insurance Company Visiting Nurse Service (1909-1953), *Public Health Nurs* 5(4):235-240, 1988b.

Hine DC: *Black women in white: racial conflict and cooperation in the nursing profession, 1890-1950,* Bloomington, 1989, Indiana University Press.

Jennings CP, Jennings TF: Containing costs through prospective reimbursement, *Am J Nurs* 77(7):1155-1159, 1977.

Knight W: *Managed care: what it is and how it works,* Gaithersburg, Md, 1998, Aspen.

Lewenson S: *Taking charge: nursing, suffrage, and feminism 1873-1920,* New York, 1996, National League for Nursing.

Lynaugh JE, Brush BL: *American nursing: from hospitals to health systems,* Malden, Mass, 1996, Blackwell.

Nightingale F: *Notes on nursing: what it is, and what it is not,* New York, 1858/1969, Dover.

North FH: A new profession for women, *The Century Magazine* 25(1):38-47, 1882.

Petry L, Vreeland EM: Nursing education, *Higher Education: Semimonthly Publication of the Federal Security Agency* 8(16):181-186, 1952.

Pfefferkorn B, Rovetta C: *Administrative cost analysis for nursing service and nursing education,* Chicago, 1940, American Hospital Association and National League of Nursing Education.

Reverby S: *Ordered to care: the dilemma of American nursing, 1850-1945,* Cambridge, UK, 1987, Cambridge University Press.

Roberts MM: *American nursing history and interpretation,* New York, 1954, Macmillan.

Wald LD: *The house on Henry Street,* New York, 1915, Henry Holt.

Wald LD: *Windows on Henry Street,* Boston, 1934, Little, Brown.

Wurzbach ME: Managed care: moral conflicts for primary healthcare nurses, *Nurs Outlook* 46(2):62-66, 1998.

How a Managed Care Organization Works

Francesca Losito

KEY LESSONS IN THIS CHAPTER

- Health plans use case management processes to facilitate and monitor medical care to their members in both the hospital and the community.
- Managed care organizations monitor quality in a number of ways, including state oversight, federal oversight, voluntary accreditation, standardized performance indicators, and mandates from employers and business sectors.
- The Medical Management operations of the managed care organization should receive regular feedback on provider and member satisfaction through periodic satisfaction surveys.
- Managed care organizations are accountable to industry, the legal system, external regulatory agencies, and the marketplace.
- The National Committee for Quality Assurance (NCQA) is a private, not-for-profit organization dedicated to assessing and reporting on the quality of managed care plans.

Managed care organizations (MCOs) use a variety of strategies to manage patients from both a clinical and a financial perspective, including medical management, case management, quality management, and utilization management.

This chapter describes how managed care works from these perspectives and how these functions are applied within the context of a healthcare plan. The following are described:

- *Structure:* what and who makes up the department(s)
- *Process:* how a member or provider navigates within the structure
- *Desired outcomes:* the goals of the organization and how they are measured

STRUCTURE: MEDICAL MANAGEMENT

The monitoring of all members, in or out of the hospital, takes place in the department usually known as Medical Management (MM). The MM department consists of Medical Management operations (MM Ops), case management (CM), and quality management (QM).

Medical Management Operations

The individuals who are considered "operations" within this department generally are not clinicians. The department may consist of an Operations Manager or Business Manager who is responsible for the development, assessment, and maintenance of effective and efficient daily operations. Daily operations include processes and procedures performed by the MM department staff, who provide a high level of service, accommodate growth, and are sensitive to changing customer needs. The health plan may use project managers, who are responsible for identifying, investigating, planning, and implementing process and system enhancements for the department. They provide system development, process development, project management, and analytical support for the MM department.

Medical management analysts provide research and analytical support for the MM department. Responsibilities include developing and continually improving reports that analyze the productivity of staff members. Medical management coordinator/customer service associates (MMCs) assist members and providers with all aspects of utilization management programs. MMCs receive incoming telephone inquiries; complete authorizations for all elective admissions, diagnostic services, and ambulatory surgery; and refer the member or provider to the appropriate nurse case manager. MMCs gather and record demographic information and serve as the first line in quality member service delivery.

A health plan uses case management to facilitate and monitor medical care to its members both within the hospital and in the community. Historically, MCOs targeted their efforts on patients with catastrophic, complex illness or injury, who were frequent users of healthcare resources. Today MCOs continue to manage complex members, but the trend has shifted to sophisticated disease management programs that focus on prevention. Prevention becomes particularly important for members who may have preexisting conditions that can exacerbate if not monitored. This shift in focus has been due largely to the National Committee for Quality Assurance (NCQA) standards (NCQA, 1996) and the enrollment of Medicare and Medicaid populations in managed care plans. Most MCOs focus their case management programs on the 3% to 5% of the population that consumes the greatest amount of resources. Originally, case management focused largely on patients with catastrophic illness or injury. The NCQA standards have forced MCOs to rethink their case management strategies. The use of case management for catastrophic illness or injury still occurs, but programs have begun to focus more intensely on more prevalent conditions (Sajdak, 1998).

A common disease management program focuses on a chronic illness such as congestive heart failure (CHF). An individual with CHF would be enrolled in the program and would be monitored by a set of clinical guidelines established by the plan. The goal of the program would be to prevent unnecessary hospital admissions while helping the member maintain a better quality of life in the community. Strategies to meet these goals would include interventions such as using community-based visiting nurse services, who evaluate the patient at home, monitoring vital signs, assessing lung sounds, checking for evidence of edema, providing patient education, reporting responses to existing therapy and medication regimen, and evaluating the member's ability to remain compliant with the treatment plan.

Claims

Historically, claims is a "back office" operation in which information entered by the MM department is used to process claims, so providers can be paid for services rendered. It sounds simple, but in reality it is a complex and technical process. In the provider relations department, the staff are able to discuss the ways in which case management can reduce unnecessary readmissions and improve quality of life through the various programs set up by the health plan. The claims department needs to have strong links to the provider relations department, since it depends on accurate information and communication for claims to be processed in a timely manner. For example, if MM makes a decision regarding an extracontractual benefit, this needs to be documented accurately in the computer system. When this process is overlooked or when MM has a backlog of data not yet entered, the claim will not be paid correctly, if at all. Additionally, if a claims processor is unable to differentiate between a diagnosis and procedure, this also will result in a delayed payment. To optimize efficiency, health plans need to use clinical resources within the claims department and provide oversight and clarification when necessary. Ideally, claims processors should be assigned to a designated number of case managers, who sit next to this group and from whom questions and clarification of documentation can be discussed and decided in "real time." In this way, the plan can improve the speed with which they are able to process and pay a claim.

Case Management

The term *case management* is frequently used when describing an approach for managing complex medical care. In 1996 the Commission for Case Manager Certification defined case management as " . . . a collaborative process which [sic] assesses, plans, implements, coordinates, monitors and evaluates the options and services to meet an individual's healthcare needs using community resources available to provide quality and cost-effective outcomes" (Commission for Case Manager Certification, 1996). This definition describes a complex, multidisciplinary process that requires the input and support of many players in the healthcare delivery system, including patients, their support systems such as family and friends, all care providers, and vendors or other suppliers to the healthcare system (Sajdak, 1998). The success of this approach depends strongly on the collaborative effort of the interdisciplinary team(s) with shared goals for the patient.

The health plan may also use social workers who are valuable as case managers, especially with patients who have complex illness or injury and who are socially or economically unable to provide for themselves. Social workers can provide CM department staff with consultations and identification of community resources needed to enhance the quality and scope of services to members.

There are various types of case management that differ from one organization to another. The type of approach depends on the structure of the organization and its desired outcomes. A well-run CM program is organized and staffed with nurse case managers, has well-developed policies and procedures and an internal evaluation mechanism, and links appropriately to other departments, such as provider relations, claims, and member services (Sajdak, 1998).

An example of the case management process includes the following steps (Sajdak, Gerbarg, and Zachary, 1998):

- *Case management identification process:* In this step, the case manager identifies patients in need of case management based on high-risk criteria such as multiple medications, functional deficits, and multiple admissions.
- *Case management assessment process:* The case manager conducts an assessment to determine the patient's specific needs and the level of case management intervention necessary based on the assessment.
- *Case management implementation,* including the treatment plan.
- *Benefit plan extension process* (i e , extracontractual benefits): In this step, the case manager may determine that the patient's plan does not cover needed services and that an extension or adjustment must be made.
- *Attending physician, family, and patient communication:* Ongoing communication is critical to the success of the case management process.
- *Documentation* continues throughout the process.
- *Patient outcomes evaluation:* The patient's progress is monitored against the outcomes identified by the guidelines in use.
- *Patient and provider satisfaction:* An ongoing part of the evaluation process.
- *Interface and communication with other MCO departments,* ongoing as needed.
- *Case management closure process:* The case is closed when the need for case management intervention is no longer there.

The nurse case manager-to-member ratio differs from plan to plan. Medicare members historically have required a lower case manager-to-member ratio because of the intensity of this particular patient population, whereas commercial or Medicaid populations can be run effectively with higher ratios. A fair industry ratio standard is generally a 1:5000 to 1:7500 for Medicare members and a 1:10,000 to 1:15,000 for commercial and Medicaid populations.

Today's CM programs have evolved from earlier programs that primarily managed healthcare utilization, which have existed for more than 20 years. These early efforts focused on reducing the number of inpatient admissions and eliminating unnecessary hospital days. To achieve this objective, health plan administrators reviewed the hospital admission for medical necessity before the admission (precertification) and determined the need for ongoing care (concurrent review). For cases that were not part of the concurrent review process, the process was applied retrospectively (i.e., after the patient was discharged from the hospital) (Sajdak, Gerbarg, and Zachary, 1998).

The majority of health plans today include the process for precertification before admission, as well as concurrent review, to determine clinical necessity and appropriateness in terms of site of care. Precertification would be applied before the use of any services across the continuum, including hospital, outpatient, or home care. The set of protocols, guidelines, or clinical pathways a case manager uses to determine medical necessity differs from plan to plan. The nurses performing this function must be trained and certified in the use of the specific protocols applied by the plan. The medical directors also must have a working knowledge of the plan's specific clinical protocols, since they may be needed to resolve a dispute when the provider disagrees with the plan's case management decision to not cover a particular level of service.

The following are two nationally recognized standards that a health plan may use:

1. InterQual (InterQual, Inc, 1998), a criteria-based tool that assesses the following three criteria:
    - Intensity of service—the specific resources used in patient care
    - Severity of illness—the specific clinical signs, symptoms, and test results
    - Discharge screens—clinical outcomes to be met for a safe and appropriate discharge.
2. Milliman & Robertson's *Healthcare Management Guidelines* (Doyle and Schibanoff, 2001), is used by providers and payers to determine a *goal length of stay* for an episode of illness. The *Healthcare Management Guidelines* consist of seven different volumes to help determine appropriateness. The seven volumes cross the continuum of care and are applied based on the patient's current care delivery setting. They include inpatient and surgical care, return-to-work planning, ambulatory care, home healthcare, primary and pharmaceutical care, recovery facility care, and workers' compensation.

In reviewing the patient's condition, the plan case manager reviews each *day*, not in terms of a "clock day" (24 hours), but rather in terms of a *phase* or *stage*. It is conceivable that a patient can remain on "day 1" for 5 days, depending on the patient's condition and inability to progress.

Regardless of the specific guidelines used by the plan, these preestablished guidelines, along with the plan's policies and procedures, assist the CM and medical staff in evaluating each individual in terms of treatment plan and/or the need to move the member through the continuum of care to reach the desired outcomes.

The success of these processes depends on good communication with all internal and external customers. Each discipline needs to support the other's efforts and share the same goals and desired outcomes.

Quality Management

Another component of MM is quality management. Quality assessment and management methods include reviews carried out by physicians. Usually this process is performed by a group of physicians whose collective judgment is better than that of the individual. The process tends to be informal and does not rely on the use of written criteria and standards, although case selection may follow sophisticated identification techniques. The explicit review process applies specific criteria to the medical record or uses a process of observation of actual care delivery.

A good QM program is one in which the health plan has made a conscious decision to place quality as its main priority for managing its members' care and quality of life. Paris and Silberman (Carefoote, 1998) have identified a few of the drivers that have influenced this need, including the following:

- *State oversight:* The states regulate health maintenance organizations (HMOs) and other forms of managed care, usually through their insurance department. Although the states look at a variety of variables such as enrollment and utilization review (UR), they also monitor quality. Most states ask HMOs to have specific quality assurance plans and to take corrective action when problems are noted.
- *Federal oversight:* The U.S. Department of Health and Human Services also has the responsibility for overseeing specific MCOs, including federally qualified HMOs and plans enrolling Medicaid or Medicare enrollees. The comprehensive set of benefits that HMOs must provide is outlined in the federal statute, as well as specific requirements for the HMO, including reporting on utilization patterns, availability, and accessibility. For those plans that participate in Medicaid managed care arrangements, the Health Care Financing Administration (HCFA) sets out additional requirements that must be part of any contract with MCOs, such as formal written QM programs. The contract is intended to stipulate compliance with the QM program, which usually entails independent external quality reviews and focused studies on clinical care and delivery systems, as well as an examination of both underutilization and overutilization.
- *Voluntary accreditation:* Although most MCOs are not required to obtain formal accreditation, the competition from other accredited organizations often compels them to do so. In the area of voluntary accreditation, there are three primary associations: (1) NCQA, (2) the Joint Commission on Accreditation of Healthcare Organizations (JCAHO), and (3) the Utilization Review Accreditation Commission (URAC).

Additional information on each of these follows.

Standardized Performance Indicators

The Health Plan Employer Data and Information Set (HEDIS) contains more than 60 performance measures and is a renowned indicator of quality in managed care today. Responsibility for HEDIS currently resides with the NCQA. HEDIS was designed to provide MCOs with a standardized reporting format for identifying quality improvement indicators. It also enables MCOs to track their performance over time. Similarly, HEDIS provides employers and purchasers of healthcare with meaningful information for comparing the value of managed care products. The latest version of HEDIS has an increased emphasis on outcomes, and it is used to assess performance in the commercial population, as well as the Medicare and Medicaid populations (Carefoote, 1998).

HCFA and the Kaiser Family Foundation initiated the development of a standardized Medicare report card based on the HEDIS model. U.S. Healthcare and U.S. Quality Algorithms, Inc (USQA) have used their expertise to develop a population-based method to assess quality of care measures, access and satisfaction measures, and utilization statistics. The impact and use of the Medicare report card in managed care is not yet known, especially now that HEDIS has broadened its scope to include QM in the Medicare population (Carefoote, 1998).

Employer and Business Mandates

Historically, employers have evaluated health plans based on costs alone, but that is changing. Beauregard and Winston (1997) have identified at least four reasons why large employers are moving away from evaluations based on costs alone to evaluations that include financial efficiency and quality components. First, employers want to ensure that they are receiving value for their healthcare dollar. A plan that costs less may result in higher claim costs due to poorer quality. Second, the development of standard performance indicators such as those found in HEDIS enables employers to compare health plans in meaningful ways. Third, employees are better educated about quality healthcare and are asking their employers about the quality provided by health plans before they choose one. Finally, some employer groups are hiring benefits managers with clinical backgrounds, recognizing that a relationship exists between effective clinical management and low claims costs. These clinically driven benefits managers are clearly interested in the quality provided by a health plan, especially in the area of health promotion and wellness activities.

Using a formal request known as a Request for Information (RFI), purchasers of healthcare are demanding that MCOs respond to specific questions about their performance so that they can make meaningful assessments about the value of different health plans. Often the questions will address HEDIS measures and the plan's performance over time (Carefoote, 1998).

Competition

MCOs now find themselves competing for business not only on the basis of cost, but on the quality of care and service they currently provide and on their past performance. MCOs that cannot prove their effectiveness through performance indicators will find themselves trying to join the ranks of those organizations that have implemented HEDIS just to remain competitive. It is no longer acceptable to "ride the wave" of a long-standing relationship— MCOs must be able to prove their value to healthcare purchasers, and they must have existing documented QM programs.

The core competencies of any successful QM program will have the following characteristics (Carefoote, 1998):

- Clear mission and goals
- Active leadership
- Defined structure and accountabilities
- Coordinated activities
- Effective planning
- Comprehensive scope of services
- Focus on improvement
- Data-driven decision making
- Sound policies and procedures
- Adequate resources

Most health plans are committed to promoting quality healthcare for their members by delivering efficient and effective utilization management and monitoring the quality of their health services. The MM department contributes to these goals through its quality control procedures and system of referrals to the QM and network delivery departments.

Utilization Management: Quality Control

To ensure the quality of utilization management activities, the health plan maintains clearly documented policies and procedures, systematically monitors review activities, and collects data to ensure the following:

- Staff adherence to MM policies and procedures
- Provider compliance with MM requirements
- Effective and appropriate MM activities
- Identification of utilization trends and problems to be addressed
- Member and provider satisfaction with the MM program

A four-step cycle of continuous quality improvement for all of its quality control activities is as follows:

1. *Monitoring:* Assessing staff, providers, and health services using computer data, feedback mechanisms, screening criteria, and other sources of information to look for incidents or patterns that may indicate a quality problem.
2. *Problem identification:* Evaluating facts to determine the nature and cause of the problem.
3. *Corrective action:* Identifying and implementing steps needed to resolve the issue or problem.
4. *Follow-up:* Ensuring that the corrective action is being followed and has the desired effect.

Quality Improvement Components

The following activities support continuous quality improvement initiatives:

Quality Assessment of Staff

The MM department monitors the quality of individual staff activities and performance through regular assessments. These include routine auditing of case loads, telephone monitoring, auditing of files for necessary documentation, and appropriate communication with all parties involved.

Utilization Review and Auditing

Annual review of criteria and rectification of specific guideline(s) or protocol(s) adopted by the health plan are done. Certification is issued only to reviewers who demonstrate the ability to apply the protocol correctly and consistently.

Program Evaluation

Utilization management activities are reviewed and updated on an annual basis in response to new healthcare delivery technologies, program evaluation, and changing patterns in local health services delivery.

Confidentiality Policies

All member information collected by the health plan is kept confidential and used solely for the purposes of utilization and quality management. Summary data used in program reporting does not contain identification of individual patients.

Member/Provider Satisfaction

The health plan is obligated to follow up on all complaints received on its utilization management activities. Complaints are logged and investigated. MM should receive feedback on provider and member satisfaction by periodic satisfaction surveys. The results of these surveys are evaluated for identification of problem areas and resolution.

PROCESS: NAVIGATING THE STRUCTURE

How Members Connect with the Managed Care Organization

Most MCOs have a general "800 number" or a locally designated number that the member can use to speak with a customer service representative, who determines where the customer needs to be directed. Any call by a medical professional (physician, hospital, or ancillary facility) that is clinical or refers to precertification, benefits, medical policy, out-of-network specialist exceptions, or case management is transferred to the MM department. For more complex medical issues regarding emergency room (ER) visits or inpatient hospitalizations, members also are transferred to the MM department, where they can speak with a nurse case manager.

When Members Need to Call

Members will call to verify their benefits or to change their primary care physician (PCP). In most instances, members need to access the health plan's healthcare system when they have a question about their benefits. Although they may have the information at hand, it is hard for most people to know exactly which benefits are covered. For example, if a member uses the ER for treatment, he or she must notify the health plan within the timeframe listed in the members' certificate. Failure to notify the health plan could result in the member having to pay out-of-pocket for the ER visit for not adhering to the plan's policies. If the ER visit is not life- or health-threatening, the member should notify the health plan before visiting the ER so that the plan can divert the member from the ER to an urgent care center or the PCP's office when appropriate. Members also call their health plan to file a complaint. Some examples of complaints include the following:

- Administrative problems (e.g., referral or billing issues)
- Communication or rapport (e.g., the provider was rude or failed to return phone calls)
- Access to care (e.g., the member spent a long time waiting for an appointment or there was no covering doctor)
- Quality of care (e.g., the treatment plan appears questionable for member diagnosis and/or perceived problems)

DESIRED OUTCOMES: GOALS, MEASUREMENT, AND ACCOUNTABILITY

Managed Care Organization Goals

The MCO's primary goal is to coordinate healthcare resources to achieve positive outcomes specific to patient needs. In addition, the MCO designs case management and other processes to empower the medical team to be proactive, decisive, accountable, and committed to the provision of optimum patient care in a cost-effective manner. Future trends in managed care case management should continue to have a strong focus on the education and empowerment of the patient household. Programs such as disease management, on-site concurrent review, complex case management, home care, discharge planning, social work, and high-risk case management are a constant evolving and improving process designed to reach optimal recovery, thereby reaching optimal outcomes.

Outcomes Measurement: Monitoring Utilization Management and Customer Service Indicators

MM monitors and reports on several key indicators. These indicators provide an objective means of measuring department performance in providing customer service and quality healthcare. They allow the health plan to set goals for improvement in specific utilization and customer service areas. These indicators are as follows:

- Average length of stay for inpatient admissions
- Bed days per 1000 member months for inpatient admissions
- Denials per 1000 member months
- Complaints per 1000 member months
- Rate of overturned denials based on complaints
- Percent of calls abandoned
- Calls per 1000 member months
- Total calls
- Average speed to answer
- Percent of calls transferred from customer service department.

MM programs focus on service delivery and maintenance of high levels of customer satisfaction, often surveying members about their satisfaction with care, the process used to arrange care, and the vendors who provided the care.

Indicator Monitoring

Quality management includes monitoring indicators that have been selected based on accreditation/regulatory requirements and organizational priorities. Indicators are typically focused on resource utilization, quality of care, access, and member satisfaction.

Patient/Provider Satisfaction Surveys

Surveys of both patients and providers are conducted periodically to determine how the organization can improve its service. Results are forwarded to those responsible for responding to the results.

Medical Record Review

Medical record review, using established parameters, can be used in peer review or in support of credentialing and recredentialing activities.

Medical Evaluation Studies

Performance information from other medical record review or claims data is analyzed to further determine appropriateness of care.

Committee Support

Utilization and quality issues are addressed, solutions are identified, and progress is monitored through interdepartmental committees, which vary by number and type according to the complexity of the organization. MM staff typically provide support and information for the committee work (Sajdak, 1998).

Managed Care Organization Accountability

Gosfield (Sajdak, Gerbarg, and Zachary, 1998) writes that managed care accountability mechanisms can be conceptualized as falling within the following four prominent categories, which serve as the framework for outlining medical management oversight activities.

Industry

Within the industry, self-regulation has been evident from the beginning of the managed care era. This category includes health practitioner regulations, the use of contracts to regulate healthcare providers, and accreditation programs, which originally were voluntary but have become increasingly mandatory over time.

Legal System

Accountability for quality often comes from tort verdicts, in which liability for damages resulting from poor patient outcome lawsuits can have a dramatic affect on the behavior of the industry as a whole. Although case law holding MCOs liable for bad patient outcomes has been relatively limited, a current trend exists that confirms MCOs' legal responsibilities for patient care (Sajdak, 1998).

External Regulation

Two primary entities regulate the quality and service utilization of MCOs—the federal and state governments. The number of Medicare and Medicaid beneficiaries enrolled in managed care plans has experienced unprecedented growth since 1993, and with over 18 million Americans enrolled, HCFA is now the single largest purchaser of managed care in the United States (HCFA Press Office, 1997). Through these stringent regulations and enforcement activities, HCFA has proceeded to take all steps necessary to ensure its beneficiaries are protected.

Marketplace

When consumers demand more information, when they demand certain services, or when they select one health plan over another, they directly influence the behavior of MCOs.

Collectively, the marketplace has begun to examine more closely the inner workings of managed care. Much of the interest has been stimulated by the negative stories printed in the popular press, and much of the marketplace's efforts have focused on measuring the performance of health plans across a variety of dimensions (Sajdak, Gerbarg, and Zachary, 1998).

Accountability Mechanisms

Provider Contracts

MCOs rely heavily on their networks of providers to be accountable for the care and service they provide. To this end, they have developed elaborate provider contracts that stipulate the following:

- Criteria to be used for appointing and credentialing practitioners
- Cause for terminating practitioners who do not meet "quality" standards
- Adherence to the plan's quality improvement efforts
- Use of clinical practice guidelines and standard medical record-keeping systems

These are but a few of the clauses that can be found in provider contracts. In recent years MCOs have put more emphasis on these contracts and are more conscientious in using them for accountability purposes (Sajdak, Gerbarg, and Zachary, 1998).

Accreditation

There are a variety of agencies and commissions that serve as accrediting bodies for providers and/or MCOs, some of which are as follows:

- NCQA: The NCQA is a private, not-for-profit organization dedicated to assessing and reporting on the quality of managed care plans (Carefoote, 1998). In 1991 and in response to a need to standardize information about the quality of these organizations, NCQA began accrediting MCOs. To be accredited, an MCO must meet approximately 50 standards that focus on the delivery of services and continuous improvement of the quality of care.
- URAC: URAC was founded in 1990 as an educational corporation with the goal of establishing minimum UR standards that serve to encourage efficient review processes and to provide a method for evaluating and accrediting UR programs. The first standards were published in 1991, with significant revisions in 1994. URAC has two accreditation programs: one for companies performing UR and one for preferred provider organization (PPO) networks (Carefoote, 1998).
- JCAHO: JCAHO is the primary accrediting body for healthcare organizations, and it is now playing a greater role in accrediting MCOs. Since 1994, JCAHO has accredited HMOs according to the standards outlined in the Accreditation Manual for Healthcare Networks. The conceptual model underlying these standards focuses on the improvement of organizational performance (Carefoote, 1998).

Federal and State Requirements

The U.S. Department of Health and Human Services has a responsibility to provide oversight to all MCOs that are licensed to provide care to Medicaid and Medicare enrollees.

Medicaid managed care participants are required by HCFA to provide formal written QM programs. The primary oversight mechanism outside of regulations are peer review organizations (PROs) (Fried, 1996). Most states regulate HMOs and other forms of managed care through their insurance department, although some states shift some or all of this responsibility to the department of health. A majority of states do the following (Carefoote, 1998):

- Prohibit HMOs from issuing any materials that are false, misleading, or deceptive
- Require adequate access to personnel and healthcare facilities
- Require plans to have specific quality assurance plans and to take corrective action when problems are found
- Mandate that HMOs have specific grievance procedures
- Require plans to collect, analyze, and report certain utilization, enrollment, and grievance data to the state
- Mandate that certain information be provided to enrollees and the public at large, including the enrollee's financial obligations, covered and excluded services, and procedures for obtaining services and filing complaints
- Have mechanisms to solicit enrollee participation in HMO policy decisions
- Have a system to ensure the HMO's financial solvency and to hold the enrollee harmless for a carrier's failure to pay the provider
- Have a variety of enforcement mechanisms to ensure that HMOs comply with their statutory and regulatory requirements

Accountability for the delivery of quality services and utilization in managed care is now the responsibility of many. Health plans now find themselves barraged by a variety of stakeholders yearning to enhance the visibility of oversight mechanisms and tighten the rules under which health plans operate.

FUTURE CHALLENGES FOR MANAGED CARE ORGANIZATIONS

Consumers and purchasers demand healthcare services that are outcome-based and cost-effective. Current accountability mechanisms have yet to satisfy the purchasers and consumers. In 1996 alone, more than 1000 measures aimed at tightening the regulation of HMOs (Weber, 1997) were being debated in legislation, which indicates the need for more stringent oversight for managed care plans. Future and proposed accountability mechanisms serve to enhance MCO oversight through more comprehensive and far-reaching regulations with stronger enforcement strategies; mandatory accreditation that encompasses quality, access, utilization, satisfaction, and outcome standards; and reliable and comparable data that measure performance across plans (Carefoote, 1998). The future holds significant challenges for MCOs striving to meet the increased oversight demands placed on them by both purchasers and consumers.

REFERENCES

Beauregard TR, Winston KR: Value-based formulas for purchasing: employers shift to quality to evaluate and manage their health plans, *Manag Care Q* 5(1):51-56, 1997.

Carefoote R: *Medical management: quality management,* 1998, URL Managed Care Resources, Available online: www.mcres.com/MCR.

Commission for Case Manager Certification: *CCM certification guide,* Rolling Meadows, Ill, 1996, The Commission.

Doyle RL, Schibanoff JM: *Healthcare management guidelines,* New York, 2001, Milliman & Robertson.

Fried BM: *Overview of managed care,* 1996, Available online: www.hcfa.gov/pubform.htm.

Healthcare Financing Administration Press Office: *Fact sheet: managed care in Medicare and Medicaid,* Washington, DC, 1997, Healthcare Financing Administration Press Office.

InterQual, Inc: *ISD-AC: acute care adult,* Marlborough, Mass, 1998, InterQual.

National Committee for Quality Assurance: *NCQA: an overview,* Washington, DC, 1996, The Committee, Available online: www.ncqa.org/pages/communities/news/jointrel.htm.

Sajdak M: *Case management: medical management "signature series,"* 1998, URL Managed Care Resources, Available online: www.mcres.com/MCR/mcrmm0.6.htm.

Sajdak M, Gerbarg MD, Zachary B: *Medical management: utilization management "signature series,"* 1998, URL Managed Care Resources, Available online: www.mcres.com/MCR/mcrmm0.2.htm.

Weber DO: Second thoughts: can managed care be ethical? *Healthcare Forum J* 40(4):17, 20-25, 1997.

Fundamentals of Managed Care

Lauren Hoffmann

KEY LESSONS IN THIS CHAPTER

- Although managed care plans date from 1919, the rapid growth of managed care accelerated greatly during the 1980s and 1990s.
- Managed care is not a single health insurance model but rather a complex system that coordinates and provides health services and benefits.
- When evaluating the quality of services provided by managed care plans, nurses must weigh the relative importance of the diverse variables that combine to create a comprehensive and high-quality product.
- Managed care plans vary greatly in the types of services they cover for plan members, as well as how they control access to those services.
- Managed care plans that seek accreditation demonstrate their commitment to provide quality care and service to their members.

American experimentation with managed care plans began in 1919 when Thomas Curran and James Yocum, two physicians from Tacoma, Washington, transformed their clinic into a prepaid group plan to provide care to local mill workers for a fee of $0.50/month (Theodosakis and Feinberg, 2000). Ten years later, 1500 schoolteachers in Baylor, Texas, formed a group plan that covered an enrollee for up to 21 days of hospital care for an annual premium of $6, and the Ross-Loos plan provided similar coverage for residents of Los Angeles, California (American Association of Health Plans, 2000; Theodosakis and Feinberg, 2000). In the late 1930s, a physician named Sidney Garfield began providing prepaid care to 5000 employees of the Kaiser Corporation working on the California Aqueduct, and by the mid-1940s, Kaiser moved from the construction business to the healthcare business. It was another 20 years after the Kaiser Corporation's move from construction to healthcare, however, that a physician named Paul Ellwood developed the concept of a healthcare system consisting of private healthcare companies called *health maintenance organizations* (HMOs), which operated in open markets but were regulated by the government (Theodosakis and Feinberg, 2000).

Despite growing interest in this concept of prepaid comprehensive healthcare, the United States experienced rapid growth of indemnity, or fee-for-service, plans, which provided medical benefits without cost controls throughout the 1950s and 1960s, leaving managed care plans with a small segment of the health insurance market. Currently, indemnity plans cover only 10% of Americans with healthcare benefits, but as recently as 1988, more than 70% of Americans were covered by indemnity plans (American Association of Health Plans, 2000). This figure may be somewhat misleading, however. In fact, the growth of managed care plans rose sharply, beginning in the 1980s and continuing unchecked throughout the 1990s. Only 15 million Americans were enrolled in managed care plans in 1984, but by the year 2000, more than 65 million Americans were enrolled in managed care plans (Kaiser Family Foundation, 1999; Theodosakis and Feinberg, 2000).

Managed care plans are now unquestionably the dominant players in the health insurance market. Although frustrations with limits placed on access to care have made managed care bashing a national pastime, American consumers owe a debt of gratitude to the managed care industry. In 1993 the Congressional Budget Office predicted that the United States would spend nearly 20% of its gross domestic product (GDP) on healthcare by the year 2000. In fact, largely due to medical cost-control measures implemented by the managed care industry, the healthcare percentage of GDP has been held to 14% since 1992 (Scott, 2000). Furthermore, the managed care industry fueled the development and implementation of medical practice guidelines that set national standards for the management of specific conditions and improved the overall quality of patient care.

COMMON CHARACTERISTICS OF MANAGED CARE PLANS

Managed care is not a single health insurance model but rather a complex system that coordinates and provides health services and benefits. Several models of managed care plans exist, as described in the following sections. Nevertheless, all managed care plans share the following characteristics:

1. Managed care plans maintain oversight of the medical care provided to plan members.
2. Managed care plans enter into contractual relationships and organization of providers delivering medical services to plan members.
3. Managed care plans tie covered benefits to rules and restrictions set by the plan.
4. Managed care plans require plan members to receive care from providers affiliated with the plan or to bear a greater burden of the cost of care received.
5. Managed care plans cover more preventive care services than do fee-for-service plans.

6. Managed care plans do not require plan members to file claim forms for medical services they receive from plan providers.

Preferred Provider Organizations

Although preferred provider organizations (PPOs) are a relative newcomer to the managed care industry, enrollment in PPOs has grown at nearly twice the rate of HMO enrollment in the past 7 years (Theodosakis and Feinberg, 2000). In 2000 PPO enrollment surpassed HMO enrollment by roughly 3 million covered lives, with 80.9 million Americans covered by HMO plans and 84.5 million covered by PPOs (Kaiser Family Foundation, 1999).

PPOs closely resemble traditional fee-for-service indemnity plans. PPOs contract with providers who accept a discounted FFS to provide medical services to plan members. PPOs allow plan members to self-refer to specialists, including those outside the PPO network. When plan members select out-of-network providers, however, they must meet an annual deductible before coverage begins and must also pay higher copayments than when they select providers within the network.

Physician hospital organizations (PHOs) and exclusive provider organizations (EPOs) are variations on the PPO model. PHOs are alliances between hospitals and physician groups to provide care to plan members. EPOs are alliances among a variety of healthcare providers to provide care to plan members, usually under profit-sharing arrangements. Both PHOs and EPOs are recent entries into the managed care industry, and little information is available about their structure or the experiences of their plan members.

Health Maintenance Organizations

HMOs are businesses that sell prepaid healthcare services to consumers (Steinberg, 1997). HMOs receive a fixed premium each month for each enrolled HMO plan member. Plan members receive comprehensive healthcare in return for paying their monthly premiums and must select a primary care physician who acts as a gatekeeper to coordinate the plan member's access to medical services. Of all managed care plans, HMOs are the lowest-priced for the plan member.

Staff-Model Health Maintenance Organizations

HMOs, like any other business, can be structured in different ways. A staff-model HMO hires physicians and other providers, such as pharmacists and therapists, as employees and pays them an annual salary. Staff-model HMOs are usually one-stop shop providers for the plan member's healthcare needs (Roberts, 2000; Theodosakis and Feinberg, 2000). The staff-model HMO may own the buildings, equipment, and offices, which can make this model attractive to the elderly and the chronically ill by making it possible to receive multiple services, such as diagnostic testing, prescription filling, and consultations with specialists, in the same location. This one-stop shop approach not only makes this the managed care plan that places the strictest controls on providers and plan members but also makes staff-model HMOs the bargain basement of managed care plans, with the lowest plan member premiums and copayments in the managed care industry.

Staff-model HMOs are often for-profit organizations. Roughly 10% of all HMO members in the United States, or 6 million individuals, participated in staff-model HMO plans in 1996 (Steinberg, 1997). As a general rule, staff-model HMOs place more emphasis on PCPs and set limits on both the selection of and access to specialists. In addition, employee turnover is often high in staff-model HMOs, which means that plan members are unlikely to nurture long-term relationships with their primary care providers.

Group-Model Health Maintenance Organizations

Group-model HMOs provided medical benefits for nearly 15% of all HMO patients in the late 1990s (Steinberg, 1997). These HMOs contract with physician groups to provide medical services to plan members. Primary care providers in group-model HMOs are most often compensated through profit-sharing arrangements in addition to salary. Providers in a group-model HMO may maintain some private-practice patients in addition to plan members. This HMO model is similar to the staff-model HMO in that it tends to place the heaviest emphasis on primary care and limits access to specialists.

Nevertheless, providers in a group-model HMO are self-governing. In other words, it is the medical group that hires, fires, promotes, and provides incentives for providers and not the HMO.

Independent Practice Association Health Maintenance Organizations

An independent practice association model HMO, or IPA, blends characteristics of the group-model HMO with those of a traditional fee-for-service indemnity plan. IPAs are groups of providers in private practice who form an alliance to provide medical services to members of one or more managed care plans, usually under capitated arrangements. Unlike other capitated arrangements, however, providers in IPAs not only may contract with more than one HMO but they also may maintain private patients under fee-for-service arrangements. The IPA sets fewer restrictions on plan members by offering a much broader selection of providers than most other HMO models.

In an IPA, the IPA receives money from an HMO to provide medical services to its plan members. The IPA pays primary care physicians a fixed fee, or compensated rate, for each plan member who selects them for primary care. Specialists in an IPA model receive a discounted fee-for-service, which means that providers in IPAs often engage in *cost shifting*, or charging more to their fee-for-service patients to compensate for any losses in revenues suffered from treating managed care plan members (Theodosakis and Feinberg, 2000).

Network-Model or Mixed-Model Health Maintenance Organizations

The network-model HMO combines components of the staff-model HMO, group-model HMO, and IPA, making it by far the most complex HMO structure in the managed care market. In fact, the structure of a network-model HMO is so complicated that even network providers may not clearly understand it (Theodosakis and Feinberg, 2000). Individual providers and provider groups in a network-model HMO are linked by contracts to an organization that may provide care in more than one state. Individual providers may be members of more than one provider network, and the HMO generally also contracts with hospitals and clinics. Thus plan members may not have to switch primary care physicians when they change health plans. In addition, network-model HMOs offer a larger number of specialists for plan members to select from (Roberts, 2000).

Providers in network-model HMOs are often compensated under a capitated arrangement, but they may also be salaried or compensated under a discounted fee-for-service structure, thus making it difficult to determine how compensation structure impacts quality of care in network-model HMOs.

Point-of-Service Plans

HMOs developed point-of-service (POS) plan options in response to consumer dissatisfaction with limitations placed on provider choice and access to specialty care (Theodosakis and Feinberg, 2000). These plans also were an attempt by HMOs to compete with the growing popularity of PPOs. In several ways, POS plans are the HMO version of an indemnity plan. Primary care physicians in a POS plan generally make referrals to other providers in the HMO network. Nevertheless, plan members can refer themselves outside the plan and still receive some coverage for medical services. If a network provider makes a referral to an out-of-network provider, the POS plan pays all or most of the plan member's bill. Plan members in POS plans not only pay the highest premiums of any HMO plan members, but if plan members exercise their option to refer themselves to an outside provider, they must not only meet their annual deductible but also pay a larger copayment (Agency for Healthcare Policy and Research, 1997).

Although POS plan members express high satisfaction with their option to self-refer to out-of-network providers and still receive coverage for medical services, few plan members exercise this option. In fact, one study of more than 145,000 POS plan members in the midwestern and northeastern United States found that more than 90% of POS plan members do not exercise their option to self-refer out-of-network during the contract year (Forrest et al, 2001).

EVALUATING THE QUALITY OF MANAGED CARE PLANS

Many variables impact the quality of care plan members receive under any given managed care plan, making it difficult to state authoritatively that one particular managed care model provides better customer service or better clinical outcomes than others. Evaluating the quality of a managed care plan requires a series of checks and balances (Agency for Healthcare Policy and Research, 1997).

When evaluating the quality of service provided by managed care plans, nurses must weigh the relative importance of the diverse variables that combine to create a comprehensive and high-quality product. Some of the factors that impact the quality of a managed care plan are as follows:

1. The caliber of the network providers
2. The benefits covered
3. Customer service

4. Patient satisfaction with all aspects of care and service
5. Programs such as wellness, prevention, and disease management
6. Limits and barriers placed on access to care
7. The method used to compensate providers
8. The amount set for monthly premiums, deductibles, copayments, and coinsurance
9. The amount set for lifetime caps on medical coverage
10. Accreditation status

PAYMENT MODEL USED TO REIMBURSE PROVIDERS

Managed care revolutionized the manner in which healthcare providers receive compensation for their services. Managed care plans use a number of provider compensation strategies to reduce medical costs. One important consideration in weighing the overall quality of a managed care plan is the mechanism the plan uses to compensate providers and how that reimbursement method may impact the quality of care received by plan members.

Capitation is a common method of provider compensation used by many managed care plans. This method secures a fixed dollar amount that the managed care plan pays its providers. Capitation saves the insurance company money, but it may create an adversarial relationship between the provider and the patient/plan member (Steinberg, 1997). Under a capitated contract, providers receive a set amount each month for every plan member assigned to them. For example, a physician may receive $10/month for every managed care plan member assigned to him or her by the managed care plan. This means that the physician receives $10/month for each individual plan member whether or not the physician provides any medical services to the plan member. It also means that if a plan member remains healthy and comes into the office only once or twice during the course of the contract year, the physician receives $120 for spending an hour or less with the plan member. If the plan member develops an illness requiring multiple visits, however, the physician's hourly rate begins to drop dramatically. Capitation often has the unintended effect of forcing physicians to ration plan member access to care. Providers are in effect at-risk for the services they deliver because they receive the same fixed compensation regardless of the number of services delivered. In other words, under this compensation method, providers usually make money on healthy plan members and lose money on plan members with chronic conditions, such as diabetes and asthma (Roberts, 2000).

Contact capitation is a relatively new provider compensation method. Under this compensation strategy, providers are paid a fixed amount per qualifying plan member rather than per their entire assigned member population. Contact capitation contracts may pay providers either a global fee for an entire episode of care for a qualifying plan member or a monthly payment for the period of time a qualifying plan member is diagnosed with a specific condition. In general, this compensation method places less risk on the provider and places greater risk on the managed care plan than do traditional capitated arrangements.

Most managed care plans that use a capitated model to compensate providers for their services require plan members to pay a copayment for each provider visit. Steinberg (1997) cautions that when copayments are set too low, plan member demand for provider services increases, which may further strengthen the adversarial relationship between the plan member and the provider by inadvertently lowering the provider's annual salary and forcing the provider to maintain a high patient volume to keep his or her practice economically viable.

Some managed care plans, specifically staff-model HMOs, pay providers an annual salary. Physicians may also receive bonuses, stock options, or profit-sharing arrangements. Providers who are on salary to a managed care plan are tightly restricted by the plan in terms of what treatment options and services, such as referrals to specialists, they are able to offer plan members (Theodosakis and Feinberg, 2000). Providers in staff-model HMOs have few financial incentives for limiting the services they provide, however, since their annual income is not dependent on the quantity of services they deliver to plan members.

The discounted fee-for-service model is most often used by IPAs and PPOs. Under this system, physicians, particularly specialists, receive a lower payment for managed care plan members than they receive for private patients. This method of payment differs sharply from capitation in that the physician only receives payment when a plan member receives his or her services. However, Theodosakis and Feinberg (2000) argue that although the discounted fee-for-service method of compensation is very different from capitation, it has a similar effect in that physicians must rely on high patient volume for their practices to remain economically viable.

A fee-for-service, or indemnity, system reimburses the provider after he or she provides medical services for a plan member. Fee-for-service reimbursement methods offer the provider the most freedom in terms of treatment options. This model also provides a strong incentive for providers to offer high-quality medical care, since they must compete for patients based on their reputation for service and quality (Steinberg, 1997). The fee-for-service method was also responsible for the skyrocketing medical costs that spawned the rapid growth of managed care in the 1990s. Fee-for-service is in effect the opposite of managed care.

How providers are compensated for their services impacts whether or not they benefit financially from their decisions to provide medical services to plan members. Most experts (Steinberg, 1997; Roberts, 2000; Theodosakis and Feinberg, 2000) believe that a discounted fee-for-service compensation method provides plan members with the highest quality of medical care and the widest range of treatment options. Conversely, they argue that capitated compensation methods are the most restrictive for both plan members and providers and are therefore the least desirable.

PREVENTIVE SERVICES AND OTHER COVERED BENEFITS

Most managed care plans provide basic medical coverage that includes preventive care. Managed care plans vary greatly in the types of services they cover for plan members, however, as well as how they control access to those services.

Nurses evaluating the quality of a managed care plan should determine how the plan defines and addresses the medical services listed as follows:

- Physical exams and health screening
- Physician office visits
- Vision care
- Dental care
- Referral to specialists
- Hospitalization
- Emergency care
- Prescription drugs
- Mental health care
- Substance abuse counseling and rehabilitation
- Obstetrical and gynecological care, including the schedule of prenatal visits
- Schedule of well-child visits
- Immunizations
- Ongoing care for chronic conditions
- Physical therapy and rehabilitative care
- Home health, nursing home, and hospice care
- Chiropractic and other alternative care, such as acupuncture
- Experimental treatments
- Health education and wellness programs
- Demand management
- Case management
- Disease management

Finding the managed care plan that offers the best fit for an individual consumer depends greatly on the individual's specific health needs. A young healthy adult will have very different health needs than an older adult with one or more chronic conditions. An effective method for comparing managed care plans to determine which one best suits the needs of an individual is to list medical services that the individual received in the past year and medical services that the individual will need in the coming year and compare how each managed care plan addresses those services (Agency for Healthcare Policy and Research, 1992, 1997).

COST VERSUS BENEFIT

Managed care plans vary greatly not only in the services they provide for plan members but also in terms of the restrictions and conditions they place on how plan members access those services. Therefore it is important not only to compare the medical services provided by managed care plans but also to compare the limits placed on each service and any barriers placed on accessing those services. These issues impact both the overall quality of the healthcare provided by the managed care plan and the satisfaction of plan members with the plan's performance.

Questions nurses should answer when evaluating the quality of a managed care plan include the following:

1. Is the plan accredited by a nationally recognized accreditation agency?
2. What are the qualifications, accreditation status, and licensure and board certification status of plan providers?
3. What is the size and composition of the provider network?
4. How are providers compensated for their services?
5. Does the plan provide incentives to providers who limit plan members' access to care?
6. Are plan members assigned a primary care physician, or may they select their own from among physicians in the provider network?
7. How heavily does the plan use nonphysician primary care providers?
8. Does the plan place gag rules on its providers?
9. How strictly must providers comply with clinical pathways and practice guidelines developed by the plan?
10. How long must plan members wait to schedule sick visits with their primary care providers?
11. How long must plan members wait to schedule routine visits and physicals?
12. How long past their scheduled appointment time must plan members wait in their physicians' offices?
13. What is the average time providers spend with plan members during an office visit?
14. How far must plan members travel to see providers?
15. How restrictive is the plan's drug formulary?
16. What is the process for referring plan members to specialists?
17. What is the process for accessing a specialist not available through the managed care plan?
18. What is the process for accessing emergency services?
19. What is the process for providing continuing care for life-threatening or long-term conditions?
20. What deductibles, copayments, and coinsurance costs must plan members pay?
21. What is the annual limit placed on plan member utilization of services, such as physical therapy, occupational therapy, mental health care, and home health care?
22. Are there annual limits set on services such as diagnostic tests?
23. What is the maximum annual out-of-pocket expense for the average plan member?
24. What is the lifetime limit on medical coverage for plan members?
25. What is the plan's grievance and appeals process?
26. Does the plan allow independent review of cases under appeal?
27. How does the plan maintain confidentiality of patient records?
28. How often and by what methods does the plan communicate with plan members?
29. How easy is it for plan members to access customer service?
30. How long must plan members wait for answers to their questions about plan benefits?
31. What is the process for accessing medical care for plan members who are vacationing or out of town on business?

The weight nurses place on the answers to each of these questions depends on their individual definitions of quality medical care and their personal views on issues such as the use of nurse practitioners as primary care providers.

COMMITMENT TO QUALITY OF CARE AND SERVICE

Clearly the quality of a managed care plan is difficult to measure. In general, however, a managed care plan that does the right things for plan members at the right time with positive outcomes provides quality healthcare to its plan members. Nurses do not have to rely solely on their own evaluations to determine the quality of a managed care plan. Each state has a department of insurance that reports on managed care plans operating in the state and provides information on the number and type of complaints filed by plan members. In addition, several accrediting agencies and consumer advocacy groups provide detailed data on managed care plan performance, including accreditation status.

Managed care plans that seek accreditation demonstrate their commitment to provide quality care and service to plan members. The accreditation process is both costly and lengthy. To become accredited, managed care plans must demonstrate compliance with performance standards set by the accrediting agency. Three organizations currently accredit either managed care plans or specific programs and services of managed care plans, such as demand management, utilization management, and case management programs.

The National Committee for Quality Assurance (NCQA) sets performance standards for and accredits managed care organizations. In addition, NCQA issues report cards on managed care plans, which are available to the public. The Health Plan Employer Data and Information Set (HEDIS) performance measurement tool developed and implemented by NCQA is used by more than 90% of American managed care organizations (Families USA, 2001).

The American Accreditation Healthcare Commission/Utilization Review Accreditation Commission (URAC) sets performance standards for and accredits healthcare organizations, including PPOs, utilization review organizations, case management programs, and Internet healthcare sites. The District of Columbia and 25 states currently recognize URAC standards and accreditation, and several states have mandated URAC accreditation as a prerequisite for certain types of healthcare organizations to conduct business in the state.

The Joint Commission on Accreditation of Healthcare Organizations (JCAHO) also sets performance standards for, accredits, and reports on the performance of healthcare organizations, including PPOs and managed behavioral healthcare organizations.

All three organizations publicly report on the accreditation status of managed care plans that seek accreditation. Nurses can access performance report cards for specific managed care plans on the agencies' Websites listed in Appendix 4-2 at the end of this chapter.

In addition to accrediting agencies, nonprofit consumer watchdog groups also report on the performance of health plans. The Foundation for Accountability (FACCT) collects and reports on managed care plan performance data. The goal of consumer advocacy groups, such as FACCT, and accrediting agencies, such as NCQA, is to ensure plan members receive adequate, appropriate, and safe medical services and that consumers select the managed care plan that best satisfies their needs.

NAVIGATING THE MANAGED CARE ENVIRONMENT

The dawn of the managed care era ushered in a new way of thinking about healthcare delivery and with it a new way of talking about the delivery of healthcare services. Healthcare professionals must familiarize themselves with the language of managed care to navigate smoothly through today's managed care environment. Appendix 4-1 at the end of this chapter provides basic definitions of common managed care terminology that all healthcare providers should understand. Many government agencies, professional associations, and private organizations provide general information on managed care issues, as well as information on the performance of specific managed care plans. The organizations listed in Appendix 4-2 provide useful managed care resources for both healthcare professionals and consumers.

REFERENCES

Agency for Healthcare Policy and Research: *Checkup on health insurance choices,* Rockville, Md, 1992, The Agency, AHCPR Publication No. 93-0018, http://www.ahrq/consumer/insurance.htm.

Agency for Healthcare Policy and Research: *Choosing and using a health plan,* Rockville, Md, 1997, The Agency, AHCPR Publication No. 97-011, http://www.ahrq.gov/consumer/hlthpln1.htm.

American Association of Health Plans: *Individual choice model of health insurance,* Washington, DC, 2000, The Association.

Families USA: *What consumers need to know: Families USA on managed care,* Washington, DC, 2001, Families USA.

Forrest CB, Weiner JP, Fowles J, et al: Self-referral in point-of-service health plans, *JAMA* 285(17):2223-2231, 2001.

Kaiser Family Foundation and Hospital Research and Education Trust: *Employer health benefits 1999 annual survey,* Menlo Park, Calif, 1999, The Foundation.

Roberts SS: Health maintenance organizations part 1: kinds of HMOs, *Diabetes Forecast* 52(11):59-61, 2000.

Scott JS: Thank you, managed care? *Healthc Financ Manage* 54(12):26-27, 2000.

Steinberg AJ: *The insider's guide to HMOs: how to navigate the managed-care system and get the healthcare you deserve,* New York, 1997, Penguin.

Theodosakis J, Feinberg DT: *Don't let your HMO kill you: how to wake up your doctor; Take control of your health and make managed care work for you,* New York, 2000, Routledge.

APPENDIX **4-1**
Glossary of Managed Care Terms

A

accreditation: Systematic review of a managed care plan by an accrediting agency. Recognized managed care accrediting agencies include the National Committee for Quality Assurance (NCQA), the Joint Commission on the Accreditation of Healthcare Organizations (JCAHO), and the American Accreditation HealthCare Commission/Utilization Review Accreditation Commission (URAC). Accrediting agencies evaluate how the managed care plan compares to established standards in specific performance areas, such as credentialing of healthcare providers and consumer satisfaction. If a managed care plan meets the agency's standards, it becomes accredited.

actual charge: Cost imposed by a provider on a plan member or a managed care plan for a specific medical service or product.

actuarial: Calculation used to estimate the financial risk for a managed care plan of enrolling an individual or group of individuals. Managed care plans establish eligibility criteria and insurance premiums based on these calculations.

adverse selection: Circumstance in which a managed care plan's members are older or sicker than anticipated and are likely to incur higher medical expenses than expected for the managed care plan.

allowable charge: Amount a managed care plan determines appropriate to pay a healthcare provider for a defined medical service or product.

alternative healthcare: Products and services, such as acupuncture, homeopathy, nutrition therapy, and massage, that may complement the services provided by physicians and hospitals.

ancillary services: Any service including imaging, such as x-rays and CT scans, and laboratory services, such as blood and urine testing, provided to a plan member to assist with diagnosis and treatment.

appeal: Review of a decision by a managed care plan to limit or deny a medical service provided to a plan member.

assignment of benefits: Process by which a healthcare provider, such as a physician or hospital, accepts payment for a medical product or service directly from the managed care plan. Assignment limits the amount the provider may collect from the plan member in addition to the allowable charge determined by the managed care plan.

at-risk: Situation whereby a healthcare provider receives a fixed, predetermined sum of money to care for an individual or group of individuals and risks losing money if total expenses for care exceed the fixed amount paid.

authorization: Approval by a managed care plan for a plan member to receive a medical service or product, such as a specific surgical procedure or diagnostic test.

B

balance billing: System that allows a healthcare provider to collect the difference between the provider's actual charge and the plan's allowable charge from a plan member. If a provider's actual charge for a service is $100 and the plan's allowable charge is $80, of which the plan pays 80%, or $64, then the provider collects the difference between the actual charge and the plan's payment ($100 to $64), or $36 from the plan member. If the provider accepts assignment of benefits, however, then the provider only collects the difference between the plan's allowable charge and the plan's payment ($80 to $64), or $16 from the plan member.

behavioral healthcare: Products and services that diagnose and treat mental and emotional illnesses.

benchmark: Industry measure of best performance for a defined process or outcome.

beneficiary: Individual, or the individual's dependent, who enrolls in a managed care plan and is entitled to receive coverage for medical products and services covered by the individual's contract with the plan.

benefit limits: Limits on how much the managed care plan pays for specific medical products or services or the quantity of services a consumer is eligible to receive.

benefits package: Set of medical products and services covered by the contract between a managed care plan and the purchaser of care.

C

capitation: System used by managed care plans to pay providers in which the provider receives a fixed, predetermined amount of money, often on a monthly basis, from the managed care plan to care for the entire population of plan members.

carve out: Product or service provided by a managed care company that specializes in a specific service, such as mental healthcare.

case management: Coordinated professional process used by managed care plans to review, plan, and assure delivery of care provided to a plan member. Case management ensures that plan members receive the appropriate service from the appropriate provider in a timely and cost-effective manner that produces good clinical outcomes by assessing the plan member's care needs and developing appropriate treatment plans.

case rate: Payment system in which managed care plans pay healthcare providers an all-inclusive fee to provide care for a plan member, based on the member's diagnosis or the specific medical treatment or surgical procedure provided to the member.

certification: Decision reached by a managed care plan after utilization review that a reviewed medical product or service meets the clinical requirements established by the managed care plan for medical necessity and appropriateness.

chronic care: Ongoing, supportive care provided for an ongoing or lengthy illness. Chronic care includes diagnosis, treatment of complications, and patient education designed to minimize complications and maximize the plan member's health status and quality of life.

clinical pathway: Medical diagram that helps providers identify the most appropriate course of treatment for a specific plan member based on the member's clinical diagnosis.

closed panel: Group of physicians who work for a managed care plan and only treat plan members.

COBRA (Consolidated Omnibus Budget Reconciliation Act):   Federally mandated program that converts existing healthcare coverage through an employer to a private plan after a qualifying event, such as employment termination or disability, that results in an employee's inability to perform his or her job.

concurrent review: Review conducted during a plan member's course of treatment. A concurrent review determines medical necessity and appropriateness of healthcare services provided to a plan member.

coinsurance: Portion of healthcare costs not paid by the managed care plan, for which the individual plan member is responsible.

contact capitation: A capitated payment system based on experience. The managed care plan pays providers a capitated amount per qualifying patient/ plan member rather than the entire plan member population. Providers are paid either a global fee for the entire episode of care or a monthly payment for the time period during which the patient/plan member is referred to and cared for by the provider.

contract: Legal agreement between a managed care plan and either an employer or an individual that describes the monthly premiums due to the managed care plan, the healthcare services provided by the plan, and how much the plan pays for each service. Managed care companies also sign contracts with providers to care for plan members for negotiated fees.

contract year: Twelve-month period covered by the agreement between the plan and the employer, individual, or provider.

contracted provider: Hospital, physician, or other healthcare provider, who enters into a legal agreement with a managed care plan to care for the plan's members for negotiated fees.

coordination of benefits: Process between two or more managed care plans that cover the same individual plan member to ensure that the plans do not make duplicate or unnecessary payment for services.

copayment: Defined sum of money a plan member pays each time he or she receives a covered service from a plan contracted provider.

cost sharing: Responsibility of an individual managed care plan member to pay a portion of the cost for care the plan member receives. Cost sharing arrangements include copayments, deductibles, and coinsurance.

cost-based reimbursement: Payment system in which managed care plans pay providers based on the actual costs of services provided to plan members.

coverage: Process that identifies the services and products that are benefits under the plan member's contract with the managed care plan.

covered expenses: Costs of medical products or services eligible for payment by the managed care plan.

credentialing: Process of verifying aspects of a provider's professional education, background, credentials, licensure, and litigation history to ensure competent, safe care for plan members. Managed care plans set defined requirements providers must meet for education, licensure, service availability, and accessibility before their inclusion in the managed care plan's provider panel.

current procedural terminology (CPT) codes: Five-digit codes used in claims submissions for billing professional services.

customer service: Resource provided by managed care plans to answer member's questions, resolve disputes or complaints, and explain the operations of the managed care plan.

D

deductible: Cost-sharing arrangement in a managed care plan that requires the plan member to pay a fixed dollar amount of covered expenses each year before the plan begins to pay its share of the member's medical costs.

demand management: Program provided by managed care plans or providers to monitor initial member requests for clinical information and services.

denial of care: Refusal by a managed care plan to cover a specific test or treatment.

diagnosis-related group (DRG): Clinical groups based on a plan member's diagnosis, procedure scheduled, age, sex, and discharge status in a classification system related to body organ systems and surgical procedures.

direct contracting: Legal relationship between a managed care plan and an employer in which the managed care plan agrees to provide a specific set of healthcare benefits for employees for a specified premium.

discounted fee-for-service: Payment system in which a managed care plan pays a provider a negotiated fee for each medical service provided after the service is provided to the plan member.

disease management: Organized program of healthcare and patient education services designed to help patients with a specific diagnosis, such as asthma or diabetes, improve their overall care, health status, and quality of life by preventing complications associated with their disease. Disease management programs also measure effectiveness by monitoring utilization, total medical costs, patient outcomes, and plan member's satisfaction with care.

disenrollment: Process of ending membership in a managed care plan.

drug formulary: List of prescription drugs covered by a managed care plan.

drug utilization review: Systematic evaluation of prescription medicines used by managed care plans to assess costs, prescription patterns, and the appropriateness of drug therapies.

E

ERISA (Employee Retirement Income Security Act): Federal law that regulates the pension, health, and welfare benefits provided by employers to their employees. ERISA exempts some employer group health plans from state laws and regulations that govern insurance.

evidence of coverage: Detailed description of the medical benefits available to a member of a managed care plan provided to members after they enroll in the plan.

exclusion: Medical product or service a managed care plan will not cover.

experience rating: Premium rating system that adjusts the rate of the insured group based on past utilization experience and other factors specific to the group.

experimental care: Medical product, service, or treatment not proven to be therapeutically beneficial to the satisfaction of the managed care plan. Products or services determined to be experimental are excluded from coverage by the managed care plan.

explanation of benefits: Statement sent to a plan member that shows the actual charges levied by the provider to the plan member, the managed care plan's allowable charge for the medical service, the plan's payment for each service, and the amount owed to the provider by the plan member.

F

fee schedule: List of prices a managed care plan agrees to pay for specific medical services or products provided to a plan member by providers.

fee for service payment: Payment made by a managed care plan to a provider after the provider delivers care to a plan member.

first dollar coverage: Managed care plan benefits that do not require the plan member to meet an annual deductible before the plan coverage begins.

first-level review: An initial review of a request for benefit coverage.

G

gag rules: Contractual agreement between managed care plans and providers that restrict the providers' ability to discuss with plan members the range of testing and treatment options available to members through the managed care plan. Gag rules may also restrict the provider's ability to discuss the financial relationship between the provider and the managed care plan.

gatekeeper: Primary care physician who controls the managed care plan member's access to certain tests, treatments, and consultations with specialists.

grievance: Complaint brought by a plan member to the administration of a managed care plan. Complaints may address a plan coverage decision, quality of care, or a dispute over how much the plan has paid for a medical product or service.

guaranteed issue: Coverage provided to a plan member by a managed care plan regardless of prior medical history or preexisting condition.

I

indemnity insurance: Health insurance that pays for care after plan members receive it. Payment is usually on a fee-for-service basis, with little effort to monitor or evaluate the cost or appropriateness of care.

indicator: Defined, measurable variable used to evaluate the quality or appropriateness of care delivered to plan members.

L

level of care: Treatment alternatives on a continuum of care that includes inpatient, partial or day hospitalization, outpatient, and long-term residential treatment.

lifetime cap: Maximum dollar amount of benefits available to a plan member in a managed care plan.

M

managed indemnity insurance: Indemnity insurance plan that contains limited managed care features, such as utilization review, to help control costs.

mandated benefits: Medical products or services offered in managed care plans that are required by either federal or state law.

maximum dollar limit: Highest amount of money a managed care plan agrees to pay for claims within a defined period of time.

Medicaid: Joint federal and state program that provides health insurance to low-income individuals who meet eligibility requirements.

Medicaid HMO: Managed care plan approved by a state government to enroll individuals eligible for Medicaid in that state.

medical loss ratio: Amount of money spent on medical care for plan members by a managed care plan.

medical underwriting: Process used by managed care plans to evaluate the level of risk posed by an individual or group of individuals, based on data such as age, sex, race, family health history, and personal health history. Medical underwriting determines the health insurance premiums the managed care plan charges the individual or group.

medically necessary: Healthcare products or services the managed care plan deems appropriate and indicated to assist in the diagnosis or treatment of disease.

Medicare: Federal health insurance program that provides medical benefits to individuals over age 65 who receive Social Security benefits or individuals who are disabled and meet eligibility requirements. Medicare Part A provides coverage and payment for hospital care. Medicare Part B provides coverage for physician services.

Medicare HMO: Managed care plan that meets federal standards and is eligible to enroll individuals receiving Medicare benefits.

Medigap: Supplemental health insurance for individuals covered by Medicare that pays for some of the deductibles and coinsurance for which Medicare beneficiaries are responsible. Medigap plans also may cover additional services not covered by Medicare Part A or B.

monthly premium: Amount paid to a managed care plan each month by an employer or individual to receive coverage from the plan.

N

noncancellable (guaranteed renewable) policy: Policy that guarantees plan members who pay their monthly premiums continue to receive insurance benefits.

O

ombudsman: Individual who assists managed care plan members resolve problems or complaints with the plan.

open enrollment: Defined period of time during which individuals are able to choose and enroll in or to disenroll from a managed care plan.

open panel: Physician or physician group that cares for patients from many managed care plans and other payers, such as Medicare.

outlier: Case where length of stay or cost of care exceeds the defined limits of a specific diagnosis-related group (DRG).

out-of-plan (or out-of-network): Providers who do not contract with the managed care plan.

out-of-pocket expenses: Cost of medical services or products that plan members must pay for themselves. These costs include deductibles and copayments, as well as products and services not covered by the managed care plan.

outcome: Result achieved through treatment or other intervention.

outcome data: Information gathered by a managed care plan that describes the result of care provided to its members.

oversight: Monitoring and direction of activities in an effort to achieve desired outcomes.

P

participating provider: Hospital, physician, or other healthcare professional, who signs a contract with a managed care plan and agrees to care for plan members for negotiated fees and conditions described in the contract.

payer: Insurer, such as a managed care plan, that covers and pays for a defined set of healthcare benefits for a plan member.

per-member-per-month (PMPM): Graduated sum paid by a managed care plan to a provider who delivers care for plan members under a capitated arrangement. The term also refers to the premiums paid to managed care plans by employers, as well as the method Medicare uses to pay Medicare HMOs that enroll Medicare beneficiaries.

pharmacy and therapeutics committee: Group of healthcare professionals, including physicians and pharmacists, who review new drugs and biotechnology products and decide which ones the managed care plan will cover, under what circumstances, and at what cost to the managed care plan and its members.

pharmacy benefit manager (PBM): Managed care plan that distributes and manages prescription drugs for managed care plan members.

plan member: Individual, or his or her dependent, who enrolls in a health plan.

practice guidelines: Suggestions for how physicians should manage patients with a particular symptom or diagnosis to achieve the best outcome.

practice profiling: Process used by managed care plans to measure how well physicians who treat plan members perform compared to financial and clinical criteria developed by the managed care plan or national standards.

preexisting condition: Medical condition or disease for which a managed care plan member was treated during a defined period of time before enrolling in the plan. If a plan member has a condition treated during the defined time, the managed care plan, depending on state and federal laws and the contract terms, may limit coverage for care delivered for costs related to the preexisting condition.

preadmission certification: Approval given by a managed care plan to admit a plan member to a hospital for medical treatment, testing, or surgery.

preauthorization: Approval given by a managed care plan for a plan member to receive a medical treatment, test, or surgical procedure on an outpatient basis.

preventive healthcare: Medical products and services designed to delay or prevent the onset of illness or injury.

primary care physician: Physician who controls a plan member's access to other plan services, such as diagnostic testing or consultations with specialists, for the managed care plan.

prospective review (or precertification): Review of medical necessity or appropriateness conducted before a plan member receives a medical service or is admitted to the hospital.

provider: Qualified, licensed professional or institution that delivers medical services to managed care plan members under a contractual relationship with the managed care plan.

Q

quality assurance: Program used by providers and managed care plans to evaluate the care provided to plan members and identify and correct care delivery problems.

quality review: Evaluation of a managed care plan member's medical records to assess that care delivered was appropriate and medically necessary.

R

reconsideration: Request for additional review of a utilization review that resulted in a decision not to certify. The peer reviewer involved in the initial decision performs this review using additional information provided by the plan member or provider or peer-to-peer discussion with the provider.

referral: Authorization by a managed care plan or primary care physician for a plan member to access other services, such as diagnostic tests, care from a specialist, or physical therapy.

report card: Data used to evaluate and report how well a managed care plan performs on financial and clinical performance measures compared to other managed care plans or national standards.

retrospective review: Review of medical necessity or appropriateness conducted after services are delivered.

risk management: Program designed to reduce or prevent medical costs resulting from illness or injuries to managed care plan members. Risk management programs generally include identification, analysis, and evaluation of issues leading to potential loss and implementation of measures to reduce incidents that may result in loss.

S

secondary payer: Additional insurance plan an individual enrolls in. The second plan coordinates with the primary payer to cover services not paid for by the primary payer.

second-level review: Appeal of a request for benefit certification denied by the initial review conducted by a clinical peer.

shared financial risk: Payment arrangement, such as capitation, in which providers share risk with managed care plans on the services they provide to plan members.

stop-loss insurance: Insurance that limits financial risk for providers who accept capitated payments to provide services to managed care plan members. When a plan member's expenses reach a defined amount, the stop-loss insurance pays bills to limit further financial losses for the capitated provider.

T

technology assessment: Evaluation of a new test, surgical procedure, treatment, drug, medical device, or biotechnology product by a managed care plan to determine which of these the plan will cover, for which patients, and at what cost to the plan and plan members.

therapeutic substitution: Replacement of a drug prescribed by a plan member's physician with a similar or equivalent drug.

third-level review (expedited appeal): Request for an additional review conducted by a second peer reviewer not involved in the original decision.

third-party administrator: Managed care plan or payer that processes claims, pays bills, and manages contracts with providers for self-insured health plans.

triage: System used by managed care plans or providers to prioritize plan members so that members with the greatest need receive care first.

U

underutilization: Failure to provide appropriate or necessary services to a plan member, or provision of an inadequate quantity or quality of services to a managed care plan member.

usual, customary reasonable charge: Amount a managed care plan considers an appropriate fee to pay for a defined medical product or service in the geographic area in which the plan operates.

utilization: Measurement of the quantity of defined medical services used by a given plan member or group of members in a defined period of time. This figure is usually expressed as the quantity of services, such as hospital admissions or emergency room visits, used per year per 1000 plan members.

utilization management: Evaluation and determination of the appropriateness of the utilization of medical products and services and the provision of assistance to providers or patients to ensure appropriate future use of medical products and services.

utilization review: Formal evaluation of the medical necessity and appropriateness of medical care services and treatment plans.

W

waiting period: Period of time during which a managed care plan member is not covered by the plan for a particular medical condition.

withhold: Portion of fees paid to providers by managed care plans held back by the plan until the end of the contract year. Providers who meet defined plan criteria often receive the withheld money in the form of a bonus at the end of the contract year.

APPENDIX **4-2**
Directory of Organizations Providing Managed Care Resources

American Accreditation Healthcare Commission/ Utilization Review Accreditation Commission (URAC)
1275 K Street, Suite 100
Washington, DC 20005
(202) 216-9010
www.urac.org
This organization sets performance standards for and accredits healthcare organizations, including preferred provider organizations (PPOs), utilization review organizations, case management programs, and Internet healthcare sites. The District of Columbia and 25 states currently recognize URAC standards and accreditation, and several states have mandated URAC accreditation as a prerequisite for certain types of healthcare organizations to conduct business in the state. Information on accredited organizations is available on the Website.

Agency for Health Care Research and Quality (AHRQ)
Executive Office Center, Suite 600
2101 E. Jefferson Street
Rockville, MD 20852
www.ahrq.gov
This government agency supports research into quality of care issues. Research briefs, clinical practice guidelines, and other useful resources are available on the agency Website.

Alliance for Health Reform
1900 L Street NW
Washington, DC 20036
(202) 466-5626
www.allhealth.org
The Alliance publishes position papers on managed care issues.

American Association of Health Plans (AAHP)
1129 20th Street NW
Washington, DC 20036
(202) 778-3200
www.aahp.org
This is a trade organization for health maintenance organizations (HMOs). The AAHP has more than 1000 HMO members representing more than 140 million covered lives. Information on selecting managed care plans and current issues in managed care are available on the Website.

American Association of Managed Care Nurses (AAMCN)
4435 Waterfront Drive, Suite 101
Glen Allen, VA 23060
(804) 747-9698
www.aamcn.org
This is a professional association for nurses working in managed care environments. The AAMCN offers managed care certification, education opportunities, and other resources for nurses.

American Association of Preferred Provider Organizations (AAPPO)
PO Box 429
Jeffersonville, IL 47131
(812) 246-4376
www.aappo.org
This is an alliance of PPOs and other open-access healthcare networks. AAPPO provides market research and other information on this segment of the managed care industry.

Employee Benefits Research Institute (EBRI)
2121 K Street NW
Washington, DC 20037
(202) 659-0607
This organization publishes findings on employee benefits and compensation arrangements, including health benefits.

Families USA
1334 G Street, NW
Washington, DC 20005
(202) 628-3030
www.familiesUSA.org
This consumer protection group provides consumer resources on managed care and conducts research on managed care quality issues.

Foundation for Accountability (FACCT)
520 SW 6th Street
Portland, OR 97204
(503) 223-2228
www.facct.org
This organization collects data on managed care plans and reports on their performance.

Foundation for Taxpayer and Consumer Rights
1750 Ocean Park Blvd., Suite 200
Santa Monica, CA 90405

(310) 392-0522
www.consumerwatchdog.org

The Foundation provides a wide range of consumer news, fact sheets, and other resources on a variety of issues, including healthcare and health insurance. The nonprofit group also provides consumer advocacy services.

Health Care Financing Administration (HCFA)
7500 Security Blvd.
Baltimore, MD 21244
www.hcfa.gov

This is the government agency that oversees Medicare and Medicaid programs. The agency Website also provides general information on managed care issues.

Health Insurance Association of America (HIAA)
1025 Connecticut Ave.
Washington, DC 20004
(202) 223-2599
www.hiagg.org

The HIAA has more than 294 health insurance company members representing more than 123 million covered lives. Information on all aspects of the health insurance industry is available on the association's Website. A complete listing of consumer insurance counseling hotlines for each of the 50 states and the District of Columbia is available on the Website.

Joint Commission on Accreditation of Healthcare Organizations (JCAHO)
1 Renaissance Blvd.
Oakbrook Terrace, IL 60181
(708) 916-5790
www.jcaho.org

The JCAHO sets performance standards for, accredits, and reports on all types of healthcare organizations, including PPOs and managed behavioral healthcare organizations. Information on the accreditation status of organizations is available on the Website.

Managed Care Online
1101 Standiford Ave., Suite C-3
Modesto, CA 95350
(209) 577-4888
www.mcareol.com

This Internet-based managed care resource company publishes online newsletters and free online managed care fact sheets. Managed Care Online also compiles a variety of data on managed care available from several national databases in a user-friendly format.

National Association of Insurance Commissioners (NAIC)
2301 McGee, Suite 800
Kansas City, MO 64108
(816) 842-3600
www.naic.org

NAIC is the organization of insurance regulators from all 50 states, the District of Columbia, and the four U.S. territories. Its primary responsibility is to protect the interests of insurance consumers and coordinate regulation of multistate insurers.

National Committee for Quality Assurance (NCQA)
2000 L Street NW, Suite 500
Washington, DC 20036
(202) 955-3500
www.ncqa.org

NCQA sets performance standards for and accredits managed care organizations. In addition, NCQA issues report cards for managed care plans. The Health Plan Employer Data and Information Set (HEDIS) performance measurement tool developed and implemented by NCQA is used by more than 90% of American managed care organizations. Information on the accreditation status of health plans and other plan performance issues is available on the Website.

Patient Advocate Foundation
753 Thimble Shoals Blvd., Suite B
Newport News, VA 23606
(800) 532-5274
ww.patientadvocate.org

This organization provides consumer information on managed care and assists individuals in the appeals process.

The Business of Managed Care

5

Strategies for Operationalizing Managed Care: A Case Study

Laurel Nadler

KEY LESSONS IN THIS CHAPTER

- An initial key strategy in implementing managed care systems is to set up a dynamic patient education process.
- Organizations should identify an employee who can serve as an "education coordinator" for their managed care enrollees.
- Information technology can serve as an important adjunct in operationalizing managed care and in streamlining the process, creating reports, and tracking authorizations.
- The staff in any organization need to learn managed care principles to support the change process.
- A need for data and information is implicit in any managed care system.

In the United States before managed care, society was accustomed to providing, financing, and consuming healthcare in certain well-established ways. Consumer habits and attitudes had developed over lifetimes, shaping expectations of doctors, nurses, hospitals, and insurance companies. Providers also had firm expectations of the healthcare system. Their training taught them professional codes of conduct, sets of values about patient care, how to interact with patients, what was important or even sacred in their professional lives, and what was to be ignored. These learned codes of conduct formed a part of their pride in their profession. All of this was perfectly appropriate, and no one ever expected it to be challenged (Shi and Singh, 1998).

Then managed care arrived, bringing many changes that were strenuously resisted because of these firmly held values and expectations. In this chapter we set aside any judgments about the merits of managed care versus indemnity-based healthcare because much is still unknown about the effects of managed care on healthcare and society.

WHAT DOES *OPERATIONALIZE* REALLY MEAN?

Some may take the attitude that managed care is here to stay, leaving no alternative for providers or consumers but to accept managed care and adjust to it, at least for now. This chapter discusses operationalizing managed care. In this context, *operationalizing* refers to changing the current systems and processes in provider institutions such as hospitals, physician's offices, and clinics to respond positively to this significant change in care delivery and reimbursement. It also means building new systems and processes for care delivery, patient education, and financial operations, among others, so that managed care can be accommodated. It refers to proactively preparing our organizations for changes in the ways we think and do business.

In addition to changing systems and processes, operationalizing managed care also influences the attitudes of consumers and providers and helps them accept and adjust to managed care. Changes in people's attitudes are less concrete than changes in paperwork and procedures, but it is difficult to change one without changing the other. Changes in both employees' and consumers' attitudes are imperative for successful changes in the ways we structure and provide care in our emerging care delivery systems (Knight, 1998).

Some of the topics discussed in this chapter are patient education; provider education; managing enrollment, referrals, and authorizations; ensuring access and continuity, credentialing providers; developing information systems and analyzing data; and managing relationships with managed care plans. Patient education programs provide an infrastructure in which to support positive attitudinal change. Process changes help healthcare organizations survive, from both a patient satisfaction and a financial perspective.

PATIENT EDUCATION

Patient education, in this context, involves the education of consumers and family members to work with and in managed care infrastructures and to navigate through them. The following strategies describe successful tips for operationalizing managed care in any organization.

Getting the Word Out

In a city where a large portion of the Medicaid population was expected to enroll in managed care, a hospital prepared a written plan to educate the patients. Keeping in mind the advertising principle that consumers need to receive a message seven times before it makes an impression, the hospital's plan included a number of different devices and strategies to get the message across.

According to the plan, a managed care information booth was set up on the main floor of the Outpatient Department, near the patient waiting areas and clinics. It was decorated with appropriate signs, colorful posters, and displays holding brochures from managed care organizations (MCOs). A new position was created for an Education Coordinator to staff the booth. During the most critical 2-year period, while the public was informed of the upcoming changes and given a chance to enroll in the plans of their choice, the Education Coordinator spent almost 100% of her work time being visible at the booth and ready to assist patients with their questions.

The selection of a person to fill the position of Education Coordinator was a fortuitous one. The hospital chose a qualified person who received a promotion from a clerical position in the Outpatient Department. Given the multicultural nature of the patient population, it was important that she was bilingual in a language spoken by a large proportion of the patient population. Many patients already knew her from her previous position or at least knew her by sight, which gave her an important measure of credibility and neutrality and helped distinguish her from the enrollment representatives of individual plans who might also be on the premises approaching patients on the same subject. Because she recognized that her previous position could be an asset, she used it to her advantage. She wore her hospital ID prominently and started a conversation with a patient by giving her name and stating that she is an employee of the hospital. For patients, the new government requirement that they join a managed care plan had created understandable insecurity and distrust. It was reassuring to have someone familiar, who was also a representative of the hospital on which they relied, to explain the new rules. With the addition of the language and cultural identification, the Education Coordinator was extraordinarily effective in communicating information and gaining trust.

The Education Coordinator was well trained and well informed, and she spoke to patients about many aspects of managed care, including the new, mandatory government requirements that patients choose a plan; the concept of a primary care provider (PCP) and the choice of a PCP at the hospital; the problems inherent in not taking action to choose a plan or a PCP; the possibility of exemptions for certain patients from enrollment in managed care; the need for referrals and authorizations for certain services under managed care; and the benefit packages offered by the various plans. Assistance was individualized, and the discussions could mention the special health needs or preferences of the patient and various family members if the patient wished. At her booth, the Education Coordinator could access the hospital's appointment system, as well as its managed care database, which is described later in the chapter. Doing so individualized her discussions with patients by providing certain key information, such as the name of the patient's current physician (if the patient had forgotten it or could not spell it well enough to later write it on a managed care enrollment form).

Patients' relationships with the Education Coordinator could extend over long periods of time as they first considered enrollment, then later joined a plan, and even later encountered and overcame obstacles involving referrals, transportation arrangements, or the healthcare and managed care needs of other family members.

Many patients approached the Education Coordinator, attracted by the signs, the activity around the booth, and her welcoming attitude. If she was not busy at a particular time, the Education Coordinator would walk around the nearby patient waiting areas to introduce herself and strike up a conversation or telephone patients at home for follow-up. Nevertheless, the hospital wanted to stimulate contact with an even wider group of patients. To increase the flow of patients seeing the Education Coordinator, the staff hung colorful cloth banners near the building entrance with text that challenged patients to "ask us" about managed care. More signs were provided that directed patients from the entrance to the managed care information booth. Finally, thousands of 4" × 7" cards were printed on brightly colored paper. The cards were handed to appropriate patients by the finance staff, who checked in patients before each visit. As time went on, different cards (on different-colored paper) were developed for various insurance and managed care situations. For example, an orange card was used for Medicaid patients who might be eligible for Medicaid managed care, and a blue card was used for uninsured patients who might be eligible for Child Health Plus. The cards directed patients to the managed care information booth for more information, which increased the flow of people visiting the booth.

When the flow of patient traffic to the managed care information booth seemed to lessen, the hospital made small variations by changing the color of the cards or the type of sign. This approach worked for a time, since patients took notice of the changes and decided to act by seeing the Education Coordinator. At one point, attractive colored signs, which included an enlarged reprint of the managed care enrollment form and some instructive text, were placed around the Outpatient Department.

Promotional items (small address books purchased at about $1 apiece) were ordered and were available for the Education Coordinator to distribute to patients who came to speak with her. The promotional items had space to write in the name of the patient's PCP, so that the patient could take away a written record of the PCP's name to refer to at time of enrollment.

It should be noted that the hospital offered a choice of plans and permitted the plans' enrollment representatives onsite to market the plans to patients. Not every hospital may want to do this, although it was an important step for this hospital because the Medicaid population was being mandated to join managed care plans, and if the hospital's patients were not well-informed, they could inadvertently join or be assigned to other providers, thereby eroding the hospital's client base.

Under the circumstances, contracts were signed with a wide variety of plans that covered Medicaid managed care patients, and many of those plans were invited to be on-site on a rotating basis. From a patient education viewpoint, the bottom line was that patients, required by the government to make a choice of plans, wanted to have a number of plans to choose from at the hospital where they received their care. It was important for them to hear that the hospital was not allied with any one plan but rather had a number of plans from which to choose. Actually the benefit packages of the various plans were quite similar, possibly indistinguishable one from another, but that did not matter. The concept of choice and the presumed independence and neutrality of their hospital were what seemed to matter to the patients.

From an operational perspective, therefore, it is important to have available reference personnel and information for patients. In addition, it is important to remember that patients prefer choice as they go through this process. Information and choice are key to successful operationalization and will ultimately result in retention of patients to the hospital system.

Patient Satisfaction Groups, Direct Mail, and Community Education

In a newer initiative, the hospital is currently experimenting with patient satisfaction groups. The Education Coordinator invites patients, especially managed care patients, to a 30-minute discussion group in which refreshments are served. The Coordinator asks a few preselected questions about patients' satisfaction with their care at the hospital and with their choice of MCO. She also questions their knowledge of certain key concepts, such as where to seek care if they are sick during the night. Patients come and talk about their satisfactions and dissatisfactions. A report is written for management to review. Through the groups, the hospital hopes to learn more about how patients feel and to give patients a sense of participation and community with the institution that serves them and wants to serve them even better (Krowinski and Steiber, 1996).

The hospital is also experimenting with direct mail to both patients and the general public as a way to educate them on the subject of managed care offerings and hospital and outpatient services.

To reach even further than a patient education program, a provider or provider institution may decide to engage in community education in managed care. This approach can win new patients to the practice and can create a stronger tie between the members of the community and their hospital or physician's office. Providers can use current contacts or develop a list of local community-based organizations, social service agencies, religious institutions, schools, and day care centers. Contacting them to determine the needs of *their* customers is a first step. Depending on how great the need for managed care education is specifically and how receptive the community is to this subject, the managed care topic can be combined with other topics. For example, a church might permit a hospital representative to speak to parishioners about the hospital and the variety of services offered, including accepted managed care plans. Also, a nurse could deliver a series of well-baby lectures at a social service agency, with some added information about managed care for the family.

Common Themes in Patient Education

Finally, to see how the patient education strategies discussed in this chapter could be used in smaller institutions, such as group or faculty practices or individual physician offices, it is useful to identify some of the themes in patient education. One central theme is *the close relationship between the patient's ability to negotiate the healthcare or managed care system and the patient's health and well-being.* This relationship is a primary goal of patient education. Admittedly, this theme represents a broad-based approach to this issue, which is not held by everyone. Look at it this way: a patient may arrive for a doctor's visit, which could potentially provide excellent quality healthcare. If a managed care-related problem exists, however, such as a question about eligibility or the status of a referral, that visit may not take place, or it may occur only after the patient has become upset and confused over the managed care problem presented by the staff. Unfortunately, patients typically find out about a managed care problem at the office visit or moments before a scheduled surgery or admission, when they are most vulnerable. Staff may decide to call them later at home, work with them on their next visit, or somehow attempt to resolve their managed care problems without their presence—anything but bother the patient at that difficult moment.

Staff in the provider office or institution *could* say in effect to the patient, "We can treat you here for your sore throat or your cancer, but please settle these managed care problems on your own, with your plan." To do so is to compartmentalize integrally connected problems and issues. Barriers to healthcare access will eventually equal no healthcare. Is it the responsibility of the provider or the provider institution to assist the patient, perhaps compensating for the deficiencies of the patient's MCO? Offering patient education for managed care represents a significant expense for any provider. Each practice or institution will make its own decisions in this regard, but one argument in favor of delivering patient education and assistance in the physician's office is that the patient is often at the office and has a relationship with staff who have prior experience in this area. Also, the provider institution is supposed to *care* for the patient.

Another theme in patient education is *the use of the "personal touch"* to educate patients and surmount managed care problems. As described earlier, the selection of a staff member who individualized her discussions with patients was central in developing a positive and effective relationship with them. Choosing staff who are familiar and respected to serve as advocates for managed care education can be adapted to even a private practice. Creating a welcoming environment where the patient can feel comfortable discussing these issues is important as well.

Experimenting with *many forms of communication*—visual (signs, banners, inexpensive printed cards, and booths), one-on-one interviews, focus groups, direct mail, and so forth—is also something that could be adapted on a smaller scale for an individual practice. Communication should stress the positive. Instead of hanging a sign saying, "You are responsible for knowing your own copayment," stress the positive in some way, such as "We welcome members of many managed care plans. Please ask us for a list of our plans." Then use the "personal touch" to explain one-on-one about the need to remember the MCO's ID card, which records the copayment.

At all times, the institution should be sensitive to the individual's ability to learn, readiness to learn, and potential barriers to learning, such as language or cognitive difficulties. As the Patient Education Coordinator identifies such patients, she or he should refer these patients to a social worker or an RN for further intervention and assistance.

Patient education should be a limited affair. When done correctly, patient education will build patients' knowledge and resources about the system and enable them to negotiate the system on their own in the future. Thus the need for assistance in this regard will decrease.

PROVIDER EDUCATION

Patients must acclimate to managed care and so must staff. To respond to this need, another new key position was created for a Managed Care Nurse Liaison. The Nurse Liaison is a highly experienced, highly skilled RN with superior communication skills and technical knowledge. In an apparent repeat of the fortuitous choice of the Education Coordinator, a nurse was chosen for this position who was very well known and respected among the nursing staff and physicians of the Outpatient Department. This connection helped overcome the resistance and resentment of staff toward the changes and inconveniences brought about by managed care (Cohen and Cesta, 2001). Whereas the Education Coordinator presented a familiar and reliable face to managed care for the hospital's patients, the Managed Care Nurse Liaison humanized and legitimized the subject of managed care for the nursing staff and physicians. She worked directly with staff and was available to teach them and answer their questions. In both cases, the "personal touch" helped overcome barriers to managed care, which is sometimes thought of as an impersonal and inhumane system. It enabled both patient and staff education to take place.

The Managed Care Nurse Liaison's responsibilities included educating staff about managed care procedures; developing and monitoring processes for the smooth flow of referral paperwork through the system; obtaining authorizations for services as required by the MCOs; interfacing with individual physicians on managed care issues; working with the Medical Directors and the quality staffs of MCOs on a variety of issues; serving as backup for the Education Coordinator; and working directly with managed care patients when there were more complex clinical needs or when the administrative issues depended on the clinical issues (as in the case of exemptions from managed care). In point of fact, the Education Coordinator and the Managed Care Nurse Liaison worked closely together on a daily basis.

The Managed Care Nurse Liaison provided informal day-to-day contact with staff as a type of on-the-job training. A more formal training program also was established. Over a few years, presentations on managed care were given to staff throughout the hospital, including physicians, nurses, physical therapists, social workers, administrators, and clerks. Training programs were individualized to the target audience so that they could relate to the content.

As time went on, it became obvious that the more informed staff began to serve as liaisons themselves. In this way the education became a "train-the-trainer" program. Well-informed staff were better able to educate patients and families and to continue to provide a positive environment for them.

Also, attractive and easy-to-use written materials were developed as tools for staff. Among these was a look-up chart that helped clinical and financial staff throughout the hospital determine what the approval procedures were for specific services by specific plans (Table 5-1). The services and procedures, such as angiograms, endoscopy, and outpatient mental health, were listed down the left-hand side of the page, and the contracted MCOs were listed across the top. The grid beneath indicated which service or procedure (if any) was needed. In addition to this chart, the Managed Care Nurse Liaison developed a binder with flow charts and fact sheets describing administrative procedures under managed care; information about the contracted managed care plans and their policies and procedures; and special types of information, such as emergency department notification procedures under managed care. The binder was distributed widely throughout the hospital, and updates were frequently issued. An example from this binder, "A Quick Guide to a Managed Care Plan," is shown in Figure 5-1.

Early bitterness and complaints from staff about the new managed care systems became muted with the passage of time. Through ongoing educational programs, the staff learned whatever new procedures were associated with managed care, and familiarity brought acceptance. The early days, when only a small percentage of the patient population belonged to managed care plans, were the hardest. Then, it seemed that all the fuss and bother over managed care was hardly worth it. Later, when large numbers of patients had joined managed care plans, it was apparent that the new procedures were important. By then, the processes had been at least partially mastered.

TABLE 5-1
Authorization/Referral Guide for Managed Care Plans at Saint Vincent's Catholic Medical Centers—St. Vincent's Manhattan, New York

Service/Procedure	Plan A	Plan B	Plan C	Comments
Admission (inpatient)	Auth	Auth	Auth	
Allergy services	—	—	Auth	
Ambulance	Auth	Auth	Auth	Except 911
Ambulatory surgery	Auth	Auth	Auth	
Amniocentesis	Ref	Auth	Ref	
Anesthesia services	Auth	Auth	Auth	
Angiogram	Auth	Auth	Auth	
Artificial eye	Auth	Auth	Auth	Needs letter of medical necessity (all plans)
Audiogram	—	Ref	Ref	
Audio screening	—	—	—	Needs nothing if part of physical examination
Aural rehabilitation	Auth	Auth	Auth	
Baer	Ref	Ref	Auth	
Barium enema	—	—	Ref	
Behavioral health	Auth	Auth	Auth	Plan A call Case Management Services, Plan B call PCP

From Saint Vincent's Catholic Medical Centers—St. Vincent's Manhattan, New York.
Auth, Requires authorization; *PCP,* primary care provider; *Ref,* requires referral.

For physicians and other providers, their own intellectual curiosity, professional pride and competence, and interest in their patients also helped them overcome some of their distaste for managed care. They became interested in how to care for people under a different system, and they became engaged with that system. For example, one physician in the Outpatient Department wanted to carefully control referrals for his patients. If he referred to a specialist for a one-visit consultation, he wanted it kept to one visit until he reviewed the case. He disapproved of the behavior of his specialist colleagues who were trying to operate in premanaged care fashion by asking patients to return for follow-up specialty visits without his review and approval. Note that in this case, there were no personal financial disincentives for the specialists if they treated patients without appropriate referrals because the patients were moving from primary care to specialty care within one provider system, and physicians were compensated by the hospital, not directly by the plan. This physician was just doing what he felt was right by advocating for patients' continuity relationship with their PCP, in the absence of a specific identifiable need for specialty follow-up. His attitude, which perhaps had predated the advent of managed care, nevertheless placed him in the position of being an ally of the new system. In pursuit of his own philosophy of patient care, he found himself upholding managed care policy.

How to Contact Plan A	In each category, fill in information about the plan.
Specialty care	
Preauthorization	
Labwork	
X-rays, mammograms, sonograms	
Ob/gyn	
Audiology	
Ophthalmology and optometry	
Home care	
Elective ambulatory admissions and surgery	
Mental health and substance abuse	
Prescriptions	
24-hour coverage	
Emergency services	
Appointment availability policy	
Dental	
Transportation	
How a member obtains information	
How a member changes PCP	
How a member disenrolls	
How a member makes a complaint	

Figure 5-1 A quick guide to a managed care plan. (From Saint Vincent's Catholic Medical Centers—St. Vincent's Manhattan, New York.)

In other cases, key physicians were asked to provide representation on committees formed by MCOs. The physicians began advocating for the hospital and its patients on certain issues. They were working within the new system, and they were engaged with that system. They may have fought managed care at one time, but now they were still fighting—this time from within the system.

Staff education can range from detailed, such as how to complete referral forms, to general, such as recent trends in managed care. This education provides the tools staff members need to do their jobs. It also helps them move from resistance to acceptance. Given training and time, it is possible for staff to acclimate to new ways of delivering patient care and doing business.

MANAGING ENROLLMENT, REFERRALS, AND AUTHORIZATIONS

The following are the basics of managed care operations: (1) managing the enrolled population, (2) managing the flow of referral paperwork, and (3) managing authorizations. *Managed care operations* refer to the additional checks and balances imposed by MCOs. They are the first things that need attention when an operation is either new or new to managed care.

Enrollment

Enrollment refers to the list of patients assigned to the physician by each MCO. In many types of managed care, a patient chooses a PCP. The PCP provides the gatekeeping function for the patient and controls and manages that patient's access to all other healthcare services. The PCP determines whether the patient needs to see a specialist or needs any additional services. Since this is intended to be a permanent relationship, the provider needs to know which patients belong to his or her enrolled population, which is critical financially when reimbursement for primary care is on a capitated rather than on a fee-for-service basis (Mullahy, 1995).

In a capitated environment, the physician receives a fixed amount of reimbursement each month, regardless of how many times the patient may access his or her services. When capitation is the payment method, each patient's enrollment status with the plan and choice of PCP ideally should be verified at each visit, since it can change at any time. Should care be rendered to a patient who is not a member of the plan or who has chosen another PCP in that plan, the provider should not expect payment to be rendered by the MCO.

MCOs provide monthly membership rosters for their PCPs. Some MCOs can guarantee that the members whose names appear on the PCP's monthly roster are in fact enrolled to that PCP. Nevertheless, membership status sometimes can be adjusted retroactively for legitimate reasons beyond the control of the MCO. To the extent that the MCO cannot guarantee the validity of the monthly roster, a provider may decide to confirm membership and PCP affiliation on a visit-by-visit basis by means other than or additional to the roster. Such confirmation can be done by telephoning the MCO to confirm each patient's status, but it is time-consuming. Online and third-party systems are also available for this purpose and can be effective. Nevertheless, they may confirm membership but not PCP affiliation. A provider can ask contracted MCOs for recommendations on how to confirm enrollment to their plan and to the individual PCP.

The rosters are also useful for management of the patient population. Physicians like to review the rosters to uncover potential problems, such as adult patients on the pediatrician's roster (the MCO should be notified here) or patients with whom they are unfamiliar. In the latter case, sending a welcome letter to the patient with an invitation to make an appointment for a baseline physical is most appropriate.

Later in this chapter, "Developing Information Systems and Analyzing Data" discusses a method for producing comprehensive rosters that contain the names of all the practice's managed care patients, including various plans.

Referrals and Authorizations

Many MCOs require that when a referral is made to a specialist physician, the referral be made in a format specified by that MCO. This format may be a particular paper form or some form of electronic communication. Both the specialist and the MCO receive notice of the referral. Each plan has its own format and its own rules, such as those specifying which services require a referral, for how long the referral is valid, or how many visits may be authorized on the referral.

Authorizations, in contrast, require a higher level of reporting to the MCO. *Authorizations* refer to the process of obtaining prior approval from the patient's MCO for a particular service before it is delivered. Authorizations are generally required when services are especially costly or have historically and indefensibly high utilization rates. For an authorization, the provider (or a representative such as a nurse or a clerk) must communicate to the plan (by telephone, fax, or some other method), provide information about the service required, and receive an authorization number, which constitutes the plan's agreement that the service is covered and the plan will pay.

Plans differ on which services require referrals, which require authorizations, and which do not require either. Each plan's paper referral form looks different, requires slightly different information, and has the carbon copies (for PCP, specialist, plan, or so on) in different colors and in a different order. Organizing all the information and all the paperwork needed to process referrals and paperwork is an operational challenge. The larger the practice or the greater the number of plans offered, the more complex the paperwork.

The Outpatient Department provided structure and organization for referrals and authorizations in the following way. Specialized staff were designated to oversee the process, particularly the Managed Care Nurse Liaison. The Managed Care Nurse Liaison researched all the rules and requirements of the various plans and organized the information in easy-to-use documents for staff reference. (See previous discussion in this chapter for detailed information on her authorization chart.) Although all staff (including nurses and clerks) were responsible for completing routine referrals, the authorization function was centralized in the Managed Care Nurse Liaison. She requested and obtained authorizations from the MCOs, and in the process developed useful relationships with the utilization management staff at the various plans and became deeply familiar with the plans and their procedures.

She could handle multiple authorizations requested from a single plan at one time. Also, she was more likely than a staff nurse to be available when an MCO called to provide an authorization number or request more information.

Some aspects of the referral process also were centralized. For example, the many pieces of different-colored referral paperwork going to different places tended to be mixed up by busy staff interacting with patients. Staff were instructed to place completed referral paperwork into labeled baskets. The Managed Care Nurse Liaison, the Education Coordinator, and the managed care group's secretary all took responsibility for sorting and routing the various papers. Additionally, patients who arrived for specialty visits without appropriate referrals presented a special, immediate problem. In such cases, the Education Coordinator or the Managed Care Nurse Liaison was contacted to resolve it.

Some MCOs have set up paperless systems in which referrals are recorded and processed electronically, either by telephone, the Internet, or a third-party system. Such systems hold some promise for reducing the workload.

Other MCOs are recognizing that their systems of referrals and authorizations may not accomplish much in terms of cutting down on inappropriate use of services and saving money. Given all the work involved, it may not be worth the effort. With the possibility of some flexibility in this regard, it may be worthwhile for a provider to negotiate with the MCO for a relaxation of the rules. This negotiation process should take place at the management level at the time of contract negotiations between the provider facility and the MCO. For example, where there is a network of health centers or practices, the MCO may be willing to waive the requirements for documented referrals when they take place within that network.

ENSURING ACCESS AND CONTINUITY

Managed care plans set certain standards for providers. Sometimes MCOs' insistence on these standards can force providers to make positive changes. Such changes have occurred in two areas in particular—patient access to care and continuity of care. In these cases, significant operational changes may be necessary for the provider (Shi and Singh, 1998).

The MCO is concerned with access to care, that is, whether its members can get the healthcare they need when they need it. The MCO may set certain standards for access. For example, a member must be able to get an appointment for urgent care within 24 hours or an appointment for prenatal care within 1 week during the third trimester, and so forth. The plan will investigate complaints from members who report that these standards have not been met.

To meet standards for access, a provider or provider institution must ensure that patients can successfully reach them by telephone or in person to make appointments and that appointments are available. Inadequate telephone and appointment-making systems and poorly-trained staff are typical provider problems. Fitting patients who need urgent care (some of whom may be walk-ins) into a busy schedule poses another challenge.*

---

*Of course, innumerable other potential barriers to access exist, including language barriers and transportation problems. These barriers will not be discussed here.

Self-Test Access

A provider or provider institution may wish to test itself regarding access. Telephoning the practice is a good way to start. How does it feel to be a patient negotiating the system? If the telephone system is automated, are the prompts, such as "Press 1 for appointment, press 2 for laboratory results," easy to understand, and do they yield the desired results? Is the caller cut off, forwarded to the wrong extension, or left hanging? If the system is not automated, or in those parts of an automated system that eventually lead to a customer service representative, are staff respectful and informative? Can the caller get an appointment?

Another good self-test for access is an anonymous patient survey. A brief (two or three-question) paper survey can be handed to each patient during his or her visit. Questions might include, "On a scale of 1 to 10, did you find it easy to make an appointment with our office?" or "How helpful was the staff when you called to make an appointment?"

Also, telephoning other providers to see how their systems work can be useful. What ideas can be gleaned about how to organize the telephone system and train the staff?

After the self-assessment, it is time to plan access changes. At this hospital, consultants were hired to help set up a call center for making outpatient appointments, which brought very satisfactory results. If a provider needs to design or redesign a telephone system and cannot afford to hire consultants, it will be important to do as much research as possible in both the literature and the field before attempting it.

Staff training and organization also are key to achieving access goals. Managed care now expects more from staff, who need to be acquainted with the practice's managed care plan affiliations (which may differ by physician), referral procedures, and appointment standards. Provide as much training, attention, and close supervision as possible to appointment-making staff. Training should include telephone etiquette, customer service, managed care principles, access standards, and which managed care plans are accepted. Organize appointment-making personnel so that they can work closely with designated nursing triage staff to give appropriate appointments to sick patients. Develop a policy on how to handle walk-in patients, and ensure that it accords with state and federal law.

Continuity of care is another area in which managed care has stimulated some positive changes that require operational adjustments by providers. *Continuity of care* refers to the patient being cared for by the same provider over time. For primary care, the relationship with the PCP should be a permanent one. For specialty care, the patient's relationship with the specialist is expected to last at least over one episode of care (Knight, 1998).

Operational adjustments that bring about continuity of care may need to be made by larger provider institutions such as hospitals or even large group practices. They are generally not required for individual physician practices, where continuity of care is inherent in the way the practice operates.

Large teaching hospitals particularly need to make adjustments to offer continuity of care to patients. In such hospitals, outpatients may be treated by resident physicians supervised by attending physicians. The resident physicians rotate through various departments, and the attending physicians in a given specialty may take turns covering outpatient department sessions. This situation can potentially undermine continuity of care.

When resident schedules cannot be changed because of teaching requirements, continuity of care should ultimately be the responsibility of attending physicians. Because of managed care, it may no longer be possible for attending physicians to share responsibility for a given outpatient session, take turns, or treat the schedule as secondary to other, more pressing responsibilities. Having the same attending physician in the specialty session regularly to see patients for follow-up visits is required to ensure continuity of care. This situation may mean compensating attending physicians differently to recognize the increased responsibility required under managed care.

CREDENTIALING PROVIDERS

Credentialing is the process by which a managed care plan decides whether a provider can participate in its plan. By engaging in the credentialing process, the MCO seeks to facilitate the provision of quality healthcare by appropriately trained and qualified providers. The credentialing process follows policies and procedures set by the plan. Many plans seek accreditation by the National Committee for Quality Assurance (NCQA) and are guided by the rules they set for credentialing.

During credentialing, the MCO examines the provider's completed application form and attached documents. A typical application calls for information about the provider, such as education and training, board certification status, work history, and malpractice history and coverage, as well as information about the provider's practices, including location, hours, coverage arrangements, procedures, and use of laboratories. The provider must also answer confidential questions on a variety of subjects, such as illicit drug abuse and history of loss or restriction of license. Documents or copies of documents that must be submitted along with the application may include the provider's diploma, board certificates, license and registration, Drug Enforcement Agency (DEA), malpractice face sheet, curriculum vitae, and letters of recommendation from colleagues. MCOs conduct primary and secondary source verification on many of these documents.

MCOs focus on the credentialing of physicians but also may agree to credential nurse practitioners—usually as PCPs—and midwives. Nurses other than nurse practitioners are not required to be credentialed to provide services to members of managed care plans, although they may be involved in the administrative process at a provider institution or an MCO.

The credentialing process has been bitterly and universally criticized because it is so repetitive and time-consuming and because providers are uncertain about what the MCOs are trying to accomplish. The frustration of providers and administrative staff involved in completing the application forms and assembling the documents cannot be underestimated. A physician may need 10 or 15 MCOs for business reasons. Each MCO offers its own form and has its own rules about documentation and submission. Recredentialing takes place every 2 years, and the MCOs have their own separate (although shorter) forms for this purpose. Over and over, similar information must be written out in different formats on applications for credentialing and recredentialing.

Problems also may occur after the application is mailed to the MCO. MCOs can be inundated with provider applications and may have internal delays in processing them. Applications can be lost. Even when the MCO has the application and has every intention of processing it, the wait can seem interminable. In this author's experience, a 3-month wait is the minimum, and a 6-month wait is typical. (The NCQA guideline is 180 days, which is not good for the provider.) Sometimes applications go unprocessed for a couple of years before they are processed. By then, all the documents are out of date, and the provider must furnish new ones. Of course, providers also share the blame for delays, since they frequently submit incomplete application packages or outdated documents.

Aside from the repetitive, duplicative nature of the credentialing process and the inefficiency of that process, providers also are unsure what credentialing actually accomplishes. Most providers apply to plans and expect to be admitted. The credentialing process does screen out some providers. The MCO may refuse to credential or recredential certain providers or may terminate other providers after they are credentialed. The MCO may follow certain established quality standards, such as only credentialing physicians who are board-certified or board-eligible in their specialty or refusing to credential physicians with troubled malpractice histories or physicians facing disciplinary charges.

The results still are poorly understood, however, and to the provider community, the large amount of work involved in credentialing appears to have a small payoff in terms of selectivity of providers. In the future, it will be interesting to see if the managed care industry can streamline or centralize its procedures for credentialing by eliminating the duplication of applications and documents. It also would benefit the industry to provide a better explanation of how its members (patients) benefit from the credentialing process. MCOs are guided in their conduct of credentialing by NCQA and by contracts they may have with government entities or employer groups, so a given MCO may not be free to act alone to make major changes in the credentialing process. Nevertheless, the plans' cost of doing business is driven higher by the stringent requirements for credentialing. Organizing would help bring about change in this arena.

In the meantime, the challenge for providers and provider institutions is to keep the work to a minimum while credentialing the providers. This goal can be accomplished by negotiating with the MCOs for certain key changes in the credentialing procedures and also by establishing efficient and effective systems and procedures.

The following are some tips for providers and provider institutions for managing the credentialing process:

■ If asked, some MCOs will accept application forms that are different from their own. One example is a standard form issued by another party. (The HMO Council of New York State publishes a standard form that is accepted by some plans there.) If a provider can get a number of plans to accept a standard form, the provider will need to fill it out only once. Then it should be kept on file, and a photocopy of the completed form should be signed and dated by the provider for each new plan. If an MCO agrees to this, it still will require the provider to sign and date the plan's own attestation and release form.

MCOs also have been known on occasion to accept copies of forms issued by other plans. Therefore if a provider fills out Plan A's application form, it can be photocopied later, the name "Plan A" can be crossed out, the provider's original signature can be affixed, and the form can be sent to Plan B with the provider's original signature and date. This procedure is uncommon, but MCOs may be receptive to it when they are under pressure to credential providers in a certain locale or with a certain specialty. The use of a standard, accepted application form for multiple plans supplemented by each plan's own attestation form (as described previously) has the bigger payoff, however, and should be pursued assiduously.

- Providers should organize as much of the paperwork as possible to be done by support staff rather than by physicians themselves. Clerical or administrative staff can fill out applications or at least certain limited parts of applications. Then, parts of the application that must be completed or signed by the physician should be tagged or highlighted. Files with copies of the physician's standard documents, including the DEA, registration, and letters of recommendation, should be maintained and kept up-to-date. Having the receptionist photocopy the physician's framed diploma for the application is not the best approach. It also produces a poor photocopy that may not be accepted by the MCO.

- In large provider institutions such as hospitals, there may be times when documentation on hundreds of physicians must be assembled at once for submission to plans. Limited parts of the application can be prefilled by clerks without access to individual physicians or their files. For example, information about the practice, such as location, hours, and use of laboratories, may be known. Before submission to the provider or the support staff in the provider's department, a cover sheet should be affixed that contains a good explanation of why the application needs to be completed, what the deadline is, where it should be sent on completion, and any special instructions. Administrators who organize such efforts should take care to communicate at every opportunity with all concerned, including providers and other administrative staff. To get them past the angst of the credentialing process, it is helpful to issue frequent reminders of the importance of being credentialed or to provide explanations of the efforts being made to streamline and improve the process. It is also helpful to thank everyone for their efforts.

- Keep detailed records on the status of individual applications. A simple database created using spreadsheet software is adequate for operations with hundreds of providers and numerous MCOs, and it produces useful reports. With the help of the database, it is possible to track the movements and status of individual applications in process—the date the application was sent to a provider's department or secretary, the date the application was received back and whether it was complete, the date the application was sent to various MCOs, any additional information required by MCOs, and finally, the date the provider was credentialed by each MCO. Such a system affords excellent follow-through.

- More complex automated solutions exist, such as database software that maintains information on physicians and can produce applications in the format required by various selected MCOs. An operation would need to be quite large to justify the effort required to customize the software and maintain the database.

■ Finally, for large provider institutions such as hospitals, there *is* a way to avoid having to submit applications to MCOs altogether—delegated credentialing, in which the MCO permits the institution to credential its own providers. Hospitals routinely credential their own providers anyway. The MCO reviews the written policies and procedures of the institution that show how its credentialing and recredentialing are done to ensure that these policies and procedures are acceptable to the plan and will yield the same results as if the plan was doing the credentialing itself. Then, the plan conducts a predelegation audit of the institution's process (to be followed by annual audits). In delegated credentialing, the MCO retains overall responsibility for the process, while the provider institution conducts the credentialing activities. Some MCOs are reluctant to sign delegated credentialing agreements because it means that they are ceding their responsibility for credentialing activity to another organization. If that organization fails to comply with all the agreed-upon rules and regulations, it could place the plan's NCQA accreditation status in jeopardy or cause them to be in violation of contracts they have with government agencies or employer groups. Where delegated credentialing is possible (the institution has its own credentialing process in place or is large enough to develop one) and the MCO is willing, it will save a great deal of time, money, and aggravation. This method is worth pursuing.

DEVELOPING INFORMATION SYSTEMS AND ANALYZING DATA

A need for data and information is *implicit* in a managed care system because in managed care, the emphasis is on management, and data and information are vitally needed to manage effectively.

The following example illustrates this need. You are an administrator of a large healthcare practice that has just signed a capitated contract with a managed care plan. The practice will provide a wide range of services to enrolled members, with capitation reimbursement. Certain services cannot be provided by the practice but nevertheless are included in the capitation, so the practice is at risk; your physicians will refer patients to subcontracted groups for these services. As the contract was negotiated, your actuarial consultants analyzed the utilization expected from this population and compared it to costs. How will this scenario work in reality? When the contract goes into operation, will you have the information systems needed to track and report on utilization and costs and to compare to capitation reimbursement so that you can understand whether or not the practice is making money?

Generally speaking, the greater the amount of risk assumed by the provider organization (such as partial or full capitation), the greater and faster the need for information. Also, the larger the provider organization, the greater the need for information.

An important part of operationalizing managed care is to assess the current information system capabilities of the provider organization, especially systems for finance, billing, and patient accounts, to determine what data they can provide to satisfy managed care needs. Which managed care functions that cannot currently be performed are vital? What needs to be done immediately in terms of information systems purchase or development to acquire these capabilities? What will be needed in the future?

Although by no means inclusive, the following is a list of information system functions that may be needed to properly operationalize managed care. When an administrator draws up a similar list tailored to a particular institution, decisions can be made about which items are highest in priority, so that time and money can be allocated to these first.

- Track the number of outpatient visits completed by a member against the number authorized on the original referral. Alert the member or provider when a new referral is needed.
- Track authorization numbers provided by MCOs so that the numbers ultimately are recorded on the bill for the service.
- Reconcile the capitation payment received from the MCO against expected payments based on age, gender, disability, or other factors that figure into the capitation.
- Track the emergency room visits of members, and provide PCPs with member names and telephone numbers for follow-up.
- Track utilization of all services provided to members, with associated charges or costs.
- Provide information to PCPs on specialty visits made with and without referrals.
- Report on hospitalized members.
- Analyze appointment availability by PCPs.
- Report on after hours telephone calls.
- Report on PCP panel membership and size.
- Analyze members' PCP changes.
- Produce profiles of specialty providers.
- Report to MCOs on state-mandated preventive care such as immunizations.
- Provide encounter data to MCOs for capitated, nonbillable services.
- Report on patient satisfaction indicators.
- Make information readily available on individual providers' managed care plan affiliations, specialties, languages, and so forth.

In a large provider organization such as a hospital, an assessment about managed care-related information systems needs will be an interdepartmental effort that may include representatives from finance, information systems, managed care, medical records, admissions, and operations. Input from upper management is vital; the organization may feel it needs various capabilities and resources, but the desire to make the requisite changes or large investments ultimately may be lacking.

In addition to making assessments about large systems, there probably will be a need to develop smaller-scale, local systems and databases to fulfill the operational needs of those working in managed care. In the hospital previously discussed in this chapter, a database application was developed to track enrollment and utilization of managed care members. The hospital had worked closely with its MCOs to get their commitment to sending monthly enrollment rosters on electronic media (either diskette or e-mail) rather than paper. Each month, the various files were assimilated into the database. For each member, an historical record of membership was built, showing not only the member's current plan and PCP but also prior month-by-month affiliation.

The system was online for access by certain individuals and departments. For those who did not have online access, a monthly paper roster displaying an alphabetic listing of members was printed and distributed. Even for those without online access, this A to Z roster of all plans combined represented a huge improvement over the previous system of multiple rosters from various managed care plans and for various PCPs.

Each month, this system reached into the hospital's own information systems to cull utilization data on the patients who were indicated as managed care members. Then, this managed care information application could report on utilization of primary care and specialty services, emergency department services, ambulatory surgery services, and inpatient services.

MANAGING RELATIONSHIPS WITH MANAGED CARE PLANS

Providers' relations with managed care plans can be strained. It is most helpful for providers to counteract this trend by creating a sense of partnership with their MCOs. Some pointers for doing so are as follows:

- Providers can designate a particular staff person (or in a large institution, perhaps a group of persons) who will serve as an operational liaison to MCOs. Over time, this person or persons will develop relationships with the provider relations personnel at MCOs, which will prove invaluable.
- Providers might persuade their MCOs to meet with them, either regularly or from time to time, depending on the volume of business. They can set agendas for the meetings and address operational problems.
- Conflict can be averted by taking a collegial (rather than confrontational) approach with MCOs. Providers might bring issues to the MCOs' attention and give them reasonable time to address these issues before taking further action.

The operationalization of managed care encompasses a variety of activities. A knowledge of managed care principles is required, as is a good understanding of the provider institution's operations. The administrator in charge of an effort to operationalize managed care will find much of interest and challenge.

REFERENCES

Cohen EL, Cesta TG: *Nursing case management: from essentials to advanced practice applications,* ed 3, St Louis, 2001, Mosby.

Knight W: *Managed care: what it is and how it works,* Gaithersburg, Md, 1998, Aspen.

Krowinski WJ, Steiber SR: *Measuring and managing patient satisfaction,* Chicago, 1996, American Hospital Publishing.

Mullahy CM: *The case manager's handbook,* Gaitherburg, Md, 1995, Aspen.

Shi L, Singh DA: *Delivering healthcare in America,* Gaithersburg, Md, 1998, Aspen.

Wall Street and Healthcare: Understanding Our New Partner

Elizabeth Corso Falter, William A. Falter, and Laura A. Kukowski

KEY LESSONS IN THIS CHAPTER

- In the United States healthcare services traditionally have been thought of as a right rather than as something earned.
- Healthcare is represented on Wall Street by industries such as pharmaceuticals and medical equipment.
- As Wall Street continues to grow, the for-profit sector of healthcare plays an increasingly prominent role.
- In some instances, the whistleblower laws have had significant negative impact on the value of healthcare stocks.
- Healthcare delivery institutions find themselves balancing profit margins against the delivery of first-rate clinical services.

The Dow is up 200 points. The Dow is down 100 points. The Dow reaches 11,000. The Dow is expected to hit 12,000 by the year 2002. What does this have to do with healthcare? It is a good question and, until recently, had very little to do with healthcare. When we think of healthcare, we use terms like *patient needs,* focusing on cures, not costs, and we certainly do not think of profits. Some may think, too, of religious and charitable institution-affiliated hospitals, a great many of which are not in the best areas of town, serving the needs of the poor. Profit is the domain of Wall Street, where every day the New York Stock Exchange chronicles the success and failure of profit-oriented businesses. For over 100 years, the Dow Jones Industrial Average (DJIA), an index of the stock prices of 30 of the largest corporations in the United States, has told us whether business as a whole is doing well or poorly (Mayo, 1994). As Calvin Coolidge once said, "the business of America is business." This is best typified by that imposing edifice on Wall Street, the New York Stock Exchange. Although it may be difficult to conceive, Wall Street is playing an increasing role in healthcare, becoming a partner in the delivery of critical healthcare services to the American public.

TRADITIONAL HEALTHCARE DELIVERY MODEL

Historically, in the United States, healthcare services have been delivered very differently than most other services. For the most part, healthcare services have been evaluated in a social context rather than in an individual one, meaning that although the actual delivery of services has been uneven, access has been perceived as a right rather than as something earned. Generally speaking, the profit motive typically has not been associated with healthcare providers. Most providers have operated at the other end of the spectrum, as not-for-profit institutions. *Not-for-profit* means that the organization is exempted by the IRS from paying income taxes on any of its revenue. Any income over and above revenue is simply added to the organization's reserves. Equally important, donations to the organization can be taken as a tax deduction by the donor. Not-for-profit companies generally are formed exclusively for religious, charitable, scientific, testing for public safety, literary, or educational purposes. Any company that does not meet these criteria is defined as a *for-profit* company. The tax status of most traditional healthcare providers was clearly a function of their social commitment. Were it otherwise, they would not have been granted this special status by the IRS. Healthcare providers responded to patient needs, not desires (cosmetic surgery has always been treated differently) and were compensated on a reimbursement basis. The standard of care was determined by medical need, to which in turn a cost was attached.

To the extent that the individual had insurance coverage, the costs were covered by an insurance company. Payments from organizations like Blue Cross and Blue Shield generated a reliable stream of income, allowing providers to focus on the needs of the patient as prescribed by the physician. If an individual was not covered by insurance, the system absorbed the cost through the emergency room visit. Most healthcare providers were not-for-profit institutions, many of whom were affiliated with a religious organization that accepted social responsibility for meeting the basic healthcare needs of those who were unable to provide for themselves (Rosenblatt, 1997). What this meant, economically and financially, was that the shortfall in reimbursements for services rendered to the uninsured was ultimately absorbed by private donations and public forms of financial support. This system met the needs of the majority of Americans and was what James Tallon, president of the United Hospital Fund in New York, referred to as "the most sophisticated and technically advanced healthcare system in the world" (Tallon and Rigoglioso, 1999, p 1). This system remained effective in an environment where one-on-one patient care provided by medicine and nursing was the professional norm. The advent and rapid growth of technology and pharmacology in the post–World War II era contributed greatly to the evolution of health-care as we are currently experiencing it (Rosenblatt, 1997).

CHANGE IN THE TRADITIONAL HEALTHCARE DELIVERY MODEL

Dramatic changes in the cost structure of healthcare delivery—brought on partly by the rapid and costly development of technology and new drugs—undermined the traditional financing of healthcare. Premium structures, paid largely by corporations, began to lag behind reimbursement costs for the new medical procedures and drugs. The American healthcare system was facing a crisis, not in the quality of medical care, but in its costs. The right of every American to the best medical care was threatening to bankrupt the entire system. Traditional models of reimbursement simply did not work. Reimbursements and cost structures were out of alignment—too little reimbursement and too much cost (Rosenblatt, 1997).

Unlike healthcare services in most other industrialized countries where healthcare is provided at no cost to the individual, American healthcare services are covered (before age 65) under arrangements with insurance companies. Although historically private insurance companies have always been small players in the health insurance market, large organizations, such as Blue Cross and Blue Shield and Kaiser Permanente, were not-for-profit organizations. As previously described, they were completely compatible with the traditional healthcare services model. To understand the current healthcare system, it is important to know how these insurers were paid and who paid them. As with all insurance, health insurance is paid for by those who expect to use it, based on complex calculations that determine the probability that a person will require healthcare services. For this reason, the payment, called a *premium,* is quite different for a young, single adult than it is for a family.

This discussion brings us to another unique characteristic of American healthcare. By 1999, 63% of the population was covered by private healthcare insurance, primarily as an employment benefit (Associated Press, 2000). Typically an employee pays only a part of the total cost of his or her (or the family's) healthcare; the employer picks up the remainder. These amounts are excluded from the employee's income for tax purposes, while the employer receives a tax deduction for his or her contributions. In a sense, taxpayers subsidize the healthcare system to the extent of the tax breaks. Individuals who pay taxes and do not have private insurance coverage are subsidizing those who do have private health insurance. Still, healthcare premiums are a substantial business expense for both the government employers and corporate America. Industry analysts expect premium increases anywhere from 10% to 25% across managed care plans in coming years as insurers increase rates to cover their own rising costs (Messina, 2000).

The rapid increase in healthcare costs was but one of many problems that beset American industry in the 1980s. Under severe pressure from the rest of the world—notably Japan—to become more competitive in a global economy, corporate America began to scrutinize all of its cost structures closely. To reduce costs, companies reengineered their manufacturing and other operating processes. They also looked closely at their overhead, notably employee benefits. They realized the true impact that rising healthcare costs were having on their profitability and began to see the containment of healthcare costs not just as a profitability issue but as a survival issue. They took their case to state insurance regulators whose authority extended to setting all insurance premiums. Essentially, they told their state insurance regulators to control premium increases or they would move their businesses out of state to locations more favorable to their business. Once the decision was made to place caps on the rate of increase in healthcare premiums, the healthcare delivery was committed to a path of dramatic change. The issue was simple—if premiums could not be increased, then the focus had to be on controlling healthcare costs.

The concept of managed care, not a new concept at all, was now pushed to center stage. The issue was, and remains, how healthcare costs can be contained and who is best situated to do so. The issue of cost-effective delivery of healthcare services was completely beyond the scope of understanding of most healthcare providers operating under the traditional social responsibility model.

WALL STREET ENTERS THE PICTURE

Reconfiguring healthcare delivery required not only new ideas but also new structures and new means of delivery. All of this required financial resources above and beyond what was currently available within the group of existing providers. According to Dr. Spencer Foreman, President of Montefiore Medical Center, "The number-one problem for not-for-profit institutions is capital formation" (Fine, 1998, p B1). It was this need for capital that focused healthcare's attention on Wall Street. The link between healthcare and Wall Street really has been corporate America, the group that pays the bulk of the premiums for healthcare in the United States. Collectively, corporate America was not inclined to support any kind of government healthcare program. Rather, it wanted to reconfigure the private delivery system into a more cost-effective process. Corporate America already had extensive contacts on Wall Street who were anxious to tap into the trillion-dollar business—soon to be $2 trillion—that is healthcare.

Who is Wall Street?

Although Wall Street is a physical place—several blocks long at the foot of Manhattan Island—it is more useful to understand *Wall Street* as a shorthand term to describe a place where people and institutions that have money to invest meet to decide what to invest their money in. It is also important to understand that Wall Street, although subject to regulation to protect the public interest, is not responsible to any government entity. It is a free market driven by profit motive. Investors range from large institutions, such as insurance companies and mutual funds, to individuals and include governmental institutions. Funds made available by Wall Street become the capital base of a business in the expectation that we will not only get our money back but will get something more for time, effort, and risk. It is this whole process and the mindset that goes along with it that is being introduced into healthcare. Our purpose here is not to defend or condemn but simply to look at the implications of Wall Street's emergence in healthcare to be better prepared for the dialogue that must ensue.

Wall Street is always on the lookout for new investment opportunities—more so now than ever before. To understand the current mindset of Wall Street, one need only look at the DJIA. The DJIA is a weighted average of the stock price of 30 large, publicly held companies (Mayo, 1994). The DJIA in a sense represents the bottom line for Wall Street—its growth mirrors the success of Wall Street. It took 16 years (1956 to 1972) for the Dow to go from 1000 to 2000, and it took 2 years (1995 to 1997) for the Dow to move from 4000 to 8000. In April 1998, it passed 9000, followed by 10,000 in March of 1999 and 11,000 in May of the same year. (The acceleration in the rise of the DJIA can be tracked in most major newspapers or news programs.) As its success grows, Wall Street looks for new investments to continue this growth, one of which is the healthcare industry.

Figures show that the healthcare system spent $1.1 trillion in 1997, and this figure is expected to double by 2008 to $2.2 trillion, a figure very attractive to Wall Street. Before 1990, healthcare providers appeared nowhere on the business pages of the *New York Times* or the *Wall Street Journal*. Wall Street concentrated its efforts on those who supplied providers, such as the pharmaceutical and medical equipment companies. All of that has now changed. By 1996, 12 healthcare providers appeared in the annual ranking by *Fortune* magazine of the 100 fastest growing companies in the United States (Nocera, 1998). Coopers & Lybrand's venture-capital research division also has reported healthcare start-up companies attracting 1.2 billion dollars in venture capital in 1996. This figure is twice the amount that was invested in 1995 (Jaffe, 1997). Finally, Standard & Poors, a company whose business is to evaluate the creditworthiness of other companies, now is evaluating healthcare companies. Standard & Poors ranks companies and creates indices based on those rankings. By far the most popular of their indices is the S&P index of 500 industrial companies. In the Standard & Poors list of 1000 companies, the following providers of healthcare services can be found:

- Hospital management companies   6
- Long-term care companies   10
- Managed care companies   12
- Specialized medical services   16

Wall Street is growing and is looking for places to invest. Healthcare, a trillion dollar business, is in need of fresh money (i.e., capital). Now it is easy to see how these two entities have become intertwined.

What Resources Does Wall Street Have?

In addition to financial resources, Wall Street has other resources, such as new players, new ideas, incredible speed, financial and market discipline, and the press. All of these things have an effect on the way healthcare will operate in the future, which in turn will affect each of us. The new players introduced to healthcare often have little or no patient care experience. They include actuaries, marketers, lawyers, consultants, and architects. Even the FBI and the IRS have become more deeply involved in healthcare.

These new people bring new ideas, and Wall Street is in the business of funding ideas. Because Wall Street can move with blinding speed, it provides the ingredient—cash—for rapid innovation. Healthcare is now caught up in the pace of the for-profit enterprise. This fast pace can get healthcare into trouble, however. For example, "drive-through" mastectomies were streamlined into a day surgery for cost-containing purposes. Problems arose when patients were being denied hospital stays even when their physicians felt the stay was medically warranted. The adverse reaction created by these denials was reported in the *Wall Street Journal* almost immediately. State legislatures, hard-pressed to keep up, passed laws that required that hospital stays be extended to 48 hours for this group (Johannes, 1996).

Wall Street places great value on discipline, both market and financial. Wall Street investors expect companies to understand their markets and to meet or even exceed investor financial expectations. Companies that lose track of their markets and lose control of their financial situation are quickly and severely penalized. Moreover, any surprises or circumstances that call into question the quality of those numbers (e.g., write-offs, fraud) must be immediately disclosed to the public and may cause the value of the stock to sink dramatically.

Finally, there is the press. The press has always been involved in healthcare; the community section of most newspapers publicizes support groups and education groups offered by local healthcare agencies. Contrast that with the *New York Times* or the *Wall Street Journal*. They focus upon issues in healthcare, such as mergers, acquisitions, new laws, new business strategies, and financial performance. One thing is certain—healthcare issues increasingly will be discussed in the press, visible to all.

WALL STREET INVOLVES ITSELF IN HEALTHCARE

We have already indicated that Wall Street is actually a term to describe a global group of individuals and institutions that seek to invest their money in businesses, which will yield a return consistent with the risks they are willing to entertain. For this group of individuals and institutions, the risks are expected to be substantial, and the return they are looking for is expected to be equally substantial. One common approach is for investment banking firms, acting as intermediaries, to offer investor's participation in limited partnerships whose sole purpose is to invest in promising enterprises, in this case healthcare. The next section offers an example of this approach.

Participation in Limited Partnerships: Centennial Health Care Corporation

Welsh, Carson, Anderson & Stowe VIII, LP, is a limited partnership sponsored by Welsh, Carson, Anderson & Stowe, a New York investment firm. In October 1998 it announced that this limited partnership had committed capital of $3,150,000,000 and had been formed "to acquire controlling interests in companies in the healthcare and information service industries" (Welsh et al, 1998, p C10). The company further advertised itself to be "one of the nation's largest providers of private equity with over $8 billion of capital under management." (Welsh et al, 1998, p C10). Put simply, this investment vehicle is very much like a mutual fund for institutional investors. The goals are the same as for any mutual fund investor—to turn over funds to a professional manager and to seek a return on those funds. In this case, it is only the scale of the investment that separates the two; the motives are the same.

Within days of this announcement in the financial section of the *New York Times,* Welsh, Carson, Anderson & Stowe VIII, LP, had agreed to acquire Centennial Health Care Corporation, a provider of nursing home, rehabilitation, and home care services, for $290 million. It was "taking Centennial Health Care Corporation private," (Bloomberg News, 1998, p C3) that is, buying out all of the shares owned by the public and becoming the sole owner. Why would it do something like this? The company obviously thought that Centennial Health Care Corporation was worth more than the value placed on it by its current owners. Welsh, Carson, Anderson & Stowe VIII, LP, bought out the current shareholder, fully expecting that it would be able to turn around and sell Centennial Health Care Corporation again to a new group of shareholders at a substantially higher price. The term to describe this second phase of the transaction is *going public*—that is, selling the shares of the company back to individual investors. This term is the reverse of the original *going private*—that is, buying all outstanding shares from current investors.

Start-Up Company Funding: Healtheon Corporation

An alternative strategy for the Wall Street investor, including partnerships, is to provide funds directly to start-up companies. Typically, Wall Street investment firms spend considerable effort in seeking out ideas that can be developed into profitable businesses. A classic example of this process was played out on the pages of the *Wall Street Journal.* The company, Healtheon Corporation, is an example of how the computer industry, and more specifically, the use of the Internet, may reshape the delivery of healthcare services. The company's founder, James Clark, also a co-founder of Silicon Graphics, Inc and Netscape Communications Corp, intends to offer electronic processing of healthcare claims and on-line registration for health plans, as well as link doctors over the Internet to hospitals, pharmacies, laboratories, and insurance companies (Anders, 1998a).

The principal conduit for financing this new venture has been Kleiner, Perkins, Caufield & Byers, a celebrated venture capital firm, that is, a provider of funds to support the development of an infant business (Anders, 1998a). Traditionally, it is the private Wall Street investor who finances the development of new products and ideas. Traditional financial institutions, like banks and insurance companies, may place a small portion of their funds into start-up companies, but the risk is much too great for their normal business activities. Thus it is left to *venture capitalists,* another name for Wall Street investment bankers, to find the money to support the new ideas.

Wall Street has one goal throughout the process, which is to go public. Typically, investment bankers receive a percentage of ownership in any company they support financially. This ownership is in the form of shares and/or warrants, the right to purchase shares at a predetermined price. When a company goes public, it offers its shares to the public at a price, and the goal of investment bankers, quite simply, is to sell the shares they own at a substantial premium over what they paid for them. The substantial return is a reflection of the risk that the particular venture will fail. In fact, Healtheon faced considerable difficulty with its *initial public offering (IPO).* IPO is the term used to describe the transformation of a corporation from a private, closely held corporation to a publicly owned corporation whose shares are traded on one of the major stock exchanges (New York, American, or NASDAQ). The sale of the shares to the public provides substantial cash infusion to the company to enable it to continue its development.

Initially, Healtheon filed its plans to go public in July 1998 when major stock indexes were at their peak. This market condition suggested that potential share purchases would be willing to pay top dollar for the shares of Healtheon Corporation. By August the market had deteriorated sufficiently that the offer was withdrawn (Anders, 1998b). Indicative of the crucial role of the investment bankers in this process, the *Wall Street Journal* reported that Kleiner, Perkins, Caufield & Byers and its associates would provide another $40 million in financing (Anders, 1998b). In February 1999 Healtheon went public at $8/share and by May 1999 had reached a high of $114/share in the general euphoria surrounding any Internet-based stock.

How Different the Outcome: Starbucks Versus Columbia/HCA

One example of a Wall Street success story is Starbucks coffee, whose stock has done extremely well. In March 1995 the price of a share was a little over $10. Four years later, it was in the $35 range. The object, of course, is to buy at $10 and sell at $35. How does Starbucks do it? Starbucks has grown from less than 200 stores in 1992 to 1389 stores across the country in 1998. As of March 31, 1999, the number of stores was more than 2000 (Starbucks Coffee Company, 1998). Starbucks has reached its goal and accomplished it early. It also has diversified; people can buy Starbucks coffee in their local grocery store. Starbucks grew, went national, and diversified. Today the Internet is the rage, and Starbucks is planning to "encourage its fiercely loyal customers to shop on the Web, through starbucks.com" (Gibson, 1999, p C1). Not only did Starbucks have a good idea, it has, at least to date, executed its plans well. For that, it has rewarded its shareholders well.

Columbia/HCA had an idea not so different from that of Starbucks—replicate a proven concept across the United States. It started with a small group of hospitals that it acquired and reorganized to improve efficiency. It accomplished this through an aggressive program of acquisition and caught the eye of Wall Street. Typically, Columbia/HCA would buy four hospitals and close one. In this regard, it was able to do what the healthcare industry has generally been unable to do. In Florida, 95% of the residents were within 10 minutes of a Columbia/HCA facility (The Advisory Board, 1996). Columbia/HCA quickly became a Wall Street favorite. In March 1997 it was selling at $45/share. In October 1997 its share price fell to $26, a decline of 42%. Its stock did not drop because of the poor quality of care; it dropped because of the accusations of fraud and the business practices of the referral system within the physician group.

The financial world does not wait for legal outcomes to act. Subsequent stock analyst evaluations were surprisingly favorable, indicating basically that Columbia/HCA should be able to weather the storm. Fraud is something that Wall Street can deal with. The analysts proved surprisingly accurate as Columbia/HCA successfully retrenched, divesting itself of assets and reestablishing its market credibility. Still, analyst scrutiny continued, and punishment was swift for perceived transgressions; the share price dropped almost 5% in one day on reports (unconfirmed) that "a government witness testified that three executives of the hospital chain plotted to hide $3 million worth of overbilling from a government auditor" (Hershey, 1999, p C6). This was the fourth such suit that the Department of Justice had joined in its ongoing Medicare fraud investigation of Columbia/HCA (Bloomberg News, 1999). As of November 2001, Columbia/HCA has changed its name to HCA.

What's Worse to Wall Street than Fraud: Oxford Health Plans

Oxford's big headlines came shortly thereafter. Oxford was one of the fastest growing managed care companies in the United States. In 1991 Oxford sold for $4/share. By 1997 Oxford was selling for $89/share; however, in that same year, the stock fell 63% in one day (Nocera, 1998). The stock did not fall because there was a problem with patient care. Oxford did two things that upset the analysts: (1) it did not know how much money it owed, particularly to the providers and physicians, and (2) the company did not know how much money was owed to it. Oxford attributed this to problems in setting up a new billing system. The losses that followed brought Oxford to the brink of bankruptcy, which was staved off only by an agreement with state insurance authorities and an emergency infusion of fresh funds. Oxford also has reorganized, and after hitting a low of $6/share in August 1998, it has seen the value of its shares recover to $21/share (Freudenheim, 1999a).

Led by its new management team, Oxford continued to make progress toward its goals throughout 1999 and has finally achieved a measure of success in the new millennium. In the second quarter of the year 2000, Oxford finally swung to a profit, "benefiting from administrative-cost savings, ample premiums, and medical-cost controls" (Martinez and Rundle, 2000, p B12). Its strategy for securing a comeback has rested on tried-and-true for-profit principles, including focusing on stabilizing the revenue stream (Oxford has joined others in a wholesale exodus from Medicare), identifying revenue growth opportunities, and controlling costs, particularly medical costs. Oxford's medical-cost increased only 7% in one 2001 quarter (still almost three times the current inflation rate), compared with an industry average increase of 8% and a 10% to 12% increase at a major competitor, Aetna, Inc. Oxford's stock price has stabilized in the mid-twenties as Wall Street waits and watches, yet to be assured that Oxford really has gained control of its operation (Martinez and Rundle, 2000).

Wall Street to the Rescue: The Tenet Corporation

On July 21, 1998, the *Wall Street Journal* reported, "Pennsylvania's largest nonprofit health system, reeling from losses associated with a failed expansion, said it is selling nine Philadelphia-area hospitals and will file for bankruptcy-court protection for part of its operation" (Adams, 1998, p 7). Thus began the saga of Tenet Corporation and Allegheny Health, Education, and Research Foundation (AHERF), the largest healthcare system in Pennsylvania. Wall Street investors finance many start-up companies, watch some flounder in the marketplace, and occasionally rescue others. Tenet Healthcare Corporation is a case in point. Tenet is a California-based operator of 122 acute care hospitals with 28,000 beds in 18 states, employing 117,000 and generating $10 billion in revenues and $399 million in net income in 1988 (Rundle, 1998a). A publicly traded corporation, it is second in size only to Columbia/HCA, with whom it is often compared.

Indicative of the difficulty in operating in the healthcare market, Tenet's $345 million offer to acquire eight hospitals in the Philadelphia area was accepted, then rejected, and finally resurrected again only when AHERF was on the verge of bankruptcy, a strange turn of events for a not-for-profit institution (Rundle, 1998b). Once completed, Tenet Corporation would be the first for-profit organization to provide healthcare services in Philadelphia.

The transformation of AHERF from a respected not-for-profit institution to one in Chapter 11 bankruptcy proceedings describes one of the many pitfalls of developing profit-making aspirations in the framework of a not-for-profit institution. The parent institution, organized on a not-for-profit basis, decided to set up subsidiaries that would engage in for-profit activities. To this end, it initiated an aggressive campaign to purchase both hospitals and physician groups.

The plan was to combine hospitals and physician groups with related healthcare businesses and create a fully integrated healthcare system. Total revenue reached upwards of $1 billion from, in addition to eight hospitals, a medical school and 300 physician practices. The company's downfall was paying too much for hospitals and physician practices, which it financed with large amounts of debt. High operating expenses ($1 million in salary for the chief executive officer [CEO]) coupled with reduced payment from Medicare and private insurers contributed to losses reported at as high as $1 million/day. This loss resulted in insufficient cash to pay bondholders. While Tenet Corporation was negotiating with AHERF, its eight hospitals and other facilities in bankruptcy proceedings were faced with declining patient admissions, suspicious doctors, and fierce competition (for patients) in a consolidating market. Addressing the for-profit versus not-for-profit issue directly, Jeffrey C. Barbakow, CEO of Tenet, commented, "We have a lot of work to do in Philadelphia, but success there will open up opportunities for us in many other places that aren't always receptive to investor-owned hospitals" (Rundle, 1998b, p B6).

The acquisition of AHERF was a saga itself, involving the bankruptcy court, state officials in Pennsylvania, the mayor of Philadelphia, and Drexel University School of Medicine. After a thorough review of the hospitals' operations by a team from Tenet, the offer was made. The deal almost foundered when Drexel University rejected Tenet's invitation to manage Allegheny University of the Health Sciences. Of the $345 million Tenet intended to invest, $60 million had been targeted as an endowment for the medical school, set up as a nonprofit entity. Both the governor of Pennsylvania, Tom Ridge, and the mayor of Philadelphia, Ed Rendell, prevailed on Drexel trustees to change their minds, which they subsequently did with an additional $150 million pledge by Tenet and existing creditors of the medical school. At stake were 17,000 jobs. This funding was required to cover the significant deficits, which the medical school had been running over for the last several years. The arrangement was key to the completion of the acquisition because three of the eight hospitals being acquired were teaching hospitals closely related to the medical school (Rundle, 1998b).

The question is, has Tenet had more success in managing for-profit healthcare than AHERF? The answer depends on whom one consults. To look at Tenet's earnings alone, one would have to answer yes. In the year ending May 31, 2000, Tenet Healthcare Corporation has seen its profits reach $302 million. This 20% increase has doubled Tenet's stock prices. Barbakow was able to achieve this success by streamlining operations and making staff cutbacks. John Hindelong of Donaldson, Lufkin, & Jennette, an investment banking firm, believes it is this type of successful performance that could help repair the damaged reputations of for-profit hospitals (Sharp, 2000).

Unfortunately, advocates of Tenet's for-profit healthcare system are difficult to find after this point. Union leaders and some public health advocates argue that the beneficiaries of this success have been limited to the company's CEO and stockholders. These critics believe this type of healthcare economizing has caused the demise of quality healthcare for patients. Their arguments are not without merit. As corporations acquire weaker chains, unprofitable hospitals are closed or sold. These closings force patients to travel farther for care, as well as force urban hospitals to absorb more emergency room costs. Confirmed reports of Tenet hospitals refusing medical treatments to poor and uninsured women have also surfaced, perhaps indicative of cutbacks that have run too deep (Sharp, 2000).

The community is not alone in its criticisms of Tenet. The cutbacks made by Tenet have left employees unsatisfied as well. Nurses in Massachusetts and California have gone on strike over issues such as mandatory overtime, patient care, and better pay. Rose Ann DeMoro, executive director of the California Nurses Association, stated, "Tenet consistently prolongs negotiations, provokes nurses into striking, and refuses to have discussions with us about patient care. It's almost their policy" (Sharp, 2000, p 4).

These issues have led to the accusation that Tenet is not "sharing the wealth." Employees believe that in light of its financial success, they should be afforded more control and better pay. Although Barbakow does not address these issues directly, he insists that improving performance for stockholders, as well as for patients and staff, remain his top priorities (Sharp, 2000).

Despite financial gains made by Tenet, many conflicts still remain. Wall Street's financial rescue of a healthcare company in bankruptcy is just a financial rescue. Resolving the many conflicts that have been born of managed care requires more than just the financial skills of which Barbakow boasts.

From Riches to Rags: Genesis Health Ventures, Inc.

What happens if no white knight rides to the rescue of a company in distress, even one that serves a demonstrable need in the community? For-profit healthcare companies are simply too large to be bailed out by private or public benefactors. The answer becomes a full-fledged bankruptcy proceeding.

Genesis Health Ventures, Inc, founded in 1965, had as its mission the changing of the way eldercare is delivered in America. Not unlike Columbia/HCA's approach to hospitals, Genesis entered an eldercare market characterized as fragmented at best and as chaotic at worst. Its business model was based on the assumption that providing integrated medical care to the elderly could achieve higher quality care at less cost. Through its regionally concentrated networks, Genesis provided integrated healthcare, specialty medical, and community-based services to individuals, managed care companies, and third-party providers. It addressed the needs of the elderly on a continuum—first in supporting them in an independent environment, then in an assisted care setting, and finally providing comprehensive nursing home care. Genesis grew rapidly, achieving revenues approaching $2 billion, and served more than 150,000 customers each day. In 1997 the price of a share of Genesis common stock reached $34¾ (Genesis, 2000).

On June 22, 2000, all of this came to an abrupt halt as Genesis filed a voluntary petition for protection under Chapter 11 of the U.S. Bankruptcy Code. "The company elected to seek court protection in order to facilitate efforts to restructure capital obligations" (Genesis/ Multicare Bankruptcy News, 2000).

This statement means that Genesis is using legal process to protect it from its creditors while it comes up with a plan for reaching a settlement with those creditors. The reason this situation arose was that Genesis was not generating sufficient cash flow (which is more important than earnings) to meet its financial obligations as they came due. The first hint of problems occurred in May 2000, when it was announced that Genesis was engaged in discussions with senior lenders to develop a restructuring plan. When these negotiations failed, the only recourse Genesis had was to file bankruptcy. What was the problem? Commenting on the bankruptcy filing, CEO Michael R. Walker declared, "Deep cuts in Medicare reimbursements, which far exceeded all government forecasts coupled with chronic underfunding of Medicaid reimbursements, have severely impacted Genesis' ability to service our current capital structure" (Genesis/Multicare Bankruptcy News, 2000).

Genesis will now negotiate a plan of payment with all of its creditors. Typically, such a plan results in creditors accepting less than 100% of the amounts due them. It is not uncommon that the remaining amounts due are converted to a nonsenior obligation, either subordinated debt or stock in a reconstituted Genesis. Under this scenario, owners of common stock, having only a residual claim after all senior debt holders are paid in full, are likely to see their investment disappear. Because of the potentially adverse consequences to large numbers of individual shareholders, the final approval of whatever plan Genesis and its creditors agree on rests with the federal bankruptcy court.

The Genesis experience now brings us full circle in the for-profit experience. Wall Street, attracted by perceived opportunity in healthcare delivery, has invested substantial dollars and time to establish its viability in the for-profit sector. Some have succeeded, many have stumbled, and a few, such as Oxford Health Plans, have stumbled and revived. Genesis will have an opportunity to reestablish itself and continue to serve its elderly clients. There is no certainty, however, that this will happen or that future decisions by government agencies on reimbursement policy will again throw Genesis into bankruptcy proceedings. Although this kind of travail is considered an acceptable risk in the private sector—and shareholders need to be rewarded appropriately for assuming this risk—the questions remains if this uncertainty is appropriate where healthcare is at stake.

THE IMPACT OF WALL STREET ON HEALTHCARE DELIVERY

This discussion amounts to a complete transformation of healthcare culture. A question that remains is, Does Wall Street jibe with healthcare? In an article in the OpEd section of the *New York Times*, Nocera, a *Fortune* magazine editor, described the dilemma very well: ". . . the imperative that Wall Street demands of hot growth companies—that profits increase by eye-popping amounts year after year—doesn't quite jibe with the business of delivering first-rate healthcare to the public" (Nocera, 1998, p 11). The strain between the profit motive and first-rate healthcare for the public is not by any means new. What makes it different now is that the issue is moving to center stage, yet questions remain. Is the pouring of capital providing a better product? Will new technologies raise ethical issues of who gets the better procedures or what resources will be made available to whom? For now, the market forces are not meeting the consumer satisfaction mark. In a recent Harris poll published in *USA Today*, consumers identified the bottom three of 13 industries as health insurance, managed care, and tobacco (*USA Today*, 1998).

It is important, however, to maintain perspective and express the questions and issues in the broadest possible context. Crigger, editor of the *Hastings Center Report*, observed:

The problems in American health care today are systemic and call for systemic solutions. Neither piecemeal government regulations (federal or state) nor piecemeal market responses alone will resolve the dilemmas of designing a health care system that provides equitable access at sustainable cost. Creative, interdependent responses are called for that recognize the complex ways in which regulation, market forces, and the demands of individual health care consumers shape what health care services are delivered in what ways (Crigger, personal communication, July 17, 2000).

At this point, we have only a general idea of what will not work. Early quality studies conducted by Harvard Medical School-affiliated researchers and others indicate that not-for-profit HMOs rated higher on quality indicators than investor-owned plans (Reuters Health Information, 1999). The Clinton administration's task force, although it may have been well intended, showed that a political solution on a nationwide basis was not feasible in the current environment. In the next millennium, healthcare will most likely be a hybrid of government and private initiatives.

WALL STREET AND THE HEALTHCARE PROFESSIONAL

As long as we are asking questions, we pose another: Who is going to venture an opinion on behalf of nurses, physicians, healthcare providers, and—above all—patients? We support active participation in all quality initiatives. Thus it will be important for healthcare professionals to consider implementing the following:

- Increase the nurse's patient advocacy role
- Render opinions on legislation that affect quality of care
- Define and support efforts to ensure quality outcomes
- Identify technological improvements that can improve care easily and more immediately. For example, point-of-care testing replaces a trip to the laboratory and venipuncture with a finger prick and a personal interview with an RN who can assess the patient and make treatment modifications according to protocol, education, and written computerized instructions until the next visit. Point-of-care testing takes about 15 minutes and is managed by the nurse.

- Develop business acumen to obtain better resources for nursing and subsequently for patients.
- Look for opportunities to use nurses' clinical knowledge to improve product development (e.g., in writing software for healthcare information systems). Nearly every sector of every industry directly or indirectly involved in healthcare needs the input of the clinician, primarily physicians and nurses.
- Expand the base of professional nursing skills to include not only advanced clinical skills but also resource management, finance, and computer skills.
- Partner with physicians and colleagues in other sectors to move everyone forward in healthcare.
- Support nursing's professional organizations.

Healthcare professionals, as individuals and as a group, have important input to the continuing healthcare debate. Each of us must decide how much we can do, but we must do our part.

REFERENCES

Adams C: Tenet files for bankruptcy protection, *The Wall Street Journal*, p 7, July 21, 1998.

The Advisory Board: *The rising tide,* Lecture presented at the Annual Member Meeting of the Advisory Board, New York, August 28, 1996.

Anders G: IPO roadshow still rolls: planning an IPO, *The Wall Street Journal*, pp A1, A6, October 2, 1998a.

Anders G: Healtheon cancels planned offering, will raise $40 million from backers, *The Wall Street Journal*, p B13, October 21, 1998b.

Associated Press: More Americans now have health insurance: robust economy cited as main reason, *The Journal News*, p A1, September 29, 2000.

Bloomberg News: Centennial healthcare to be acquired by Welsh Carson, *The New York Times*, p C3, October 23, 1998.

Bloomberg News: U.S. joins whistle-blower suit against Columbia/HCA, *The New York Times*, p C4, May 26, 1999.

Crigger B: Personal communication, July 17, 2000.

Fine E: Regime to get clinics giving specialty care, *The New York Times*, p B1, February 9, 1998.

Freudenheim M: Oxford health turnaround is still a work in progress, *The New York Times*, p C2, May 13, 1999a.

Freudenheim M: Medical records company announces spree of deal, *The New York Times*, p C2, May 21, 1999b.

Genesis: Available online: http://www.ghv.com.ir_overview.shtml, July 21, 2000.

Genesis/Multicare Bankruptcy News: Trenton, NJ, June 26, 2000, Bankruptcy Creditors' Service.

Gibson R: Internet froth takes on a new meaning, *The Wall Street Journal*, p C1, May 26, 1999.

Hershey RJ Jr: Dow plummets 235.23 as investors react to rising interest rates, *The New York Times,* p C6, May 28, 1999.

Jaffe G: Start-ups in healthcare are booming: change in nations medical care provides openings, *The Wall Street Journal*, p A9, May 23, 1997.

Johannes L: Managed-care group softens view on hospital stays after mastectomies, *The Wall Street Journal*, p B6, November 11, 1996.

A look at statistics that shape the nation, *USA Today*, p A1, November 5, 1998.

Martinez B, Rundle RL: WellPoint, Oxford earnings beat forecasts by holding down costs, *The Wall Street Journal*, p B2, July 27, 2000.

Mayo HB: *Investments: an introduction*, Fort Worth, Tex, 1994, Dryden Press.

Messina J: Coping with the ill effects of healthcare inflation, *Crain's New York Business*, p 17, August 28, 2000.

Nocera J: The tarnished darlings of Wall Street, *The New York Times*, p 11, January 4, 1998.

Reuters Health Information: In Medscape, July 14, 1999, Available online: http://managedcare.medscape.com/reuters/ prof/07.14/mc07149a.html.

Rosenblatt R: *How the American health system works*, Westbury, NY, 1997, Foundation Press.

Rundle RL: Tenet plan to buy eight hospitals is dealt a serious setback, *The Wall Street Journal*, p B7, October 14, 1998a.

Rundle RL: Tenet healthcare tries rescue of Philadelphia hospital, *The Wall Street Journal*, p B6, October 28, 1998b.

Sharp K: Hospital chain's critics call recovery incomplete, *The New York Times*, p 4, August 6, 2000.

Starbucks Coffee Company: Starbucks reports first quarter results, Jan 23, 1998.

Tallon J, Rigoglioso RL: Fund-staffed effort creates new quality forum: an unprecedented opportunity to improve healthcare quality, *Blueprint* Summer, 1999. (Available from United Hospital Fund, Empire State Building, 350 Fifth Avenue, 23rd Floor, New York, NY 10118-2399.)

Welsh P, Carson R, Anderson B, et al: Announcement, *The New York Times*, p C10, October 5, 1998.

Managed Care: What's Next?

Connie Burgess

KEY LESSONS IN THIS CHAPTER

- The managed care marketplace is constantly changing, and nurses must be aware of changing trends and information.
- No evidence suggests that providers will be realizing increased revenue to deliver services over the next few years.
- Managed care reimbursement can take place through capitation, case rates, or per diem payment mechanisms.
- Future organizational success will depend on the integration of payment systems with clinical processes.
- When planning a patient's care, nurses should consider consequences, discharge planning needs, availability of resources, and continuum of care issues.

For several years, managed care has been gathering new subscribers and proliferating at a rapid pace. Since about July 1999, the activity surrounding the premise of managed healthcare (MHC), the incentives and ethics inherent in the models, and the issue of patient rights has reached almost frenzied proportions. Newspapers, magazines, talk shows, and the healthcare conference and lecture circuit are full of featured speakers offering data, opinions, and predictions. Politicians evade some issues and address others, as the insurance lobby in Washington tries to stem the tide of legislation related specifically to the patient's right to sue for malpractice. In addition, employers have not realized the anticipated savings, and the cost of premiums has risen anywhere from 4% every year to 10% or more in 2000. Significant numbers of consumers/patients are reported to be upset and to lack confidence that the healthcare system will take care of them if they become seriously ill or injured. In a November 1999 series of articles, *Newsweek* reported that 61% of those surveyed were frustrated and angry with the healthcare system, and 55% felt the system would not come through for them if they were in serious condition (Cowley and Turque, 1999). In that same time period, United Health Group, the nation's second largest health insurer, covering 14.5 million people, announced that it was giving physicians the final say in which treatments it will cover. In response, Dr. Robert Blendon, professor of health policy at Harvard University, said, "It's just extraordinary. Here they are saying that there are other ways to save money without rationing care. It removes a fundamental tenet of how these plans have been operating in order to be cost-effective" (Galewitz, 1999, p A11).

THE PROVIDER VIEWPOINT

For providers of healthcare services, the turmoil is intense for some and less dramatic for others. In California 34 medical groups either closed or declared bankruptcy by November 1999, up from 31 in 1998 (Cowley and Turque, 1999). According to the Census Bureau, 44.6 million Americans, or about 16% of the population, are not covered by any health plan, and that number is rising by about 1 million per year (Cowley and Turque, 1999). Operation Restore Trust, a federal fraud program established by Medicare to crack down on healthcare abuses, has affected providers in all aspects of the industry. In 1999 hospital executives were convicted for the first time of Medicare fraud (*Modern Healthcare*, 1999).

Many healthcare providers try to cope with decreased revenue streams and effective management of the funds they do receive. After 12 years consulting nationally and helping clients redefine their clinical delivery systems based on managed care contracts, the Balanced Budget Act (BBA), and prospective payment systems (PPS), it is this author's perspective that far too many providers address the reimbursement restrictions primarily as fiscal models, with little or no attention paid to the clinical requirements. Providers assume that quality will happen automatically, and in some instances, nurses are used as generic care providers with little concern for specialization. Many leading programs that demonstrated innovative yet cost-sensitive clinical delivery systems have been dismantled in favor of traditional downsizing strategies and strict utilization management approaches. This situation might be called a *full circle phenomenon.*

Why do we continue down the path of rigid fiscal realignment and a second generation of resizing, rightsizing, downsizing, or more specifically, discarding the solutions we created in response to cost containment? Several ideas emerged in conversations with numerous nurse managers at a national meeting in Washington, DC, in November 1999. Some suggested that there is a disconnection between fiscal and clinical leadership, especially in nursing. Others said that the change in top leadership was so frequent that new programs were often abandoned when the newest leader arrived and introduced his or her brand of cost-cutting strategies. Many clinical programs had not established any measurements to evaluate the fiscal success of their redesigned delivery models, which had gone virtually unnoticed by several participants in the discussion. Case management systems previously designed to address consumers' needs while cutting costs were reported as being replaced with straight utilization management strategies, and staff often were described as merely surviving but not enjoying their work or looking forward to a future in healthcare. A few were eager to return to the "good old days" when all they had to do was take care of patients.

THE NEW "GOOD OLD DAYS"

The thought that MHC may be disappearing pleases some people. Although MHC as previously described and implemented may disappear in the next 2 to 5 years, no evidence suggests that providers will suddenly be offered more money to deliver clinical services. The positive results of healthcare reform will not be abandoned. Although the anticipated savings have not been realized to the degree hoped, patients' empowerment and accountability for their own health, prevention, and wellness strategies, and the monitoring of system abuses are taking hold. Access to information through health plans, providers, and the Internet have dramatically increased. Delivery of healthcare services has expanded into the community and is located where people live. Technology continues to grow at phenomenal rates and offers untold future opportunities for the dissemination of information, the monitoring of health and wellness, the management of disease from home, and the development of self-care capacity among the next generations. Consumers can have their cholesterol levels measured at the local pharmacy and can track all health risks and monitor all laboratory work, prescriptions, and activities that impact those risks on Internet-based programs. They can take their self-generated health record to their physician or other healthcare professionals or can locate their health profiles on a Website in their physician's office.

These are our new "good old days," and they hold a great deal of promise for a healthy community. Nevertheless, we will continue to face a number of obstacles on the way to success.

BACK TO BASICS

The feedback received from both fiscal and clinical colleagues surrounding the cost of doing the business of healthcare continues to support the need for more working knowledge of reimbursement models and their associated incentives. As the architects of clinical delivery systems, nurses must understand what it takes to keep the business going if we are to remain relevant to the process and valued as contributing decision-making members of the team.

Healthcare delivery is local and must be managed from each community's unique vantage point. An understanding of the reimbursement methods employed by each payer, including private and government payers, is essential to building effective cost and clinical strategies. One can never assume that if patients are over 65 they will receive one level of care or if they are receiving Medicaid things will look the same from county to county. Many organizations have experienced senior populations shifting from Medicare to senior health maintenance organizations (HMOs) and then back to Medicare within a year or two. Several states have adopted HMO models for their Medicaid populations but may administer them differently from region to region. Whether operating under an HMO, a private program, or a government-based health plan, existing payment mechanisms will continue to be used, and front-line clinicians must know how to manage within those parameters. Without basic benefit information and a clear understanding of how to use it for creative, innovative care and cost-management approaches, nursing or any other discipline can anticipate being viewed by executive management simply as a necessity for healthcare operations. They will not, however, have voices in strategic positioning and important decision making.

This concept has been difficult to sell to some nurses, and the educational process related to managed care offers a superficial understanding at best. If clinicians are to have any influence in the allocation of resources and how care is delivered, however, they must build on nursing's existing knowledge base. For example, nurses are patient advocates and are in the best position to facilitate care and educate patients and families toward health and wellness. This critical role cannot be fulfilled when the advocate's competencies do not include reasonable knowledge of and skill in managing fiscal resources to the benefit of both the patient and the provider.

PAYMENT MECHANISMS AND INCENTIVES

First, nurses must recognize the various payment mechanisms and learn how to work within the established boundaries of each type. Because the MHC model has been fiscally driven, insufficient energy has been spent on how to integrate the available resources with the patient's clinical needs. Some payment mechanisms lend themselves to an individual patient approach, whereas others will get better results when applied to an entire population.

For example, the first payment mechanism used to manage costs was a discount on charges. Based on a fee-for-service model, the plan called for payment of each test or treatment provided, but the actual amount paid is discounted a specific percentage, which is typically established before the delivery of service. This approach is managed on a patient-by-patient basis, and the cost for delivering care to one patient has no impact on any others or on the potential revenue flow for the facility. The incentive to providers in this arrangement is to do as many medical procedures as possible. They will still get paid, but it will be less than in earlier years and will require more patients to equal their previous revenues.

The second payment mechanism is the per diem rate, which is also a fee-for-service model. Simply stated, the provider is paid a daily predetermined rate for the care provided to the patient. Whether receiving basic nursing care or expensive tests and medications, the amount paid remains the same. Although "sliding scales" have been established for some contracts to allow more funds for the first few days of care, the basic premise that the provider will receive a set rate for each day remains. The provider's incentive is to keep the patient for as many days as possible since they get paid the daily rate for every day they are hospitalized. The payer's incentive is to move the patient out of the hospital setting to the least costly level as early as possible. This disparity in fiscal incentives can set up a conflict between the provider and payer case managers and can create a stressful environment for everyone involved.

Capitation and case rates, or risk contracts, are two cost-based mechanisms that work quite differently from fee-for-service models. Capitation offers a preset fee based on a per-member-per-month formula, which means that the provider is paid a predetermined amount and receives the same payment whether or not the patient requests care. The provider is responsible for all care and holds the financial risk for a specified number of patients. The model rewards the provider for offering less care. The fewer the treatments, procedures, or appointments, the more of the fee the provider is able to keep. This particular payment system is the most controversial and is perceived by some to place the clinician in an uncompromising situation. The fiscal incentives are clear and are considered by many to be unethical. From the pragmatic standpoint, capitation has been difficult to operationalize for both patients and providers. The best possible outcome for the patient and the provider is for the patient to remain healthy and well.

Prevention strategies have become more popular, but the HMO may only cover a subscriber for 1 year and therefore would hold minimum financial risk. Thus investment in wellness programs may be limited. Capitation is the model used by several of the senior HMO plans. Many senior risk plans have closed due to costs, and there are indications that more are moving in that direction.

The second and most promising cost-based payment mechanism is the case rate. This mechanism has possibilities for successful healthcare management because it is unlike capitation, in which the idea is to cut costs without staff ever really knowing how much. Case rates have fiscal targets to guide expenditures. When applied across a population of similar patients, there is a good chance that quality and cost can be combined into a successful clinical and fiscal outcome. Managing a case rate is not a simple, straightforward process, however, because specific guidelines must be understood and followed. The following 10-point approach can offer a better planned clinical and cost-effective operation:

1. Do not treat all patients the same way; this is discrimination.
2. Think about and assess the need for care beyond the diagnosis or you will become trapped by its limitations. Look at the consequences of what happened to this patient for comprehensive planning.
3. Individualize all patient care planning and delivery.
4. Identify each patient's salient issues (key needs) and prioritize them. What can we do to meet their needs?
5. Use multiple strategies. No single approach works for everyone.
6. Be creative. Some patients appear to be uncomplicated, classic cases and will respond well to clinical guidelines or pathways. Others with the same diagnosis will be complex and may require more than a simple or single approach.
7. Treat to the level of the patient's need but not to the limits of his or her benefits. Some patients will require less care than the benefit allows, and some care requirements will exceed the limits. Treat to the need, and the cost will even out.
8. Use a continuum of care, and move the patient to the least costly level of care at the earliest possible moment.
9. When a patient is moved from one setting to another, do not start the care planning process over again. Build on existing data.
10. Monitor and measure what works and what does not.

The next section presents an example illustrating why it is important for nurses to understand reimbursement mechanisms and incentives.

TABLE 7-1
Comparison of Three Managed Care Markets

Parameters	New York	Chicago	Los Angeles
Bed days per 1000 lives: under age 65	1200	700	500
Bed days per 1000 lives: over age 65	1800	1200	900
Percent of physician groups capitated	35%	60%	92%

Adapted from Hamer RL: *The InterStudy competitive edge part III: regional market analysis 9.1*, St Paul, 1999, InterStudy Publications.

What Makes It Work

Although much time and energy is spent in professional organizations at a national level, healthcare is a local phenomenon; every environment requires a unique, tailored approach. What makes such an approach possible is a thorough understanding of the fiscal principles involved. The drivers of today's healthcare environment (employers, costs, and managed care) have affected the country at a different pace and with varying degrees of impact. Each response to managed care has been at the local level, and it is unrealistic to believe that there are simple or automatic answers that will fix everything. Table 7-1 compares three large managed care markets.

When caught in the intense pressures generated by cost-cutting mandates, it is easy for an organization's management to try something they believe to have worked elsewhere, often without validation. For example, a nurse who does not understand how the reimbursement models and inherent incentives work recommends the use of pathways in New York because they received such good reviews in Los Angeles. If the organization in New York was able to achieve similar outcomes through the use of pathways as applied in Los Angeles, the revenue stream would drop so dramatically that everyone would be looking for a new job. As seen in Table 7-1, New York physicians were operating in a predominately fee-for-service mode, as were the hospitals. Los Angeles physicians, on the other hand, were over 90% capitated. These are two very different incentive mechanisms and two entirely different income calculations.

NEW LESSONS ON BOTH SIDES

Once clinicians know how to interpret the various fiscal mechanisms, they can build systems for cost-effective care delivery. Nevertheless, most organizations do not take the extra steps required to integrate the payment system with the clinical process to create the best possible outcomes. Insufficient time is taken to ensure that clinicians understand exactly how the payment system works so they can think through the best possible care approach.

Clinicians are not the only staff with superficial knowledge about the process. The executive team often does not recognize the potential success of a model because of the same lack of investment in time and education for themselves and some in-depth critical thinking about what is compatible with their situation. Consulting firms, many of which are fiscally based, are frequently called in to evaluate the system and make recommendations to cut more costs. The common approach is to employ a fiscal model that leads to uninformed decisions about the impact of clinical cuts on the institution's ability to meet the needs of its customers. Many of these firms have one or two nurses to answer the question of whether there is clinical representation. The problem is that this presumes that nurses are just nurses and are not educated in the fiscal mechanisms of HMOs. This oversight leads to quick-fix templates for care that treat everyone the same or another wave of downsizing that paralyzes staff, frightens patients, and still does not make the institution fiscally viable.

The problem is compounded further with rigid rules concerning where care may be delivered. Some seem to think that care is only legitimate if provided in a hospital. Others believe the continuum of care should be used but do not always cover the cost of care in alternative settings. In any given situation, some or all of these forces are pushing against each other, and the staff and patients simply do not know what to do.

The nursing profession's challenge is to rethink cost-effective healthcare delivery from a place that includes all the available talent within an organization and is visionary and pragmatic. The chief executive officer (CEO) and the clinical staff must be in the same room in a shared educational process and must work toward getting on the same team. Few organizations have taken the time to know their own inner workings, to learn how both business and clinical problems get solved, or to allow enough time for point-counterpoint discussions. Clinical staff solve extremely complex situations every day. Often, when armed with new information from fiscal and executive leadership as to how their decisions will impact the operation, they are able to reevaluate the problem and resolve it for the good of the whole. Unfortunately, most staff are never given the chance to think about it.

TAKING SOME RISKS: MOVING TO THE NEXT STAGE

The real challenge is for top leadership to muster enough courage to allow the necessary time and education for everyone to arrive at the same door. The goals of the process must be clearly defined. "We need to cut costs" or "increase customer satisfaction" do not provide clear direction for anyone to develop a workable plan. Some grass roots and in-depth analysis and planning can yield far more commitment to organizational management and growth than another consulting firm. Healthcare professionals seem so caught up in the tenets and impact of managed care that they have lost sight of the power and strength of the staff who choose to work within the organization and take pride in owning the product and the outcomes. Not every organization will have all the talent it needs to make the best, most innovative decisions. Outside advisors will not be necessary in every setting, but what an organization needs in advisors could no doubt tolerate a review. A good facilitator and coach would be ideal: someone who has the ear of executive management and clinical staff and can elicit the best ideas from people at the same time he or she is helping them accept change. Content experts from various fields might be timely now and then, and perhaps someone who has successfully been through all the changes and challenges and knows that a balance of cost and care really can work could be engaged.

SUCCESSFUL TEAMS

This author's confidence in this approach is unwavering and based on 12 years' experience working with teams of people, many of whom had to come up with the answers or start looking for work. The teams were made up of people from all disciplines and varying degrees of education and experience. Many were new graduates who had a different perspective on how the work was done but had little life experience on which to draw. Others had years of experience and well-developed skills and knowledge but were lost in the successes of their past and were not always able to transfer their rich resources to new endeavors. Still others were intelligent, intuitive, and looking for the next great challenge.

When the process first started, the teams did not know each other very well. The first steps then were to learn from one another what each valued, how they perceived the situation, and what they had to offer. Once they moved past the old perceptions and learned the details of their service's financial status and the types of managed care plans they were contracted for, they were able to develop excellent cost-effective clinical strategies. Fiscal targets were established, and they were able to redesign their clinical approach, consolidate positions, and become more relevant to patient-driven care. Most were in the field of rehabilitation and had worked as teams in the past. This process, however, suggested to many that they had only gone through the motions of being a team but had not really experienced the level of integration and collaboration found in the new approach.

As the change process began, they identified their interests and skills and selected the task forces on which to work. Some could give more than others based on other life responsibilities and commitments, and no one was penalized for lack of participation. The most dramatic transformation was the shift from each discipline believing life in the organization was only about them to a stream of energy that put the patient first, the organization second, and themselves last.

FRAMEWORK FOR THINKING AND PLANNING

This approach to care and change is sensitive to the individual needs of each patient. This sensitivity results in expansive benefits that go beyond the medical model to include initial care planning that follows patients through each step of their care and back into their community. The Salient Factors Approach to Patient Care Planning is grounded in the World Health Organization's (WHO) differentiation between the medical model, which focuses on diagnosis and cure, and the consequence model, which is based on the results or impact to the patient from the illness or injury (ICIDH, 1980). The Salient Factors model is patient driven and allows the care team to prioritize each individual's care needs based on the impact of what has happened to that person and what the individual says is most important to him or her. Once evaluated in four areas, the treatment strategy is established, and the most clinically appropriate and cost-effective treatment strategy is initiated. Some patients require straightforward treatment and benefit from clinical guidelines or pathways. Others require several integrated strategies to address their complex needs.

The Salient Factors Model

Four questions need to be answered when planning a patient's care, beginning with admission to acute care. They are as follows:

1. *The consequences:* What are the physical, psychological, social, and behavioral consequences to the patient as a result of this illness or injury? What are the clinical interventions to cure the problem or to accommodate for the resultant loss of function or ability? For a patient with a fractured hip whose life is otherwise unchanged by the experience, a pathway will work extremely well. A stroke victim's life, on the other hand, may be altered forever and will require multiple and far more complex interventions. The question here is what will it take for this patient to reach an acceptable level of functioning.

2. *The discharge plan:* Keeping in mind that home is a destination and not a discharge plan, it must be determined before treatment where the patient is going after discharge, who, if anyone, will be there, and what the patient must do to function in that setting. Is the ability to direct others in managing their care the primary goal of patients, or should they be able to meet their own physical needs?

3. *Available benefits/resources:* What healthcare benefits does the patient have, and which treatments or levels of care are covered and which are not? For example, do the benefits include outpatient or home healthcare? If not, the team must know this before care is planned so they can either prioritize care differently or work with the payer to adjust the benefits. It might be in the patient's best interest to decrease the number of inpatient days and use the money saved to include some outpatient visits. Other fiscal, human, and community resources should be included in this part of the care planning process.

4. *Treatment systems/continuum of care:* Less costly posthospital treatment settings that may be required are identified for location and accessibility early in the care planning process so unrealistic recommendations for follow-up care are not made. For example, if a patient could benefit from home care but lives 50 miles beyond any available services, an alternative should be developed before the patient is discharged.

CONTINUUMS OF CARE

Before discussing the use of care options and settings, consider the following attitudes surrounding finances, nurses, and case management.

The business of healthcare delivery and the philosophy of caring are not mutually exclusive. In fact, nurses have the ability to develop comprehensive, cost-effective approaches to people and their health planning.

It is not uncommon to read in popular case management literature that the most important aspect of the nurse's role is patient care and that the costs should never take precedence. There is something apologetic about this thinking that does not serve patients or nurses well.

We must not think less of ourselves, and therefore our colleagues, for being competent in cost management. Often when executives and nonnursing colleagues hear the "cost disclaimer," the notion that nurses do not understand business is reinforced, and our opinion is not valued. Nurses *must* be part of an organization's dialogue and influence the direction care delivery takes. Committees of administrators with physicians as the only decision makers for the clinical side is as short-sighted and unacceptable as a group of nurses determining how to perform transplant surgery. The current solutions are inadequate for these problems.

The Continuum

The medical and health continuum of care has been described in many different ways. The most common definition probably centers around the idea of a series of places, each specializing in a specific type or level of service, such as the following:

- Intensive care
- Medical/surgical
- Subacute
- Acute rehabilitation
- Home health
- Outpatient
- Hospice

Although many healthcare organizations have multiple pieces of the care continuum, each location often operates independently from the others, each with its own protocols, documentation systems, and care planning approaches. It is not uncommon to see patients move from one care level to another accompanied by a brief summary or even their entire chart, only to have the next team essentially start over with an assessment, goal setting, and a new care plan. What is lost is that the patient's goals did not change, just the persons treating the patient. This problem is an example of our old discipline- or profession-driven model that has an inherent lack of trust in our colleagues.

The comprehensive integrated care continuum is one that has a fully integrated service system and manages patients and their resources through all aspects of their care. Figure 7-1 demonstrates a single dimension of the types of services offered in various care settings.

The coordination of care and costs by knowledgeable staff and the appropriate use of the continuum are critical steps. The movement of the patient to the next care level while maintaining continuity can be hard to accomplish even in the most experienced hands. A continuum of care is a process not a place. Many settings have the pieces but lack an effective process to achieve the best possible outcomes, whereas others feel they cannot implement a continuum process because they do not have all the "locations." The leadership and clinical expertise necessary can usually be found to successfully guide patients through the appropriate levels of care to meet their needs.

The chart in Figure 7-2 shows a simplified diagram of specific activities and settings across the care continuum. Not every patient needs every service in every setting. Case management will match the need with the setting and will facilitate patient movement to the most appropriate level.

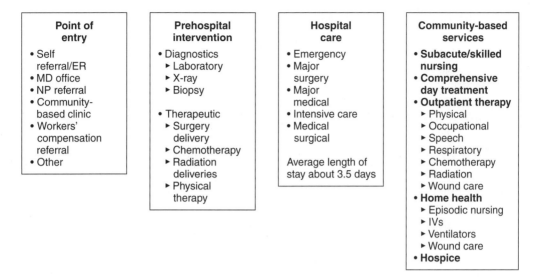

Figure 7-1   Silos of patient care service—the pieces, not the process.

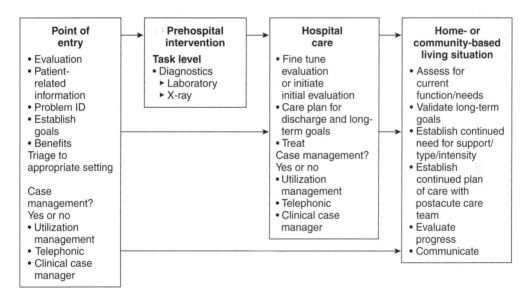

──▶ *Arrows represent case management process*

Figure 7-2   Dynamic use of care continuum.

THE FUTURE OF CASE MANAGEMENT

Many of our current processes of cost and case management have been developed over many years. What were once established as discipline- and site-specific case management programs, such as "Hospital Case Management," "Beyond The Walls," "Nursing Case Management," and "Critical Pathways," are now maturing into continuum-based approaches that can respond to the changing patient and marketplace needs. Caution must be taken, however, not to follow the most popular or trendy programs.

The next greatest challenge is the prudent use of technology, especially Internet-based health programs. Consumers have become inundated with technology and Web-based health assessments and education. The Internet, which seemed to be the answer to everything, has for some consumers become a nightmare of information that they do not know how to use, whereas for others, it is exciting and empowering. For most, technology also has introduced a new level of confusion.

Dr. David Laurence, CEO of Kaiser Permanente, noted in a speech broadcast over C-SPAN in July 1999 that HMOs and healthcare reform had demonstrated cost savings related to the use of well-integrated systems of care. He went on to say that although access to health information has proliferated, the lack of a relationship with a healthcare professional has not allowed the individual consumer of services to appropriately interpret the information. He indicated this was a significant reason for the failure of new reforms to save the projected healthcare funds, and that Kaiser would be raising their premiums by 8% to 9% that year (Laurence, 1999).

"A recent study conducted [by] Harris Interactive and AriA Marketing's research group shows that U.S. consumers want to manage their own healthcare through a combination of online, phone [sic] and nurse triage services." The research group went on to say, "We found that healthcare consumers see the Internet as a tool they can use, along with other tools and services, to communicate with caregivers and to manage their healthcare. Doctors, on the other hand, want to make sure the Internet doesn't add to their already crowded schedules or interfere with the doctor-patient relationship." The study also stated that consumers want personalized, face-to-face, or direct communication with their physicians (AHA News Now, 2000).

SUMMARY

The continued opportunities for case management and advanced practice nursing are enormous. Some people will choose not to change because they cannot adapt, whereas others will shift to more appropriate roles within the continuum of care.

Healthcare professionals should learn from the trends in business that include team approaches, staff development, and a return to increased humanism in the work environment. If we listen to what consumers want and respond with economically sound and clinically creative approaches, relevant case management will be key to the future success of healthcare delivery. The healthcare executive of the future must consider new, expanded types of leadership and create environments of exploration, thinking, and creative solutions. Our broad-based education and experience with assessment and management of people in health crises, coupled with the newfound knowledge and applications of financial principles, establish case managers as primary facilitators of health and wellness and as major contributors to solving the ongoing healthcare crisis.

REFERENCES

AHA News Now: The daily report for healthcare executives, Oct 17, 2000, Available online: www.ahanews.com.

Cowley G, Turque B: HMO hell: critical condition, *Newsweek*, pp 58-72, Nov 8, 1999.

Galewitz P: HMO gives doctors the final say, *The Press Telegram* (Associated Press), p A11, November 9, 1999.

Hamer RL: *The InterStudy competitive edge part III: regional market analysis 9.1*, St Paul, 1999, InterStudy Publications.

International Classification of Impairments, Disabilities, and Handicaps: *A manual of classifications relating to the consequence of disease*, Albany, NY, 1980, WHO Publications.

Laurence D: C-SPAN broadcast on healthcare, Aug, 1999. *Mod Healthc* (entire issue) 29(29):1-40, 1999.

P · A · R · T

III

Nursing Perspectives

8

The Impact of Managed Care on the Staff Nurse

Elizabeth A. Bonetti

KEY LESSONS IN THIS CHAPTER

- One of the most significant issues currently facing staff nurses is the need to cope with constant change.
- Staff nurses must provide complex patient care services in shorter amounts of time. Therefore effort should be placed on rapid assessment, education, and emotional support to patients and their families.
- Streamlined documentation systems will help staff nurses optimize valuable patient care time.
- Customer service is a vital component of the value-added services that staff nurses bring to patient care.
- Staff nurses will need to remain flexible as healthcare continues to evolve.

Today's healthcare organizations are operating in a world of accelerated change. Many dramatic changes in the delivery and practice of healthcare have contributed to the new realities and complexities of the current healthcare system. The social, political, economic, and global healthcare environments are now more fast paced, dynamic, information driven, and resource limited. This rapid change has resulted in greater challenges for both healthcare providers and the organizations delivering patient care. The managed care environment continues to drive healthcare practices toward a more cost-effective delivery system with emphasis on quality of care. This change also requires healthcare organizations to demonstrate greater capacity for being proactive and responsive to their respective environments. For nursing, this new arena makes past responses less effective as it changes the tasks at all levels and

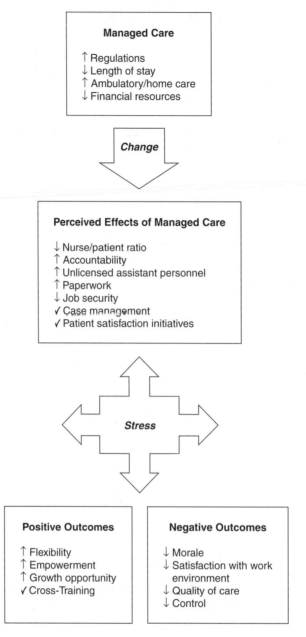

Figure 8-1   Nurses' perceptions of the influence of managed care.

encourages the search for better ways to ensure innovative problem solving. Change itself is not viewed as something exceptional but has now become the norm.

How will the nurses of today and the nurses of the next generation survive these continuing innovations in care delivery and reimbursement? The key to their future survival will be the ability to react and respond to change. Change is not one destination or one process but a series of destinations that generate new processes. Comfort with the status quo interferes with our ability to embrace change. Whether it is redesigning care to improve efficiency and customer satisfaction, adjusting schedules to meet unit needs, or implementing a new documentation system, nurses, like many other groups, often attempt to hang onto and mourn the past. Change can be a positive force by promoting creativity, diversity, learning, and growing for all persons involved. Conversely, change for the sake of change can be an upsetting and threatening force within an organization that could disrupt its functioning. Even positive change often has negative effects that must be anticipated and addressed if new strategies are to be successful.

Change is an exciting mix of opportunity and risk. Nursing professionals need to increase the opportunity and minimize the risk and unintended consequences for the bedside providers and the patients they care for. The primary goal of providing optimal patient care at the bedside remains the same, and nurses continue to advocate for patients. Although these goals have not changed for nurses, the environments in which they practice have changed. It is difficult for staff nurses to recognize that in a managed care environment, the cost of patient care becomes a driving force in all organizational strategies (Gilbert Mayer and Rushton, 1998). Nurses must be active participants in developing strategies that promote efficient, cost-effective care while maximizing the quality of care delivery and outcomes.

If bedside nursing care is fundamental to the organization, then staff nurses must be involved and become the leaders in the change processes that affect patient care delivery. The nursing profession has consistently advocated for change to improve the quality of patient care and has accepted the challenge again. Nurses are the champions for collaborative practice and care planning with the interdisciplinary team.

Figure 8-1 outlines the perceptions of staff nurses as they relate to the impact of managed care on the work environment and staff nurse responsibilities. This chapter describes the strategies used and challenges encountered by the staff nurse in the acute setting as organizations strive for excellence in a fluctuating healthcare environment.

THE CHANGING WORK ENVIRONMENT

Increasing managed care penetration with an emphasis on care delivery at all levels across the continuum, reductions in acute care beds, and strategies redesigning the delivery of nursing care have resulted in greater opportunities for nurses to work outside the hospital setting. Today nurses find themselves employed in a variety of settings, from home care to critical care. The shift in healthcare delivery to the ambulatory setting finds many medical-surgical nurses increasingly focused on acquiring new skills and knowledge that enable them to function effectively in these emerging delivery systems.

According to the American Hospital Association's profile on hospital statistics, the nurse workforce through 1994 showed strong employment, low unemployment rates, a steady decline in part-time employment, and increasing opportunities in nonhospital settings (Buerhaus and Staiger, 1996).

Starting in the early 1990s, however, employment trends among nurses began to significantly change and were most pronounced in states with high managed care penetration. For the first time in decades, the percentage of nurses employed in hospitals declined as growth in hospital employment moderated and growth in nonhospital employment increased. The decrease in growth of acute care nursing positions is reflective of a decrease in acute care beds, redesign initiatives, and the emphasis to provide care along the healthcare continuum. Many nurses have taken the opportunity to broaden their skills in the ambulatory and subacute settings (Buerhaus and Staiger, 1996).

Case manager and nurse practitioner positions also have proliferated during the 1990s. Nurse case managers are used in every care setting and are considered a valuable resource to ensure quality while maintaining costs. Nurse practitioners, as independent care practitioners, are a valuable, cost-effective alternative to physicians in providing preventive and uncomplicated patient care. These two nursing roles, although very different, have seen tremendous growth in the past 10 years

Redesigned Care Delivery

A multitude of work redesign and reengineering projects have been implemented in acute care settings. Nursing roles in the workplace have been restructured to free nurses from nonessential tasks and to increase their efficiency in delivery of patient care services. The majority of these projects have focused on the role of the staff nurse and the introduction of a variety of assistant unlicensed personnel.

The patient-centered care model (Redman, 1998) is probably the most popular redesign care delivery model, in which the role of the staff nurse is broadened to coordinate a team of multifunctional unit-based care providers. Although there are several variations on patient-centered care models, they typically include the development of new multiskilled unit-based roles and services, including the decentralization of a variety of unit support and patient care services. Services and roles are designed from the perspective of patient needs and workflow. Unit-based patient care services usually include admission and discharge activities and a variety of diagnostic and treatment services, such as selected laboratory services, pharmacy services, and respiratory therapy. Unit-based support services include environmental services, distribution of food trays, medical record administration, and patient and specimen transport.

The overall goals of patient-centered care are to increase the efficiency of care delivery, increase the quality of service, and decrease operational costs. These goals are accomplished through streamlining and simplifying processes, moving patient services closer to the patient, reducing the total number of different caregivers at the bedside by cross-training professional and unlicensed staff, increasing the functional responsibilities of unit-based personnel, decreasing service time, and reducing wait times.

In the patient-centered model, the unit staff consists of a nurse manager, staff nurses, patient care associates or technicians, unit support assistants, and administrative support associates or unit secretaries. Box 8-1 briefly describes the roles of the patient-centered unit-based staff.

Professional nurses have been unwilling to delegate tasks to others or to hold them accountable for acceptable performance. Implementation of patient-centered care models has not changed this performance; professionals are still having difficulty assigning tasks that do not require a professional nurse's direct attention and are holding personnel accountable. Although many staff nurses embrace the concepts of patient-centered care, they are unwilling to manage the personnel and the care. The staff nurse usually prefers to do it all while continuing to complain about being overworked, too busy, and very stressed. For the patient-centered care model to be successful, the staff nurse must effectively delegate and evaluate patient care outcomes for care provided by assistant personnel. Box 8-2 reviews the essentials of effective delegation as outlined by the American Nurses Association (ANA).

In addition to the patient-centered care model, improvements in system processes have also impacted bedside care delivery. Intravenous medication add-a-mixture, for example,

---

BOX 8-1
Patient-Centered Care Model: Unit-Based Roles

Nurse Manager
An RN responsible for the 24-hour management of all levels of unit staff and accountable for coordinating the development, implementation, and evaluation of quality patient care.

Staff Nurse or Patient Care Coordinator
An RN who assesses, plans, coordinates, and evaluates the care for a group of patients, with the direct nursing care delivered by the RN and a team of assistant unlicensed personnel. The RN is responsible for delegating tasks, administering medications, educating patients, and collaborating with the interdisciplinary team to evaluate outcomes.

Patient Care Associates or Technicians
Assistant nursing staff who perform delegated patient care tasks under the direct supervision of the RN, collect data for patient assessment, assist with patient hygiene needs, and carry out select nursing and respiratory treatments and phlebotomies.

Unit Support Associates
Assistant personnel who provide environmental services (e.g., cleaning and setting up patient care rooms, routine cleaning on the unit, trash removal), maintain unit supply levels, deliver and remove food trays, transport patients, and answer patient call lights.

Administrative Support Associates or Unit Secretaries
Assistant clerical personnel who provide administrative support for the unit, including general office duties, management of patient care records, transcription of physician orders, and coordination of administrative aspects of patient admission and discharge.

From Redman R, Jones, K: *J Nurs Adm* 28(11):46-53, 1998.

BOX 8-2
Essentials of Effective Delegation

The following will assist with the essential responsibilities and techniques of delegating care tasks to unlicensed assistant personnel:

- Know the state and institutional policies on delegation (the policy and procedure manual is available on each unit; for state policies, contact the state nurses association).
- Know the training and background of the unlicensed personnel.
- Clearly differentiate between nursing process and tasks. (Nursing process never can be delegated to unlicensed personnel.)
- Assess the tasks that can be safely delegated. Know the patient's needs and what he or she is at risk for.
- Know and communicate what clinical cues the unlicensed personnel should be on the alert for and why.
- Have the unlicensed personnel repeat the directions to ensure they understand.
- Make frequent walking rounds to assess the patients.
- When talking with the patient, caregiver, or unlicensed personnel, listen for cues that indicate changes in the patient's condition.
- Take frequent reports from the unlicensed personnel.
- Evaluate the unlicensed personnel's performance and the patient's response.

From Boucher MA: *Am J Nurs* 98(2):26-33, 1998.

has decreased medication administration time. The staff nurse relieved of nonnursing functions has increased time for higher level nursing activities, such as collaboration with the interdisciplinary team and patient education.

Case Management

Nursing case management in the acute care setting is a model of healthcare delivery that focuses on the coordination, integration, collaboration, and direct delivery of quality patient services and places internal controls on the resources used for care. Early assessment and intervention, comprehensive care planning, and continuum service system referrals are the emphasis in a case management model. Case management, usually an organizational care delivery model, transcends all care settings across the healthcare continuum, attempting to balance the quality components and cost of nursing service and patient care outcomes. When case management entered the hospital setting in the 1980s, nurses were recognized as the healthcare team members best prepared to manage length of stay and resource utilization.

Case management represents planned change within an institution. Case management cannot be successful without the cooperation and support of senior administration and every department and discipline within the organization. The staff nurses and case managers collaborate with the physician and interdisciplinary team to facilitate and coordinate the patient's care during the hospital stay. The staff nurses are the direct care providers, and the case manager focuses on the transition of the patient from one care setting to the next to ensure a seamless provision of care along the continuum. Both positions have their own set of complex responsibilities requiring specialized knowledge and skills. Figure 8-2 portrays the unique and overlapping role responsibilities of the physician, staff nurse, and case manager.

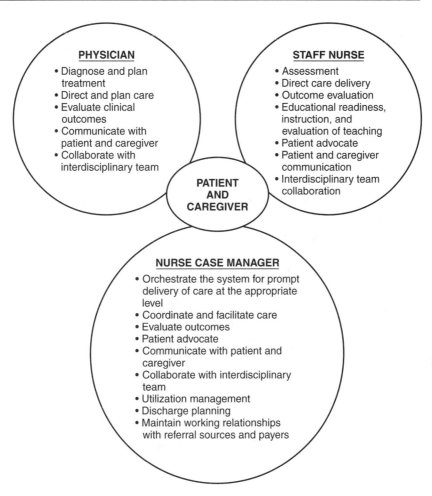

PHYSICIAN
- Diagnose and plan treatment
- Direct and plan care
- Evaluate clinical outcomes
- Communicate with patient and caregiver
- Collaborate with interdisciplinary team

STAFF NURSE
- Assessment
- Direct care delivery
- Outcome evaluation
- Educational readiness, instruction, and evaluation of teaching
- Patient advocate
- Patient and caregiver communication
- Interdisciplinary team collaboration

PATIENT AND CAREGIVER

NURSE CASE MANAGER
- Orchestrate the system for prompt delivery of care at the appropriate level
- Coordinate and facilitate care
- Evaluate outcomes
- Patient advocate
- Communicate with patient and caregiver
- Collaborate with interdisciplinary team
- Utilization management
- Discharge planning
- Maintain working relationships with referral sources and payers

Figure 8-2   Collaborative practice roles and responsibilities.

In the current healthcare environment, staff nurses must focus their efforts on assessment, teaching, and providing physical, emotional, and spiritual care to patients during a shortened hospitalization as compared with premanaged care, when patients were hospitalized for longer periods of time. Staff nurses focus their efforts on helping patients return to an optimal level of health that allows them to return to the community more quickly. Providing efficient services during hospitalization to promote a return to health are continuously in the forefront of care interventions. Nurses formulate plans that help patients help themselves and facilitate a seamless transition from the hospital to the home or to a rehabilitation or skilled nursing facility.

Staff nurses are involved in the interdisciplinary team approach to patient care. Nurses may make suggestions to improve patient outcomes and manage costs. Caring for the patient

24 hours a day, the nurse is the chief collaborator of patient care with the interdisciplinary team who facilitates patient interventions to meet the patients' needs in a timely manner. The staff nurse works collaboratively with the case manager to meet the individual care needs of each patient and his or her family.

Case management goals typically address improving organizational efficiency, increasing patient, provider, and staff satisfaction, and decreasing length of stay and cost per case. Unit-based case management is among the most common case management designs currently used in hospitals. The case manager accomplishes these goals by performing a number of complex role functions. These may include, but are not limited to, care coordination, facilitation, education, advocacy, discharge planning, utilization management, and outcome management. The nurse case manager operationalizes the role by primarily addressing coordination and facilitation of patient care, utilization management, and discharge planning.

Coordination and facilitation of patient care controls costs and length of stay while ensuring quality. Acting as a facilitator, the case manager expedites diagnostic testing, procedures, treatments, and consultations by ensuring that they are ordered and occur in a timely manner and in the proper sequence. To minimize redundancy and ensure timely services, the case manager collaborates with the interdisciplinary team on a daily basis. The case manager, through the assessment and evaluation of clinical outcomes, identifies the care setting along the continuum that is most appropriate for the patient's needs.

As utilization manager, the case manager advocates for patients with physicians, the interdisciplinary team, institutions, and payers to attain the indicated services in the appropriate setting. Outcome-based clinical pathways help the case manager advocate for quality care on behalf of the patients.

Discharge planning involves assessment, planning, and implementation with the patient, physician, and interdisciplinary team to meet the healthcare needs after the acute phase of illness. The case manager, with the interdisciplinary team, ensures that the plan is safe, appropriate, and comprehensive to address the clinical needs and identified outcomes for the patient.

Cross-Training

With escalating costs and concerns from both providers and consumers about containing costs while maintaining quality, it is important to look at the larger picture when making decisions affecting staffing at the unit level. Nursing department budgets account for approximately 50% of a hospital's operating expenses (Corey-Lisle, 1999). Thus initiatives to reduce operating expenses have direct and indirect effects on the staff nurse. Each professional nurse has an effect on the organization and its ability to provide quality care. Many initiatives have included cross-training as a means to meet staffing demands by offering education to broaden the knowledge and skills of incumbent staff.

Shortened hospital stays, fluctuations in the patient census, and unit closings create staffing dilemmas in a financially constrained environment. Staff nurses express concern about the potential to jeopardize quality patient care by having a less-specialized nurse care for the patients. Census fluctuations have sometimes resulted in nurses being asked to reduce their shifts by taking time off. Reducing shifts is acceptable as a short-term solution, but as a long-term strategy, the nurse is dissatisfied, and the organization continues to finance temporary or per diem staffing needs in high census areas.

Many maternal-child and critical care/step-down areas use cross-training of staff nurses as a strategy to gain more staffing flexibility. *Cross-training* refers to the process of educating and preparing staff nurses to work in more than one clinical area. This process offers nurses an opportunity to broaden their knowledge and skills, increases opportunities for internal re-assignment, and ultimately increases staff satisfaction. Leaving the safety of a familiar environment and venturing into possibly unfriendly clinical areas can cause resistance, but through proper preparation and education, this effect should be greatly reduced.

The keys to successful programs include a well-structured program, staff involvement in the process, a structured competency component, a clinical preceptor element, and constant ongoing assignment between the new and familiar units. Involving staff in the planning stages empowers those who are feeling powerless as a result of the redesign. Include creative, proactive, respected staff and naysayers in an attempt to create buy-in at the staff level. Clinical competencies for completion at the end of a designated orientation time frame must be identified before implementation. The resulting consequences and options for those unable to attain competence also should be prospectively defined.

The use of *preceptors,* or staff nurses with strong clinical expertise who provide one-on-one instruction and role modeling, can be an effective clinical orientation technique. Encouraging the learner to choose a preceptor or matching the preceptor and learner by personality can improve learning outcomes and satisfaction with the orientation program. Initial implementation with volunteer learners provides an enthusiastic start and develops staff champions to promote peer support. A preceptor program also fosters collegiality within the nursing staff. High peer support and peer cohesion is consistently and significantly related to the level of staff morale and stress associated with the intended change.

Many cross-training initiatives have proven unsuccessful because the recently trained staff is used only in the new clinical area when census and staffing dictate. Successful programs advocate consistent, ongoing rotation of staff to maintain skills and foster collegial relationships among the staff.

Empowerment

The power and importance of the staff nurse role is without question. The nursing process may serve as the basis for the nursing care provided, yet the most powerful intervention exists in the form of vigilance and advocacy for those patients in the nurse's care. Nurses fundamentally know that the unique needs of the patient must be met to obtain optimal outcomes. Administrators whose day-to-day work removes them from the care delivery setting need to hear and be aware of the impact of their decisions on patient care, since the patient is the organization's foremost customer. If nursing care is fundamental to the existence of an organization, then staff nurses must become empowered and accepted leaders in the change process.

Nurses who feel empowered expedite care at the unit level, contributing to high-quality patient care. The freedom to make patient care decisions and to control professional practice is critical to empowerment. Recognizing nurses' strengths and skills enables them to contribute to the organizational goals rather than obstruct the path to change.

Nursing administration must encourage the empowerment of nursing staff and bedside leadership. Nurse managers may be unable to address individualized patient care needs on the units due to increased administrative responsibilities. The nurse manager is paramount in establishing an environment that guides and enables the staff to make decisions that will improve outcomes. The unique environment and demands of today's patients and caregivers, as well as the talents and skills of the staff nurses, must be considered in fostering a learning and innovative environment at the patient-care level.

The previous examples illustrate some of the factors that nurses and nursing administrators must deal with in constantly changing care delivery systems. Change as a process is here to stay and is the only element of healthcare delivery that we can count on as we move forward. Promoting empowerment and bedside leadership is a must. Staff nurses are eager to address the challenge of becoming leaders in flexible learning environments. They also are eager to address the issues that drive inefficiency and result in decreased quality in care delivery and poor patient outcomes. Involving staff in process improvement initiatives assures champions among peers, which results in improved buy-in among the staff. Leadership fostered at the unit level, promoting optimal nursing contributions for the years ahead with improved staff and provider and patient satisfaction, guarantees creation of a healthcare system driven by the needs of the patients.

THE STAFF NURSE'S ROLE AND RESPONSIBILITIES

Nurses are privileged to care for others during a most vulnerable time in their lives. Whether holding a newborn, bringing happiness to a lonely, abused child, counseling a troubled teenager, lessening the pain of a surgical patient, seeing the loneliness of the elderly, or holding the hand of a dying patient, nurses *care* for their patients daily. Current hospitalized patients are more acutely ill, have more complex needs, and are in the hospital for a shorter period of time.

More than any other healthcare professional, nurses are directly responsible for patient care. Nurses have repeatedly succeeded in developing caring skills to complement the technological and assessment competencies at the heart of current nursing practice. Compassion, skill, creativity, and critical decision making are the ingredients nurses contribute to the quality and quantity of life for both the patient and caregiver (Miller, 1995). The patient's perception of nurses' caring is directly related to satisfaction with his or her healthcare delivery.

In addition to caring, nurses of the next millennium must exercise their intellectual skills to provide the best care possible. Nurses must continue to promote the patient's best interests and maintain their ethical obligation to ensure that patients receive the appropriate care. The role of staff nurse and case manager as patient advocate can be in direct conflict with the hospital's business mandate at times, and these issues need to be addressed to the satisfaction of all parties. Collaborating with the interdisciplinary team and nurses who constantly think, care, and advocate for their patients will provide the best care possible.

Documentation

Collaboration, coordination, and facilitation of services between disciplines are the keys to delivering a seamless continuum of patient care. Many institutions have identified the need to develop a cost-effective documentation system that reduces the amount of time the interdisciplinary team spends documenting and at the same time meets all regulatory agency requirements. The medical record previously had been very departmentalized, showing little collaboration of the interdisciplinary team. Clinical pathways and documentation by exception based on defined standards of care, clinical outcomes, and predetermined criteria for assessments and interventions have proved effective in streamlining documentation and increasing collaboration. Most hospitals that have adopted a patient-centered care model have incorporated both clinical pathways and documentation by exception. The benefits of streamlining documentation include increased accuracy; less redundancy; standardization of assessments, interventions, and evaluations; increased interaction time with the patient; and resulting cost reductions. Charting by exception is a methodology that advocates charting normal key events, assessments, and expected outcomes in a check-off fashion. Abnormal occurrences or findings are written as an exception note on the multidisciplinary progress note. If the expected outcomes are met, no further documentation is required (Mosher, 1996).

Patient Satisfaction

Superb customer service evolved as a powerful force in the 1990s, with the focus of organizations and managed care companies on exemplary customer service. Organizations realize that unmet customer expectations and inappropriate staff behaviors are bad for business and inevitably drive customers away. Most organizations use educational seminars addressing customer service and the "soft skills" necessary to improve interpersonal communication. Customer service has become a vital component of organizational strategies and involves behavioral responses, as well as the quality of services offered. Customers want to be involved in their own healthcare, to understand their diagnoses, and to be part of the decision-making process.

Customer service is a professional way of life. The nurse interacts with many "customers" on a daily basis, including patients, caregivers, physicians, ancillary nursing staff, peers, and different department staffs. The nurse must be constantly mindful that apathy, coldness, robot-like behavior, the run-around, and negativism are unacceptable behaviors. Customer service is an intellectual understanding of patient needs, listening to problems, and involving patients and caregivers as partners in their care and decision making. Customer service weighs heavily on behaviors and "soft skills" in addition to the technical competency of the nursing staff. The quality of interpersonal interactions with staff underlies the patient's evaluation of the overall quality of care. The most competent staff will rate poorly on patient satisfaction if the complementary behaviors are not evident to the customer. Everyone needs to be treated with respect, honesty, and fairness, including one's colleagues.

Superb customer satisfaction is a component of accountable practice. Intentional interpersonal skills both stimulate and reward the nurse while upholding the organization's values and mission. The confidence that comes from knowing that the nurse is meeting the customers' needs should reinforce, reward, and stimulate nursing judgment.

Patient Education

Managed care touts patient and caregiver education as a valuable process that promotes and maintains quality care while reducing costs. Patient education is one aspect of nursing care that has gained a broader scope and increased importance within the healthcare system. The staff nurse, in all settings, is the dominant healthcare team member involved in patient and caregiver education.

A patient and caregiver educational readiness assessment is done on entry into care, and educational instruction and evaluation is based on this assessment. The assessment may be done in the preoperative testing area for elective surgical admissions and in the emergency department or on the nursing unit for medical admissions. Ideally, for obstetrical cases, the assessment should be done during prenatal care in the ambulatory setting and should be available for the inpatient delivery admission, where only a brief reassessment would be indicated. Ongoing reassessment is indicated over time as the condition and educational needs of the patient and/or the caregiver change or fluctuate.

Nurses have been consistently responsible for including the patient in the planning and implementation of care. The staff nurse instructs patients and caregivers about the plan of care during hospitalization and upon discharge, medications, procedures and tests, self-care, activity limitations, and preventive care measures as indicated.

A patient pathway (Figure 8-3) is a patient education tool patterned after a clinical pathway, or a multidisciplinary action plan (MAP). Patient pathways have been developed by many institutions to outline the plan of care for the hospitalization for the patient. A patient pathway gives patients an idea of what to expect during their hospital stay and answers frequently asked questions. These tools are adjuncts to the verbal exchange between the patient and nurse and can reinforce the verbal exchange when used effectively. Patient pathways do not replace but rather supplement other educational materials discussing medications or discharge instructions. Patient pathways involve the patient and caregiver in the decision-making process and patient care. This involvement fosters empowerment of the patient and caregiver. Educated, empowered patients are more actively involved with all members of the interdisciplinary team, which is important in achieving length of stay goals without sacrificing quality. The benefits of having patients who know what to expect and what is expected of them saves the staff nurse time (Parker, 1999).

Due to shortened hospital stays, education must be across the continuum, with ambulatory setting nurses and acute care nurses working together to help the patient achieve identified outcomes. Surgical patients should be educated about their surgery and postoperative and follow-up care during the preoperative testing session. Staff nurses should actively refer patients to educational resources in the community for preventive and supportive care to continue the healthcare continuum and prevent acute care readmission. This form of patient education can serve an important purpose in helping patients work within the constraints of a managed care environment.

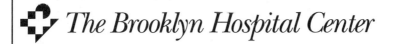

PATIENT INFORMATION
COMMUNITY-ACQUIRED PNEUMONIA

Dear Patient and Family,

    WELCOME to The Brooklyn Hospital Center and thank you for choosing our doctors and hospital for your healthcare needs. This information sheet has been developed to describe the care you will receive during your hospital stay. Created by doctors, nurses, and the healthcare team, it is an outline of important events that are necessary for your recovery.

    Especially planned for patients who have pneumonia, an infection in your lungs, this plan encourages your taking part in your care and involves you in your discharge planning. *Considering your individual needs, your treatment may change.*

    The healthcare team feels that once you have achieved the following, you are probably ready for discharge home:

    ✓ No difficulty breathing.
    ✓ A normal temperature.
    ✓ The infection in your lungs is improving.
    ✓ Tolerating your normal activity level.
    ✓ An understanding of your medications, when to call the doctor, and your follow-up healthcare plan.

Your follow-up care will be arranged before you are discharged home.
If you have any questions about this plan or your progress, please speak to your doctor or nurse.

The Brooklyn Hospital Center
4/99

Figure 8-3 Example of a patient pathway. (From The Brooklyn Hospital Center, Brooklyn, New York, April 1999.)

Continued on p. 134

THE HEALTHCARE TEAM IS HERE TO HELP YOU RECOVER!
WE WANT YOU TO BE AN ACTIVE MEMBER OF THE TEAM CARING FOR YOU.

THE HEALTHCARE TEAM	• A team of doctors, nurses, respiratory therapists, and other nursing staff will work to provide you with the best care possible and plan for your discharge home. A social worker, dietitian, and other staff are available as needed.
TESTS	• You will have a chest x-ray, if not done before admission, to show the doctor the infection in your lungs. • Blood will be taken from a vein in your arm to check the blood levels to tell the doctors how your body is fighting the infection in your lungs. • Some of your mucus from a deep cough will be checked to determine the cause of the infection in your lungs. • Other tests may be ordered during your stay or after discharge home.
TREATMENTS AND EVALUATIONS	• The nursing staff will check your blood pressure, temperature, heart rate, respirations, and general condition. • An intravenous line (IV) will be placed into a vein in your arm to give you medications to fight the infection (antibiotics) and fluids. • Coughing, deep breathing exercises, and using an incentive spirometer will help remove the mucus from your lungs. The staff will teach you these exercises, and you should do them every hour while awake.
MEDICATIONS	• You will receive medications through the IV to help fight the infection causing the pneumonia. • After 2 to 3 days the medications (antibiotics) will probably be switched to pills, which you will continue to take after discharge.
DIET	• You should be able to eat and drink. Your doctor will most likely prescribe the same type of diet that you eat at home. • Drinking extra fluids will sometimes assist in liquefying the mucus in your lungs.
ACTIVITY	• The head of your bed will be raised slightly to help you breathe more easily. • You will probably be out of bed with help within the first day or two. • The nursing staff will help with bathing or other activities, as you need them.
TEACHING	• The staff will explain all tests, procedures, and treatments. • The staff will also teach you about your medications, breathing exercises, when to call the doctor, and follow-up care. • Please ask the healthcare team any questions or discuss any of your concerns.
GOING HOME	• Your doctor and the healthcare team will plan your care to prepare for your discharge home. The staff will talk to you and your family about your home situation for special needs and support after discharge. • Many patients' health has improved, and they are ready for discharge after a 3-night stay in the hospital. • Discharge time is usually 11: 00 AM. Please arrange for someone to take you home. • It is very important that you complete all the antibiotic medication that is ordered for you to take at home. • Follow-up visits with your doctor will be arranged.

Your care may change to meet your unique needs.

Figure 8-3, cont'd   For legend see p. 133

BOX 8-3
DOs

Do read the literature and stay current on issues affecting healthcare delivery.
Do share your good ideas for process improvement with your supervisor.
Do stay patient-focused.
Do remain comfortable with change.
Do attend continuing education programs whenever you can.

BOX 8-4
DON'Ts

Don't become complacent; remain energized.
Don't expect others to always fix things for you.
Don't allow stress to affect your relationships with patients.
Don't forget why you became a nurse.
Don't ignore current changes in healthcare—stay informed.

DOs AND DON'Ts FOR STAFF NURSES

Box 8-3 provides staff nurses with some tips for working effectively in today's healthcare system. Box 8-4 provides some reminders staff nurses can use to avoid becoming negative or burning out.

LIVING WITH CHANGE: OPPORTUNITIES

Living with change should not imply insecurity but rather should represent an opportunity to develop new forms of security. In many previous nursing care models, security was based on control. It also was based on knowing the rules, knowing where everyone and everything belonged, and having categories into which to place tasks, people, or events.

In a changing, innovative healthcare environment, security stems not from domination but from flexibility. It will not come from having everything under control but from quick reaction time and being able to cut across categories to obtain the best outcomes. For innovative nurses, security will not come from staying on the same nursing unit or possibly even within the same field but from broadening their knowledge base and skills.

The nurses who will succeed and flourish in both the present and future will be those who have embraced positive change. These nurses will create a new climate to encourage the introduction of new methods and possibilities. They will encourage anticipation of and response to external pressures. They will finally encourage and listen to new ideas from both internal and external customers. Also, they will be adept at reorienting their own and others' activities in new directions to bring about higher levels of achievement that will produce innovation at the unit and organizational levels.

Staff nurses and nurses working in other care delivery settings should look for dynamic and challenging ways to collaborate on sharing information, including each other in treatment plans, and empowering the patient and family in a united front to move the patient through the continuum of care.

REFERENCES

Boucher MA: Delegation alert, *Am J Nurs* 98(2):26-33, 1998.

Buerhaus PI, Staiger DO: Managed care and the nurse workforce, *JAMA* 276(18):1487-1493, 1996.

Corey-Lisle P, Tarzian A, Cohen M, et al: Healthcare reform: its effects on nurses, *J Nurs Adm* 29(4):30-37, 1999.

Gilbert Mayer G, Rushton N: The hospital nurse's role in managed care, *Nurs Manage* 29(9):25-29, 1998.

Miller K: Keeping the care in nursing care: our biggest challenge, *J Nurs Adm* 25(11):29-32, 1995.

Mosher C, Rademacher K, Day G, et al: Documenting for patient-focused care, *Nurs Econ* 14(4):218-223, 1996.

Parker C: Patient pathways as a tool for empowering patients, *Nurs Case Manag* 4(2):77-79, 1999.

Redman R, Jones K: Effects of implementing patient-centered care models on nurse and non-nurse managers, *J Nurs Adm* 28(11):46-53, 1998.

9

Nurse Practitioners and Managed Care

Diana J. Mason and Jeffrey P. O'Donnell

KEY LESSONS IN THIS CHAPTER

- Nurse practitioners have evolved from providing healthcare to patients in limited access areas to becoming members of medical practice teams in health maintenance organizations and other managed care organizations.
- In the 1980s, state laws began to appear that entitled nurse practitioners to be reimbursed for services covered by insurance companies.
- In some managed care organizations, nurse practitioners are credentialed in the same manner as are physicians, whereas in others they are grouped under the category of "nonphysician providers."
- One of the primary, long-standing barriers to nurse practitioner practice has been physician opposition.
- Nurse practitioners as a whole must take a proactive stance and develop a multifaceted strategy to push for change as healthcare continues to evolve.

When former President Bill Clinton took office in 1993, the nursing community was expecting its efforts to support his election to pay off in ways that would open doors for nurses. His healthcare reform initiative (Health Security Act) underscored the importance of primary care, with particular emphasis on prevention. Advanced practice nurses had waited decades for this opportunity. Nurse practitioners (NPs) were known for their focus on prevention and health promotion, although many had long been providing the full range of primary care services to underserved populations. The available research suggested that NPs provided care equal to that of physicians (and sometimes better), had a high level of patient satisfaction, and were cost-effective (Office of Technology Assessment, 1986; Brown and

Grimes, 1995). Stories about NPs were appearing on the nightly news and on the front page of leading newspapers like the *New York Times.* NPs seemed to be a key element in moving the country forward on a healthcare system that was driven by costs to build a primary care infrastructure—something the country had been lacking.

The promise of a new day for NPs began to fade, however, as physicians dominated the management structures of new and growing managed care organizations (MCOs). Reports from NPs began to emerge that said MCOs were refusing to credential NPs. As managed care gained a greater share of the market in communities, patients who were previously covered by indemnity or fee-for-service plans were now looking in MCOs' directories of providers to find an acceptable primary care provider (PCP). If the NP who had been caring for them for 10 years was not listed, patients had to switch providers, unless they could afford to pay out of pocket.

NPs again found themselves fighting for every gain they needed to provide primary care to their patients. For years healthcare organizations, health policies, insurance companies, and bureaucracies had erected seemingly insurmountable barriers to NPs' ability to provide primary care. These barriers included the right to practice without direct physician supervision, prescription privileges, reimbursement, the authority to do and sign off on histories and physicals, and the right to make referrals that would be honored by visiting nurse agencies. NPs had figured out how to work around many of these barriers—sometimes in ways that were not quite legal. They had presigned prescription pads, got physicians to countersign notes after the fact, stretched the concept of *on-site supervision,* and billed under the physician's name. At the same time, they fought to make the changes needed in the laws and regulations at the state and federal level to legitimately demolish the barriers to practice.

In the midst of great gains in the legal recognition of NPs' scope of and authority for independent or collaborative practice, NPs seemed perfectly poised for managed care's move to dominate healthcare in the United States. Unfortunately, managed care erected a new set of barriers. Whereas earlier barriers arose primarily from the public sector (particularly state and federal governments), the new barriers were generated in the private sector. NPs had used their political savvy to change the public sector, but now they had to figure out how to deal with the private sector.

This chapter discusses the place of NPs in a managed care environment. After exploring the evolution of NP practice in relation to managed care, the chapter examines the extent to which NPs are included in managed care provider panels, the factors influencing this situation, and what NPs need to do to have full access to the managed care environment. The emphasis will be on primary care; however, it should be noted that managed care also opened the door for acute care NPs to arise as a more cost-effective alternative to resident physicians.

EVOLUTION OF THE NURSE PRACTITIONER IN MANAGED CARE

The role of the NP evolved from the need to provide underserved populations with primary care services, particularly health promotion and disease prevention. The role was first developed in 1965 by Loretta C. Ford, a professor of nursing at the University of Colorado–

Denver, and Henry K. Silver, a pediatrician in Denver, Colorado, with the belief that experienced nurses with advanced training could serve populations of children with limited access to care (Silver, Ford, and Stearly, 1967; Silver, Ford, and Day, 1968). The initial model for NP education consisted of a 4-month intensive theory and practical pediatric training program under the supervision of senior medical and nursing faculty. The nurses were trained to enhance their knowledge and skills in interviewing children and families, counseling parents about child-rearing practices, conducting basic physical examinations, and assessing and managing minor health problems of the well child.

The NP role emerged during a time of media attention to the unmet healthcare needs of Americans and the development of Medicare and Medicaid to reduce financial barriers to meeting these needs. As such, the role readily expanded to serve adults, the elderly, and families who had limited access to primary care services.

NPs originally functioned in settings where access to healthcare was limited, such as poor urban areas and rural locations, in both private offices and public health departments (Silver, 1968). As health maintenance organizations (HMOs) developed, NPs were perfectly suited to the team approach of the early group- and staff-model HMOs, such as Kaiser Permanente.

As the NP movement grew in size and acceptance within the nursing, medical, and healthcare communities, there was the concomitant recognition that the role had to be legitimized through laws and regulations. Initially, there was little expressed concern for nurses "practicing medicine without a license," perhaps because the role was not viewed as one that would or should ever practice without physician collaboration or supervision. By 1978, an Institute of Medicine's manpower report recommended:

Amendments to state licensing laws should authorize, through regulations, nurse practitioners and physicians [sic] assistants to provide medical services, including making medical diagnoses and prescribing drugs when appropriate. Nurse practitioners and physician assistants in general should be required to perform the range of services they provide as skillfully as physicians, but they should not provide medical services without physician supervision (Peterson, 1980, p 848).

As NPs demanded greater independence and scope of practice, nurse practice acts were rewritten, often after major battles with the physician community. Changes were needed for NPs to function legitimately in rural areas where physicians may not have been available. They were also needed in poor urban areas where there was a shortage of physicians.

NPs were also making gains with patterns of reimbursement. Initially, their services were billed under their collaborating or supervising physician's name. In the 1980s, state laws began to appear that entitled NPs to be reimbursed for services covered by an insurance company. Changes were also won in state Medicaid reimbursement rules and regulations, permitting NPs in some states to be reimbursed at 100% of the physician rate. Federal changes in reimbursement were harder to make. Nevertheless, by 1989, NPs in rural areas were reimbursed directly by Medicare for their services at 85% of the physician rate—a policy that was extended to all NPs in 1997 (Towers, 1999). Medicare also had a provision for 100% reimbursement of services provided by NPs that were "incident to" a physician's services, but the requirement of an on-site physician supervision limited the usefulness of this policy in areas where physicians were not available or where healthcare organizations were trying to control costs through efficient, unduplicated use of providers (Towers, 1999).

Of course, the reimbursement game is quite different under managed care. Theoretically, capitation payment schemes favor NPs. Capitation provides a set payment per managed care enrollee to the primary care practice or healthcare organization, thus encouraging the practice to use the most cost-efficient means possible of providing care. Although salaries of NPs improved over the past decades, they continue to be much lower than many, but not all, PCP salaries.

Although the number of HMOs grew during the 1980s, they became more popular during the 1990s, after Congress failed to pass healthcare reform legislation. Former President Clinton had made healthcare reform a major feature of his candidacy and focused on it early in his presidency. The business community was supportive of overhauling healthcare to trim costs for employee healthcare that were cutting severely into their profit margins. One of the primary features of the President's Health Security Act was managed competition, or embracing competitive free-market principles to control escalating healthcare costs (Wellstone and Shaffer, 1993). When Congress failed to pass any healthcare reform legislation, managed care and market competition became the primary approaches for addressing the escalating cost of healthcare.

One of the foremost issues of public or private reform of healthcare in the United States was building the infrastructure for primary care. Since World War II, the country had become enamored with high-tech acute care. This care was expensive and well reimbursed, but there were few rewards for primary care services. Private physicians began to flee inner city areas with a high percentage of Medicaid recipients, since the Medicaid reimbursement for a primary care visit seldom covered the costs of the service. When Clinton's Health Security Act failed to be approved, insurance companies escalated their shift to providing managed care, building primary care networks, and controlling the resources used by the credentialed PCPs. Even hospitals began to merge, consolidate services, and expand their capacity for primary care services that would serve as feeders into the now less lucrative acute care arena.

Since NPs had been providing these primary care services to underserved communities, it was anticipated that they would be welcomed into MCOs and would finally be recognized as key providers in healthcare. Many in the nursing community also believed that NPs would be eager to assume this new mantle of importance and responsibility. The medical community also saw the shift in power from acute care to primary care, however, and quickly began to retool existing physicians to practice in this arena and to shift residencies from acute care to primary care. Anecdotal reports from NPs indicated that at least some MCOs, including some large regional or national companies, refused to include NPs in their provider panels. If NPs were going to flourish, or even not lose ground, under managed care, data were needed to understand the reality of MCOs' arrangements with NPs and the factors influencing these arrangements. Studies began to appear on how MCOs treated physicians; however, few addressed NPs.

MANAGED CARE ORGANIZATIONS' ARRANGEMENTS WITH NURSE PRACTITIONERS

The extent to which NPs are included in MCO panels has received relatively little attention by researchers. As recently as 1995, researchers (Felt, Frazer, and Gold, 1994; Dial et al, 1995) reported that most HMOs did not have formal methods for estimating and reporting nonphysician providers, making it difficult to track NP utilization and credentialing. In fact, researchers indicated that NPs were not being included in MCO primary care panels and directories. When NPs were tracked, the HMOs used a nonphysician providers-to-physician ratio instead of a providers-to-members ratio, which is used for physicians. A national study of various types of HMOs confirmed that most of the HMOs did not track NPs or other nonphysician providers (Felt, Frazer, and Gold, 1994).

Where NPs are included in studies of HMO staffing ratios, they are grouped under *nonphysician providers,* a category that includes physician assistants. Weiner (1994) reported HMO staffing ratios ranging from 14.1 nonphysician providers/100,000 enrollees to a high of 26.8/100,000, with an average of 23 nonphysician providers/100,000 enrollees. This ratio contrasted with a physician-to-enrollee ratio of 119.1/100,000 enrollees. Weiner's ratios were confirmed by Dial et al (1995) in their study of 58 group- and staff-model HMOs, which found a median of 19.7 advanced practice nurses/100,000 members. Similarly, using data from 1992 and 1993, Hart et al (1997) reported ratios of 26.2 and 21.5 nonphysician providers/100,000 enrollees at two mature HMOs, noting that this expanded the overall provider ratio to 46.6/100,000 enrollees.

Even when NPs are included in an HMO's staffing ratios, they may not be included in the HMO's provider directories. In their study of group- and staff-model HMOs, Dial et al (1995) reported that slightly more than one half of NPs in these HMOs were included on provider directories. Although this finding indicates that some NPs are credentialed, the group- and staff-model HMOs are diminishing as most MCOs respond to public demand for a greater choice of providers than is usually available in these two models. In fact, in these models the NPs are usually employees of an organization that provides both financing of services and the services themselves. Felt, Frazer, and Gold (1994) studied various types of HMOs with national representation. They found that network-model HMOs did not use NPs as much as group- and staff-model HMOs did; however, this finding was complicated by the fact that not all network-model HMOs even track NPs who provide services in collaboration with a contracted physician.

The lack of available data on managed care plan arrangements with NPs led to a series of studies focusing on New York and Connecticut. These two states border each other but have different histories with managed care and have different state laws and regulations governing managed care and NP practices. For example, the full force of managed care came earlier to Connecticut than to New York. Connecticut was approved by the federal government to move Medicaid beneficiaries into managed care plans before New York. Connecticut had Medicaid managed care in place since 1995, starting with a statewide Medicaid 1915(b) waiver, which proposed that NPs and certified nurse midwives be considered as PCPs; however, MCOs were not required to list or credential them. In the face of a shortage of PCPs, the state required that MCOs demonstrate sufficient numbers of PCPs. Thus Connecticut's Medicaid managed care program included NPs and certified nurse midwives as PCPs. As of 1999, New York was still struggling to adopt Medicaid managed care statewide, even while the numbers of PCPs expanded.

In the first of the series of studies, Cohen et al (1998) conducted focus groups in which New York and Connecticut NPs reported difficulties being credentialed by MCOs. These NPs felt that they were "invisible providers" within MCOs, caring for many patients and generating considerable revenue but not being recognized for their efforts. They also noted that if they were not listed on MCO provider panels, their patients and new ones could not choose NPs as their PCPs.

At the same time, a telephone survey of executives of MCOs in New York and Connecticut was conducted (Mason et al, 1997). All MCOs listed with these states' insurance departments were contacted; 34 (53%) participated in the study. Of those participating, 15 (44%) reported some listing of NPs in provider panels, but tremendous variation existed. The number of primary care NPs listed per MCO varied from two to 200 (mean = 34; SD = 35.7; median = 15). The number of NPs in specialty care ranged from three to 200 (mean = 39, SD = 60.2, median = 11). Plans with a large number of Medicaid patients tended to credential NPs more than others; however, one of the largest MCOs in the country reported listing NPs only in areas where the MCO had no physicians as PCPs. Fourteen (41%) of the MCOs did not list NPs as either primary care or specialty providers. All of the 15 MCOs that listed NPs as PCPs also covered Medicaid patients, which represented 60% of all MCOs offering Medicaid coverage. By contrast, only four (36%) of the MCOs with risk contracts under Medicare listed NPs. Twelve (80%) MCOs listed the NPs separately as PCPs in their panel directories, whereas five (33%) listed NPs under the name of a physician or group practice, and some used both methods.

Thirteen (87%) of the MCOs that listed NPs reported that they used the same credentialing application for both physicians and NPs, yet some were unclear about their state's regulations governing NPs, such as how many a physician could collaborate with, or if a national certification was either available or required (in Connecticut) of NPs to practice in the state (Mason et al, 1997).

Whether or not the NP was a hidden provider, would the MCO monitor NP's use in credentialed physician practices? Nine (60%) of the 15 MCOs listing NPs said they did not. One Connecticut MCO reported that NPs were ". . . off the radar screen . . . and not worthy of monitoring at all" (Mason et al, 1997, p 311). On the other hand, four (21%) of the 19 MCOs that did not list NPs reported that they monitored NPs who provided care to their enrollees. In some cases, monitoring occurred as part of a physician office credentialing procedure (Mason et al, 1997).

Although MCOs routinely evaluate the outcomes and practice patterns of their credentialed physicians, would they evaluate NP practices? Twenty-two (65%) of all the MCOs evaluated NPs, although three (16%) of these did so differently than they evaluated physicians. Although there was concern about potential enrollees' impressions that the MCO was providing second rate care by using "cheaper" providers, most (82%) of the executives interviewed believed that their MCO should encourage the use of NPs, and 14 (41%) expected changes in their organizations' policies towards NPs. Of interest was the anecdotal finding that executives who were nurses were pushing their organizations to adopt models of primary care that placed the NP as a key, front-line gatekeeper. At the same time, executives who were physicians acknowledged that they or their physician colleagues on the boards of the MCOs were reluctant to see NPs practice independent of physicians (Mason et al, 1997).

How did these findings compare with the experiences of NPs? In a convenience sample of NPs attending professional meetings in New York and Connecticut, Cohen et al (1998) found that 20% of the participating NPs in New York and 48% in Connecticut reported that they were listed in at least one MCO provider directory. Because of the relatively small size of the sample that was derived using convenience sampling methods, the investigators subsequently conducted a survey of a random sample of all NPs licensed and residing in New York or Connecticut (Mason et al, 1999). With a response rate of 47%, 704 of NPs practicing in New York or Connecticut were included in the final data analysis.

Of all respondents, only 16% of New York NPs and 43% of Connecticut NPs reported to be credentialed and listed in at least one MCO provider panel; however, more than half of the NPs in this study had never applied to a MCO for credentialing and listing. While only one third had applied, this percentage was higher for Connecticut than New York (43% versus 26%; $p < 0.0001$). Combining the two states, 78% of those who applied were listed in at least one MCO, whereas 36% had been denied listing at least once. In New York, 63% of those who applied were listed in at least one MCO panel, whereas 85% of Connecticut NPs who applied were listed in at least one. These data indicate that the most important determinant of whether a NP is listed in a provider panel may be whether the NP even applies for listing. Nevertheless, the principal reason given by the respondents for why they were denied listing was that the MCO said it did not list NPs as PCPs (Mason et al, 1999).

In both this study (Mason et al, 1999) and the focus group study (Cohen et al, 1998), the majority of those studied reported being paid an annual salary that is unrelated to the number of hours worked or the number of patients seen. Only 22 of the NPs in the random survey (Mason et al, 1999) (4.2%) shared financial risks with the physicians in their practices, and 32 (6%) said they were uncertain about whether they participated in any risk sharing. Fifty percent of the respondents reported that their offices billed for their services at the same rate as the physician and under the physician's name. In the focus groups (Cohen et al, 1998), the NPs spoke of having a preference for the security of being salaried and not sharing in the risks (and potential financial rewards) of other payment arrangements that are common to physicians under managed care. This preference for security may have influenced the extent to which the NPs took advantage of the earlier gains in reimbursement policy. Less than 40% of those polled in the random survey (Mason et al, 1999) already had, or were in the process of applying for, Medicare provider identification numbers (PINs), whereas 20% saw Medicare patients without their own PINs. Less than 15% had a Medicaid PIN, whereas 37% reported seeing Medicaid patients without their own PINs.

It was expected that MCOs would require NPs to have hospital practice privileges before credentialing them, but of the 41% of the NPs who reported having hospital privileges, only 13% of these reported that they did so to meet a MCO requirement for credentialing (Mason et al, 1999).

To what extent are these findings representative of MCO arrangements with NPs across the country? As of 1999, the only other known study to examine these issues was a yet-to-be-published master's thesis that used the same questionnaire as Mason et al (1999) on a convenience sample of 96 NPs in Colorado (Scarborough, 1999). Only 27% of the NPs in this study were listed as PCPs in MCOs, and most of the others had never applied to be credentialed. Although 49% reported being the PCP for patients, 52% said the charges they generated were billed under the physician's name.

The lack of research on managed care arrangements with NPs reflects the marginalization of these providers in the current healthcare environment. Comparative multistate studies are needed to better understand the nature of the problem, the factors influencing it, and strategies that are likely to be effective for ensuring the public's access to NPs under managed care.

BARRIERS TO MANAGED CARE ORGANIZATIONS' FULL UTILIZATION OF NURSE PRACTITIONERS

Barriers to full utilization of NPs have long been rooted in public policies. Although there continues to be variation in state laws and regulations governing NPs (Pearson, 1999), managed care has erected new barriers that must be addressed in both the public and private sectors.

One of the primary, long-standing barriers to NP practice has been physician opposition, which is being enacted in new ways under managed care. As physician practice has been constrained and threatened under managed care, physician opposition to others who might replace them has escalated—and perhaps with good reason. Dial et al (1995) found that as the ratio of nonphysician providers to physicians increased, the ratio of physicians to members decreased. As recently as 1996, Anderson, Gillis, and Yoder (1996) identified lack of physician support as a major barrier to NP practice in California. Felt, Frazer, and Gold (1994) and Felt-Lisk (1996) also found the negative attitude of some plan physicians toward NP inclusion in managed care panels to be a barrier to NP practice. In the study of MCO executives in New York and Connecticut (Mason et al, 1997), two physician executives acknowledged that their physician-owned or physician-governed plans resisted including NPs in their PCP panels, even though it would benefit the plan.

On the other hand, physician support has been identified by some NPs as a factor in their applying for credentialing by MCOs (Cohen et al, 1998). Whether physician or administrator, 54% of the NPs in New York and Connecticut reported that their administrator or employer support was the primary factor influencing their applying for credentialing by MCOs (Mason et al, 1999).

State practice environments influence NP availability and MCO policies on NPs (Sekscenski et al, 1994; Mason et al, 1997). They can serve as either a barrier or a facilitator to NP inclusion in managed care plans. *State practice environment* encompasses three aspects of state policies: (1) legal scope of practice; (2) type of physician supervision, collaboration, or direction; and (3) prescription-writing authority. These policies, along with certain state insurance laws, may either explicitly or indirectly limit reimbursement and utilization of NPs (Safriet, 1992; Aiken and Salmon, 1994). Consider, for example, a legal requirement of physician supervision of NP practice. Under such a statute, a physician must usually be on-site and in some cases must periodically see the patient. The physician also might be required to countersign notes and prescriptions. This approach increases the number of persons needed to care for a patient and may restrict the NP's cost-effectiveness.

Other state and federal laws and regulations also can serve as barriers to NPs. Among the most important policies are those governing reimbursement of NPs. Before 1998, only NPs in rural areas could receive direct reimbursement under Medicare. The Balanced Budget Amendment of 1997 included other NPs and advanced practice nurses in the direct reimbursement option at 85% of the physician fee schedule. This change represents greater acceptance of and need for NPs; however, reimbursement at less than 100% of a physician's fee schedule could limit the attractiveness of NPs to group practices that want to maximize their reimbursement levels (Buerhaus, 1998; Sullivan-Marx, 1998). There is also evidence that problems exist with state implementation of the federal guidelines for Medicaid reimbursement. As of 1989, federal legislation required states to provide direct reimbursement to NPs serving the Medicaid population. In a 1992 state-by-state survey, the Physician Payment Review Commission reported that many state Medicaid programs were not covering nonphysician providers to the extent that those states' practice acts permitted (Hoffman, 1994). Although capitated managed care arrangements should facilitate the use of NPs in provider networks by providing a per capita fee to the MCO regardless of who provides the care, the continued mix of reimbursement approaches (even as determined by MCOs) makes reimbursement a continuing factor in the utilization of NPs.

The lack of both consumer and NP demand for listing were identified by MCO executives as two major factors contributing to underrepresentation of NPs on provider panels in the survey of MCOs in New York and Connecticut by Mason et al (1997). Both Felt et al (1994) and Mason et al (1997) found that MCOs were concerned that their enrollees would prefer seeing a physician. They were also concerned that "second-class care" could develop by certain groups of patients being assigned to see NPs because they are less expensive providers than physicians.

A lack of NP demand for credentialing has also been identified as a barrier. NPs who participated in the focus groups with Cohen et al (1998) reported that many of their colleagues were comfortable with being salaried employees and did not care about maximizing their opportunities under managed care. They did not want to share in either the financial risks or the bonuses that many physicians incur in group or private practices. The NP participants in the focus groups saw their colleagues' apathy as a barrier to all NPs who were fighting to be equal players in the managed care game. In addition, managed care executives noted that pressure from NP organizations was both a barrier and a facilitator to changes in policies toward credentialing and listing NPs in provider panels (Mason et al, 1997). Some of these executives clearly objected to the pressure tactics of some NP groups.

The following case study illustrates the barriers to NP practice that limit NP's opportunities under managed care. It also illustrates the power of persistent NP effort to eliminate these barriers.

Case Study: A Pediatric Primary Care Practice

Tamara* is a pediatric NP with almost two decades of advanced practice experience. In 1991 she opened her own practice, which was designed to provide the full range of pediatric primary care services to children of all ages with diverse socioeconomic status, ethnicity, and insurance coverage. She was committed to three goals: (1) practicing with a traditional NP philosophy of prevention and family- and community-oriented care; (2) providing culturally sensitive care, including bilingual services by providers and in writing; and (3) providing a site for NP students to see an independent NP practice in action.

The practice currently includes two part-time NPs in addition to Tamara. It is open 6 days a week and provides on-call coverage to over 3400 children. Tamara has hospital practice privileges in an academic medical center.

Tamara practices in a state that requires NPs to have physician collaboration for periodic review of cases and to ensure that a physician would accept the NP's referrals. She first approached physician colleagues who had hired her to practice with them or to cover their patients as needed, in one case, for over 5 years. None of these physicians would formally collaborate with her as an independent PCP.

She finally recruited a physician known to another NP in private practice to serve as her collaborating physician. This arrangement worked well until the physician's malpractice insurance company said the physician could not collaborate with a NP unless she paid $7700 per year to the insurance company or became an employee of the physician. This insurance company was a physician-owned company. Tamara filed a complaint with the state insurance department. Subsequently, the state insurance department advised the physician-owned malpractice company that it wanted collaboration with NPs to be available for all physicians without additional cost to the physician or the NP. The insurance company revised its position and issued a policy revision to allow coverage for collaboration to avoid an insurance department sanction and precedent in insurance law. This policy revision was a major victory for NPs and consumers.

Tamara also discovered that having more than one collaborating physician prevented disruption of her practice. When her collaborating physician took a job as an employee of a hospital, the hospital required that the physician be covered by the institution's malpractice insurance policy, which did not cover the physician's practice beyond the hospital. Hospitals thus were able to limit moonlighting by physicians, but it also meant that Tamara needed a new collaborating physician.

She now has three collaborating physicians, but it has not been easy to recruit them. One physician agreed on the condition that no one knew about it. It was clear to Tamara that a code within the physician community was developing to block NPs from having in-

---

*The name and identity of the NP in this case study have been changed at the NP's request.

dependent practices. It was fine for NPs to be employees of institutions or physicians but not to be on their own.

Before her affiliation with the academic medical center, Tamara had become the first NP to have practice privileges at a local community hospital. When she lost her collaborating physician, she lost her practice privileges. She then approached the academic medical center for privileges with the proactive help of the chief nurse officer, who challenged the medical center's management to state explicitly why it would not grant practice privileges to this experienced NP with excellent credentials and an outstanding track record. The chief nurse officer also got the medical center to provide a collaborating physician for Tamara. An additional factor in the medical center's support of Tamara was that it was strongly tied into the Medicaid managed care population and saw that she could bring in these and other patients. With expanded state insurance coverage for poor and near-poor children, Tamara has made sure that every patient from her practice who is admitted to the medical center is insured. She enrolls children in the state's Medicaid and child health insurance programs at her practice.

In spite of Tamara's excellent track record, as well as the record of others, the state still will not mandate that insurance companies not exclude licensed providers by type (e.g., NPs, nurse midwives, osteopaths). Tamara has been accepted into some managed care plans and has been denied by others. She has been aggressive in applying for credentialing by any and all plans in her area. Noting that it is difficult for MCOs to reject her due to her extensive experience and excellent credentials, Tamara felt strongly that she needed to be an example whom the rest of the NP community could follow. She quickly discovered that the credentialing forms used by MCOs were not suited to NP education and experience. The provider relations staff at the MCO did not know what to do with her application and would summarily reject her if she did not appeal to higher authorities. Once she was accepted into the provider panel, she found the same to be true of billing staff and secretaries in various departments. She was an anomaly who they did not know how to regard, so they often denied her consideration for credentialing or payment until she went over their heads to the highest level of management she could access. She often did so with the comment, "I'm sure you don't want your organizations being thought of as being inaccessible to providers who serve the community."

A stunningly thoughtful strategy Tamara has used with MCOs is to demand that they monitor the outcomes of her practice. She asks that they engage in quality monitoring and share the outcome data with her. She forthrightly tells them, "My goal is to force you to see that NP practice works." This statement shows confidence in her own practice and challenges the organization to begin to examine NP outcomes, which will help her colleagues as well. The first plan rose to her challenge and found that in 2 years she had only one nonsurgical hospital admission among a large caseload of children, many of whom had complex physical, psychological, and social health problems.

Other managed care plans have denied her applications for credentialing on the basis that their primary care provider panels are full, which she feels is a euphemism for "we won't list any NPs." In fact, these plans do not list any NPs as PCPs. She also has found that it is particularly difficult to get MCO consideration when the organization is in the midst of a merger.

An emerging concern is the state government's contracts for state and federally-funded insurance programs (e.g., Medicaid, Child Health Plus) with for-profit plans that exclude NPs, even though the state regulations included NPs in their definition of PCPs. The majority of these plans are owned or controlled by physicians.

Tamara realized early on that activism had to be a part of her practice if she and other NPs were going to survive. When MCOs deny her applications, she appeals to executives within the organization who can set policy. When an insurer denies her payment of a claim, she involves her attorney, who writes letters to the organization and explores other avenues to remove the barriers to her practice and that of other NPs. She lobbies not just legislators who can write better laws but the executive branch officials who are responsible for the regulations that interpret, or misinterpret, these laws. In the case of Medicaid, the federal Healthcare Financing Administration (HCFA) had required that states ensure access to NPs and certified nurse midwives several years ago. One Medicaid MCO decided to show inclusion of NPs by placing an asterisk by the physician's name and a footnote stating that the physician's practice includes NPs. When the state's Department of Health approved this method of meeting the HCFA requirement, Tamara was outraged and appealed to the responsible state administrator, as well as HCFA. The appeal is pending.

In spite of the struggles to remove barriers to her practice, Tamara believes that NPs should not be afraid of managed care.

Being a NP in this arena works. You can give good care. You can do fine financially under capitated plans. They really support NP practice—that unique relationship with patients and families, the communication and prevention focus. You have to be smart about how you deal with managed care plans, read the paper to stay abreast on changes in the managed care scene nationally and locally, and speak up for yourself. Don't let the secretary or billing staff or provider relations representative tell you [that] you can't do it! If you're going to care for your patients, you have to be a player.

SURVIVING THE MANAGED CARE ENVIRONMENT

The Application Process

The first step in today's healthcare market is entry onto the provider panels of MCOs. Contracting with an MCO to be designated a PCP allows the NP to be listed in the MCO's provider directory and to be reimbursed for the services rendered to patients of that MCO. To become a provider panel member, contact the Provider Relations department at the MCO to request an application, complete and return the application, and follow-up as necessary by telephone or mail (Buppert, 1998). Dolan states, "Winning provider contracts takes more care than you may think. And every delay or rejection can cost you a bundle" (Dolan, 1997, p 72). Apply to the MCO plans in the order of highest frequency to which your patients belong. Applications are complicated and require a significant amount of time to complete. Keep copies of applications submitted to reference if the MCO calls with a question and also so you do not have to start over again each time you complete an application. Dolan (1997) recommends requesting the application in writing.

Be sure the application is complete before submitting it to the MCO. Many practitioners leave completion of the application to another, such as the office manager. Dolan (1997) reports that the most frequent omission is a required signature within the application. Do not automatically assume that the only place you need to sign is on the last page. Be sure to enclose all required documentation, including license and Drug Enforcement Agency (DEA) certificate, and make sure they are current. Some practitioners keep commonly requested documents in clear plastic sleeves in a three-ring binder so they can be easily copied and so the original will not be accidentally sent in with an application. Unless specifically allowed, do not use "see attached" and force the reviewer to go hunting for the information. Repeat information, even if it is redundant. You want to make the reviewer's task as easy as possible. The same care that you give to your patients should be given to the application; check it twice.

Once your application has been submitted, call the plan every 2 to 4 weeks to determine where your application is in the process (Dolan, 1997; Workman and Buppert, 1998). Ensure that they have received the application, that they have everything needed, and ask for the expected decision date. If you have not heard from the MCO by that date, call to determine if there are any issues with which you should be dealing. If this is the first time your practice is applying to a particular MCO, be prepared for a site visit. The National Committee for Quality Assurance (NCQA), the primary accrediting agency for MCOs, mandates visits to a percentage of provider offices. Be prepared for the visitor to review charts, to see Occupational Safety and Health Administration (OSHA) and Clinical Laboratories Improvement Act (CLIA) handbooks, and to assess the friendliness of your office and staff toward patients. Dolan reports that they may "even inspect your refrigerator to 'make sure the urine specimens aren't next to the tuna sandwiches'" (Dolan, 1997, p 79). The site visit also provides an opportunity for the NP to show patient satisfaction survey results and to provide data on the cost-effectiveness of the practice.

Dealing with Rejection

As shown previously, not all MCOs will recognize NPs as PCPs (Mason et al, 1997). If you are rejected, attempt to find out the reason for your rejection. Does the MCO permit NPs on provider panels? If they do not, find out why. If it is an MCO policy, find out who is responsible for that policy. If the reason is due to state law, determine which law precludes NPs from provider panels (Buppert, 1998). Be aware that MCOs are not legally required to explain their rejection, so you may need to use your best interviewing skills (Dolan, 1997). Contact your state NP professional organization to see if other NPs have had similar problems with that MCO and if they can recommend strategies that have been effective either with that MCO or in general. The state NP organization may be able to assist legally. Should you be told that the provider panel is closed, attempt to find out if other types of providers are needed. You may have the qualifications for one of those panels and need only to submit additional documentation (Workman and Buppert, 1998). Should you be rejected based on your malpractice history, be sure to provide documentation to show any extenuating circumstances (Dolan, 1997).

Work with your state NP organization to demonstrate to MCOs whose policy prohibits listing and/or reimbursement of NPs the effectiveness of NP practice backed up with appropriate research. Be aware of the current Health Plan Employer Data and Information Set (HEDIS) measures required by NCQA, and demonstrate how your practice meets or improves on the standards for relevant measures (Buppert, 1999). Key primary care measures include immunization rates, smoking cessation advice, elderly health maintenance, adult cancer screening (mammogram and Pap smear), perinatal care (first trimester and postpartum within 6 weeks of delivery), chronic illness (myocardial infarction, diabetes, and mental illness) (Rustia and Bartek, 1997).

Ask your patients who are covered by that MCO to write letters requesting reimbursement for you (and for all NPs) for services rendered. These letters should go to both the MCO and the patient's employer (the MCO's actual client). Ask other providers who are listed by an MCO for their support in changing the MCO policy (Buppert, 1998). If all else fails, submit the patient's bill to the MCO and look for payment as an out-of-network provider. There is usually a large threshold amount before the MCO will cover out-of-network services, but it does not hurt to try before requesting payment from an individual patient.

Negotiating the Contract

When you are offered admission to a provider panel, you will need to negotiate a contract with the MCO covering both compensation and practice issues. Be sure to determine what services the MCO includes in primary care and the type of reimbursement, whether fee-for-service or capitation.

Capitation rate contracts need to be researched carefully to protect against catastrophic losses (Stevens, 1999). In Evergreen Re's *1998 Managed Care Indicator* (1999), "more than 30 percent of those surveyed (half of whom were physicians and the other half hospitals) admitted they really did not understand the level of risk for which they had contracted" (Stevens, 1999, p 1). Capitation is expected to grow significantly, from 40% of revenues to 51% of revenues (Evergreen Re, 1999). If the contract specifies a capitation rate, the services included in the rate must be specified. Watch for indefinite descriptions such as "primary care services"; work to have terms defined by Current Procedural Terminology (CPT) codes. Look at your past use of services to predict future use. Be aware of the product line under contract, regular patients make an average of two primary care visits per year, but Medicare patients may make an average of seven to eight visits a year (Stevens, 1999). Be sure your per-member-per-month (PMPM) rates are adjusted by insurance type. Know your patient diversity so that your fees reflect your patients. Children and seniors make more visits per year than other patients. If you are in a primary care practice, you should limit the amount of risk accepted by inserting a clause limiting out-of-pocket risk, such as hospital services, radiographic studies, and immunizations. You can reduce your risk by purchasing stop-loss insurance to cover catastrophic losses (Stevens, 1999).

Other issues in negotiating a MCO contract include turnaround time between billing and payment, office hours requirements, basis for bonuses or incentives, circumstances under which the contract can be terminated (by either party), and the directories under which the NP is to be listed (Buppert, 1998). An experienced legal counsel should be consulted to assist with negotiating terms and rates.

Managing Billing for Managed Care Services

Most MCOs will accept either paper HCFA 1500 billing forms or electronic (by computer) submission of bills for payment under your contract. Electronic submission provides quicker reimbursement through a priori checking for completeness of submission and by instantaneous entry into the MCO's payment system. In either case, both provider and patient identifying information are submitted, along with the appropriate International Classification of Diseases (ICD-9) codes and/or CPT codes and the date of service. Failure to include any of the above will result in rejection of the bill. A typical office visit consists of one or more ICD-9 codes and one or more CPT codes. Coding of services has become a specialty unto itself in the healthcare industry today. A detailed description of coding is beyond the scope of this chapter, but Buppert (1998) provides the following general guidelines:

- A billable visit requires face-to-face contact and must be associated with an ICD-9 code.
- Distinguish between new and established patients when using CPT codes.
- "History-taking, examination, and medical decision making are the key components in determining code selection" (Buppert, 1998, p 72).
- Level of care billed must be supported by medical record documentation.
- A variety of codes normally appear in a practice's billing. A preponderance of higher-level codes could lead to a charge of upcoding, which is equivalent to a false claim.
- Bill for all possible services provided.

If a bill submitted to an MCO is rejected, the NP should contact the MCO and determine the reason. It may be possible to resubmit with more information or documentation. Be sure to check payments received from MCOs as to amount.

Protecting Your Practice

Your practice should have a compliance plan to protect against accusations of insurance abuse or fraud. The compliance plan allows you to prove that you have been following the rules and regulations specified in your contract. The compliance plan can also check to ensure that bills include all services rendered and that they are accurately reimbursed (Rieder, 1999). If you are working under a capitation rate, be sure to audit the checks received against the agreed-upon rates (Dolan, 1997).

The complexity of today's healthcare market requires good information systems. Use your computer system as an information system to trend out different aspects of the practice. Doing this can help identify growth areas in which you may want to purchase new equipment or advertise your competency. Conversely, it can help you identify areas of decline in which you may want to reinvest or divest.

CHALLENGING THE SYSTEM

Managed care has had a tremendous influence over how healthcare is distributed and where this care is delivered. Whether NPs are part of this picture depends largely on the efforts of individual nurses and the nursing profession. We can easily create a public demand for MCOs to credential and list NPs by mobilizing nurses to request that their MCOs include NPs as PCPs. We still need individual NPs to challenge the system—to apply to be listed and to persist in challenging rejections.

We also need more research that describes the experiences of NPs with managed care, as well as comparative research on the outcomes of care when the primary caregiver is a nurse versus a physician.

If we believe that NPs are good for the health of the citizens of this country, then we must develop a multifaceted strategy to push for change. Such a strategy should include targeting the private and public sectors, the media, professional organizations, grass roots action, and education. There is a rich history of nurses knocking down the barriers to practice. The barriers to full inclusion of NPs in provider panels of MCOs await our attention and activism. We have done it before, and we can do it again.

REFERENCES

Aiken LH, Salmon ME: Healthcare workforce priorities: what nursing should do now, *Inquiry* 31(3):318-329, 1994.

Anderson AL, Gillis CL, Yoder L: Practice environment for nurse practitioners in California: identifying barriers, *West J Med* 165:209-216, 1996.

Brown SA, Grimes DE: A meta-analysis of nurse practitioners and nurse midwives in primary care, *Nurs Res* 44(6):332-339, 1995.

Buerhaus PI: Medicare payment for advanced practice nurses: what are the research questions? *Nurs Outlook* 46(4):151-153, 1998.

Buppert C: Reimbursement for nurse practitioner services, *Nurse Pract* 23(1):67-74, 1998.

Buppert C: HEDIS for the PCP: getting an "A" on the managed care report card, *Nurse Pract* 24(1):84-89, 1999.

Cohen SS, Mason DJ, Arsenie LS, et al: Focus groups reveal perils and promises of managed care for nurse practitioners, *Nurse Pract* 23(6):48, 54, 57-60 passim, 1998.

Dial TH, Palsbo SE, Bergsten C, et al: Clinical staffing in staff- and group-model HMOs, *Health Aff (Millwood)* 14(2):168-180, 1995.

Dolan KP: 10 mistakes to avoid when you apply to a managed care plan, *Med Econ* 74(19):72-83, 1997.

Evergreen Re: *1998 Managed care indicator*, 1999, Available online: http://www.evergreenre.com/pdfs/managedcare.pdf.

Felt S, Frazer H, Gold M: *HMO primary care staffing patterns and processes: a cross-site analysis of 23 HMOs*, Washington, DC, 1994, Mathematica Policy Research.

Felt-Lisk S: How HMOs structure primary care delivery, *Manag Care Q* 4(4):96-105, 1996.

Hart LG, Wagner E, Pirzada S, et al: Physician staffing ratios in staff-model HMOs: a cautionary tale, *Health Aff (Millwood)* 16(1):55-70, 1997.

Hoffman C: Medicaid payment for nonphysician practitioners: an access issue, *Health Aff (Millwood)* 13(4):140-152, 1994.

Mason DJ, Alexander JM, Huffaker J, et al: Nurse practitioners' experiences with managed care organizations in New York and Connecticut, *Nurs Outlook* 47(5):201-208, 1999.

Mason DJ, Cohen SS, O'Donnell JP, et al: Managed care organizations' arrangements with nurse practitioners, *Nurs Econ* 15(6):306-314, 1997.

Office of Technology Assessment: *Nurse practitioners, physician assistants, and certified nurse-midwives: a policy analysis* (Health Technology Case Study 37, OTA-HCS-37), Washington, DC, 1986, US Government Printing Office.

Pearson LJ: Annual update of how each state stands on legislative issues affecting advanced nursing practice, *Nurse Pract* 24(1):16-24, 1999.

Peterson ML: The Institute of Medicine report. A manpower policy for primary healthcare: a commentary from the American College of Physicians, *Ann Intern Med* 92:843-851, 1980.

Rieder MJ: Practice management: take a new look at old practice management strategies, *Physicians Financial News* 17(1):23, 1999.

Rustia JG, Bartek JK: Managed care credentialing of advanced practice nurses, *Nurse Pract* 22(9):90-103, 1997.

Safriet B: Healthcare dollars and regulatory sense: the role of advanced practice nursing, *Yale J Reg* 9(2):417-488, 1992.

Scarborough L: *Managed care and nurse practitioners: opportunity or barrier?* unpublished master's thesis, Denver, 1999, Regis University.

Sekscenski ES, Sansom S, Bazell C, et al: State practice environments and the supply of physician assistants, nurse practitioners, and certified nurse-midwives, *N Engl J Med* 331(19):1266-1271, 1994.

Silver HK: Use of new types of allied health professionals in providing care for children, *Am J Dis Child* 116:486-490, 1968.

Silver HK, Ford LC, Day LR: The pediatric nurse-practitioner program: expanding the role of the nurse to provide increased healthcare for children, *JAMA* 22:298-302, 1968.

Silver HK, Ford LC, Stearly SG: A program to increase healthcare for children: the pediatric nurse practitioner program, *Pediatrics* 39:756-760, 1967.

Stevens S: Getting a handle on capitation risk, *Physicians Financial News* 17(13):s4, 1999.

Sullivan-Marx E: Medicare reimbursement for advanced practice nurses: in the front door! *Nurs Outlook* 46(1):40-41, 1998.

Towers J: Medicare reimbursement for nurse practitioners, *J Am Acad Nurse Pract* 11:289-292, 1999.

Weiner JP: Forecasting the effects of health reform on U.S. physician workforce requirement: evidence from HMO staffing patterns, *JAMA* 272:222-230, 1994.

Wellstone PD, Shaffer BR: The American Health Security Act: a single-payer proposal, *N Engl J Med* 328(20):1489-1493, 1993.

Workman L, Buppert CK: Third-party reimbursement (nursing), *Nurse Pract* 23(5):11, 1998.

The Role of the Chief Nurse Executive in Managed Care

Christine Coughlin

KEY LESSONS IN THIS CHAPTER

- Io be successful, the chief nurse executive must function as a key member of the senior leadership team, working closely with the chief executive officer, the chief financial officer, and other senior members of the organization.
- Nursing practice, as promoted by the chief nurse executive, can play a vital role in promoting proper utilization of resources and reducing length of stay.
- By forming a partnership with the emergency department leaders, the chief nurse executive can promote reduction in unnecessary admissions and overutilization of emergency services.
- The chief nurse executive is central to the success of the organization by ensuring that quality of care is maintained and that the mission or vision of the organization is strategically promoted.
- The chief nurse executive can play an advocacy role by ensuring that ethical, family-focused care is delivered.

This chapter describes the evolving role of the chief nurse executive (CNE) in the current and future state of healthcare as it transitions into managed healthcare. The CNE manages the largest segment of the labor force in the hospital. The role of the CNE is to ensure that nursing is prepared to deliver quality healthcare in an environment shifting from episodic care to management of covered lives. During this time of change, quality care and the standards of nursing practice must be maintained. The nursing governance structure under the leadership of the CNE determines how flexible and quickly nursing meets the demands of the healthcare market while maintaining quality and standards of patient care. This structure is the framework for professional practice. The nursing governance structure is explored and evaluated through the case study of Montefiore Medical Center (MMC) as the institution came to manage a population of full-risk clients.

ROLE OF THE CHIEF NURSE EXECUTIVE

The standards of care across the continuum and the professional practice of nurses are the responsibility of the CNE. In the transition to a managed care environment, the CNE's primary role is to assure that quality nursing care is provided to the patients. Regardless of the method used to pay for care, professional nurses have a responsibility to their patients and families to promote health and provide care as stipulated in the Nurse Practice Act and the American Nurses Association (ANA) Code of Ethics for Nurses (ANA, 1995a). Creating an environment in which professional nurses can excel helps promote health and quality of care. An organizational culture that supports nurses in their role of patient advocate provides the infrastructure that promotes professional practice. The CNE must align with hospital administration to foster a supportive culture for professional nursing practice.

ALIGNMENT WITH THE MISSION OF THE HOSPITAL

The CNE must understand the mission of the hospital. Nursing needs to align with the mission of the hospital and with the strategies to accomplish that mission. Ideally the CNE is part of the governance structure of the hospital and has the goal of fostering the hospital's mission. In an influential role, the CNE is part of the leadership team that develops the strategic plan to achieve the mission. The team brings different imperatives to the table. The president needs to have a clear vision and to articulate that vision to the executive team. The chief executive officer (CEO) operationalizes the vision. The chief financial officer (CFO) manages costs and ensures that the revenue is maximized so that the hospital can achieve its mission and work toward its vision. An effective CFO will communicate that cost reduction is the responsibility of every member of the organization. The CNE ensures that quality professional nursing care is delivered. The CFO and the CNE must be aligned. To have a client base, the institution must promote the product—quality care. A wise CFO, although concerned with the bottom line, knows that the product must be marketable. The CFO needs to pay attention to the patient satisfaction surveys, employee morale, and market share, all of which influence the revenue stream. The board of trustees has the responsibility to oversee not only the financial statements but also patient care. Ultimately the board has oversight responsibility for the financial and clinical dimensions of the organization.

CASE STUDY: THE CHIEF NURSE EXECUTIVE AT MONTEFIORE MEDICAL CENTER

MMC is an integrated delivery system (IDS) that consists of two acute care hospitals with 1062 certified acute care beds and a network of primary care sites. It also has its own hospital-based skilled nursing facility (80 beds), a rehabilitation unit, and a home care agency.

As CNE and vice president of clinical services at this large academic medical center in the Bronx, New York, this author has experienced MMC's transition from a fee-for-service environment to a managed care environment. The contract management organization (CMO) of the institution went from 50,000 covered lives to 160,000 covered lives overnight. This increase occurred with extensive planning and preparation. In anticipation of these market changes, the organization began planning in the mid-1990s. The organization realized that early acceptance of managed care was paramount to remaining viable as an institution. The process started with discounted fee-for-service agreements with insurance companies and partial capitation, which led to global risk contracts. MMC always focused on the local population and as part of its strategy had previously expanded its primary care networks to form an IDS. Ten years ago, there were 50 primary care physicians. Today there are over 270 primary care physicians with a high primary care-to-specialist ratio. By pursuing the vertical integration strategy and developing an IDS, MMC avoided mergers with other hospitals. Managed care currently accounts for 50% of acute care revenue.

CAPITATION HAS ITS RISKS

MMC calculated its financial risks with capitation and realized that the risks would be greater with discounted fees for service. As a large academic medical center, the care MMC was providing in the hospital setting was costly and made it unable to compete on price with other institutions in the geographic area. Any savings with fee-for-service discounts were going to the insurance companies. As fierce price negotiations ensued and third-party denials of payment increased, the vision became clear. As an institution, MMC needed to be positioned to accept and manage global risk.

GRIP

The hospital developed a strategy called *GRIP*, which stands for: *Grow* the business, *Rebalance* academic programs, *Infrastructure* enhancement, and *Performance Improvement*.

As a strategy, MMC decided to take on the management of the global risk contract, giving it more control over its destiny. As of July 2000, MMC manages the Bronx Health Insurance Plan (HIP), the oldest and largest health maintenance organization (HMO) in New York City. With its IDS, MMC provides and manages care within a system.

Grow the Business

This growth strategy works for both fee-for-service and managed care populations. In the local market, a population-based approach provides a full range of care and continuity across the IDS. The focus on the local population prompted an expansion of the primary care base. In the specialty market, MMC focused on developing centers of excellence to attract specialty referrals. The Children's Hospital of MMC attracts pediatric patients who need specialty care. It is the only children's hospital in this geographic area.

Another part of MMC's growth strategy was to establish a 911 receiving emergency department (ED) at its smaller acute care hospital. This ED is responsible for 20% of all admissions. In an effort to have only appropriate admissions, MMC established a rapid care arm of the ED managed by nurse practitioners. This area provides care to patients with less serious problems and frees up the ED for patients who need acute care and extensive work-ups for diagnosis. This stratification of services ensures that all patients are seen in a timely fashion. Patients with less acute conditions no longer have to wait a long time while the patients in more serious condition are being seen.

Rebalance Academics/Teaching Excellence Versus Productivity

Academic medical centers are by their very nature resistant to change. MMC recognized the need for the organizational culture to shift direction. The practice patterns of faculty and attending physicians required assessment and change to discourage overuse of hospital services and a shift to outpatient care and other out of hospital services where appropriate. As an IDS, MMC has its own home care agency and long-term/subacute units. It also has a rehabilitation unit and an outpatient rehabilitation service. Ready access to these levels of service facilitated the necessary changes in practice patterns. The infrastructure was in place to allow the physicians to be comfortable and feel secure in changing their practice patterns. They felt that with the needed services readily available, they could discharge their patients safely to the appropriate level of care. The utilization declines were already in progress when MMC accepted the challenge of the global risk contract. The organization needs to retain savings from nonuse of expensive hospital stays while providing, maintaining, and managing care within the system.

Infrastructure Enhancement: Communication and Integration

To ensure that the highest standards of patient care are maintained, MMC established a system of communication extending outside the acute care facilities that included a new structure for professional oversight. As practice sites came under MMCs governance, the professional practice of the nurses employed at these sites and the model of care delivery was assessed. The hospital clinical nursing directors act as liaisons to the nurses in the primary care sites where the nurses report to practice administrators. This reporting structure ensures that the standards of care and the quality of care are the same. The clinical nursing directors determine whether the competencies of the staff are maintained and make sure that all regulations are upheld.

In addition, the technology infrastructure focuses on integrating the delivery system by expanding the clinical information system to integrate the IDS sites. The plan is for all practice sites to be electronically connected. A patient's record could be accessed anywhere in the system by an authorized provider.

Performance Improvement

The driving principles of managed care include actively managing patient care, improving quality, and providing appropriate care. Utilization of resources and declines in overutilization are major goals. As MMC has become accountable for the health of a defined population of patients, its focus has changed from treating illness to promoting and maintaining health, including identifying opportunities to not only promote health and better serve MMC's clients but to be cost-effective as well. Managing the care of patients with chronic conditions, maximizing their health, and improving their quality of life are prime examples of how managed care should function. As an example, the first step for MMC was to identify the patients who had frequent admissions. Their diagnosis for each admission was identified. It was no surprise that the most frequent repeat admissions were patients with congestive heart failure, asthma, and pneumonia. The next step was to initiate a disease management program to help the patients manage their disease. Disease management was identified as one of the organization's performance improvement projects. It not only promoted better utilization of resources but enhanced quality of care as well. Disease management includes teaching patients to take better care of themselves and to better understand their disease process. In addition, follow-up visits and telephone calls from MMC's care providers helped promote a healthy lifestyle for the patients.

MANAGED CARE READINESS WORK GROUPS

Four committees, the Managed Care Readiness Work Groups, were established to oversee all care issues across the continuum. As managed care increased to account for 50% of MMC's clinical economy, MMC's leaders were determined to work more effectively as an organization. To accomplish this task, the four work groups were formed. Many initiatives were already underway working on various aspects of patient care issues, and the newly formed work groups coordinated these initiatives. The purpose of the groups was not to duplicate effective efforts but to provide a forum in which all components of the IDS could work together. The charge of the work groups was to reduce patient hospital days, to prepare the EDs, to manage better use of ancillary services, and to reduce out-of-network activity referrals for specialty and inpatient acute care. In addition, a fifth work group was formed to coordinate information management services.

The first action of the work groups was to assess the current and planned actions in each area. They then coordinated these efforts throughout the medical center. The next step was to identify and put into place new initiatives in areas that needed focused attention.

Each work group was headed by a vice president and had members from throughout the medical center. Nursing was represented in all groups, including nurse executives and nurse leaders. As the CNE, this author was assigned to chair the ED utilization work group.

The first group, which focused on reducing hospital stays, identified managing and reducing length of stay as a critical success factor for the medical center. The group identified and set priorities among problem areas. Patient groups with high admission rates and long hospital stays became target populations. The group then identified the causes of the high admission rates and the long hospital stays and designed and implemented actions to reduce inpatient days. They analyzed denials by insurance companies and identified targets to either reduce length of stay or admission rates. In addition, they assessed readmission rates and decided on appropriate action steps to reduce these rates.

The second group, chaired by the CNE and the chief of emergency medicine, examined ED use. The focus of this group was to look at the unnecessary use of EDs for routine care and to reduce avoidable admissions entering the system through the EDs. The group identified avoidable treat and release visits and initiatives that could reduce ED use for these populations. It developed and improved systems to involve primary care physicians in deciding whether or not to admit ED patients. The group also looked at alternatives to acute inpatient care, as well as disease management initiatives.

Managing the pharmacy and ancillary service use was determined to be another critical success factor and therefore was the charge of the third work group. The focus of the group was to reduce the unnecessary use of drugs and ancillary services and related costs of care for hospital inpatients. Although identifying drug use reduction opportunities was already underway, the increasing cost of drugs was a major concern. The team identified initiatives that should be started or enhanced to reduce drug use. The group also looked at ancillary service use, such as imaging and laboratory tests, and they identified patterns of use. Application of quality improvement and care management processes helps measure, track, and refine practice and service use patterns.

The fourth work group, Referral Pattern Management, analyzed and made recommendations about the referral process for MMC's primary care sites. The populations serviced by MMC's primary care network required ready access to high-quality and responsive specialty care. Increasing the referrals to MMC-based specialist from MMC primary care sites and other sources was a critical success factor for the academic departments and the medical center. The acute care hospital of the MMC's IDS provided specialized care, such as open heart surgery, all-invasive cardiology services, transplant services, and high-risk obstetrical services. The primary care sites served as a referral source, and there was capacity for more referrals.

This group is currently looking at the referral process, monitoring its success, and focusing on three perspectives. The first, the perspective of the specialty departments, focuses on how the newly added HIP sites generate many incremental referrals. The measurement affects the incremental costs associated with acquiring the new sites related to the new revenue generated by the incremental referrals. The second perspective is the primary site perspective, which is measured by the response times to the referrals. How long does a patient wait for a referral to a specialist? How available are the services of the specialty? Service levels and problem areas for enrollees are assessed. In addition, specialty expenses overall are measured. These include both in-network and out-of-network expenses. Finally, the independent practice association (IPA) perspective assesses service levels and problem areas for enrollees. In addition, specialty expenses overall are measured, including both in-network and out-of-network expenses.

A final task force was formed to assess data and information systems. The availability of timely, reliable data is critical to the effectiveness of MMC's efforts to manage care, set priorities, and allocate resources. It is also essential to manage the utilization, costs, and quality of care provided under risk contracts. The four work groups need timely reports in varying levels of detail relevant to their needs. Presently the ability to provide detailed reports to support management decision making is increasing. MMC still operates a number of different systems, however, which do not communicate efficiently with each other. This group's initial focus is on clinical care systems in EDs, acute care hospitals, clinical practice sites, and throughout the integrated primary care network. The long-term plan is to include MMC business information systems.

EARLY PREPARATION FOR MANAGED CARE

To be ready for the changing economics, MMC underwent major changes and reduced leadership personnel in the mid-1990s. In 1996 the institution was faced with a serious financial challenge that was met by quickly combining operations at both the Jack D. Weiler Hospital of the Albert Einstein College of Medicine and the Henry and Lucy Moses Division and reducing leadership positions. MMC decided to move to a care center model. In this model, patients with similar needs and services were grouped together under one administrative leader. Before accomplishing this task, MMC unified two hospitals with different organizations and cultures. The Weiler Hospital was a small community hospital, with many voluntary physicians serving the middle-income community of the East Bronx. The Moses Division more closely resembled a city hospital, with a very active emergency department and a large population of Medicaid and Medicare patients.

The leadership team was established before the care center model was implemented. After the hospital unification, consultants were hired to assist in the redesign effort. Care center leaders were chosen first, and the executive team was then put in place before the redesign into care centers was initiated. Physicians were then partnered with the care center vice presidents as the model evolved.

The structure of care centers at MMC established a vice president (nonnursing role) who reports to the senior vice president of acute care. Under each vice president are clinical directors of nursing who are responsible for the daily operations of the care centers. The vice presidents and clinical directors of nursing are accountable for units at both sites. Vice presidents also have other service lines that report to them. For example, the vice president of surgery is responsible for the laboratory service lines. The size and scope of the care centers determined how many clinical directors were needed. There are two clinical directors in the surgical care center—one for perioperative and one for the inpatient surgical units, including the surgical intensive care units. The medicine care center includes both inpatient and outpatient oncology. This care center also has two clinical directors of nursing, one for medicine and one for oncology. Both directors manage inpatient and outpatient areas.

At MMC, the CNE is also the vice president of clinical services. Responsibilities include the ED, the pharmacy, social work, and the skilled nursing facility. The departments of nursing education and research, nursing informatics, CCM, customer services, and nursing quality management support the professional nursing practice. The clinical directors of the care centers report to the CNE for professional practice issues, although the CNE does not have fiduciary responsibility for the nursing cost centers in the care centers. The vice president of each care center is accountable for the nursing care budget.

NURSING GOVERNANCE

The governance structure for nursing at MMC is a shared governance model and was established before implementing the care center/service line organizational structure (Figure 10-1). The CNE is the chair of a nurse executive leadership (NEL) committee, which functions as an advisory body to the CNE and provides leadership in the strategic planning process aligned with the mission, philosophy, and performance targets of the organization. This forum coordinates and prioritizes projects, initiatives, and resources. The NEL committee consists of all clinical directors of nursing and the director of nursing education and research, the director of informatics and special projects, the director of CCM, the director of customer services and nursing quality management, and the director of the resource center. The CNE also chairs the Nursing Executive Council (NEC), the main governing body for nursing practice, whose membership consists of all levels of practicing nurses.

The charge of the NEC is as follows:

- To provide an organizational structure to ensure that patients with the same nursing care needs receive comparable levels of care throughout the medical center.
- To provide an organizational structure that has the authority and responsibility for establishing standards of nursing practice through the development of performance standards and competencies.
- To provide an organizational structure that delineates clinical privileges and credentials for professional nursing staff and nonprofessional support staff who provide patient care and report to nursing.
- To provide an organizational structure that participates in the interdisciplinary development of policies, procedures, critical pathways, teaching guides, guidelines, standards of care and physician order sets, and documentation (manual and automated).
- To provide an organizational structure to monitor, evaluate, and report the ongoing quality improvement initiatives and outcomes within care centers and in the aggregate.
- To implement and recommend strategies based on data-driven decision making for improving the nursing care delivered to the patients.
- To develop and reinforce clinical programs and educational initiatives based on organizational prioritization.
- To ensure that ethical and family-focused implications are considered when policy decisions are made.
- To provide a supportive environment that encourages and supports scientific inquiry for continuous quality improvement.
- To provide a channel of communication between the NEC, the Medical Quality Council (MQC), the New York State Nurses Association (NYSNA), and staff.
- To act as a coordinating body for communication exchange between departments.
- To fulfill regulatory requirements defined for patient-focused and organizational functions.

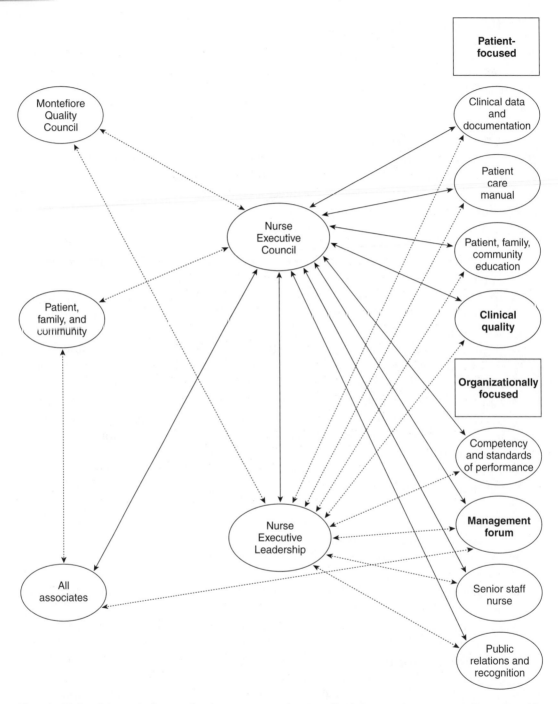

Figure 10-1 Schematic diagram for the nurse executive council structure and governance. (From Coughlin C: *J Nurs Adm* 31(3):113-120, 2001. [Created by Janet Kasoff, RNC, CNAA, MA, Director of Nursing Informatics and Special Projects, Montfiore Medical Center, Bronx, New York.])

The CNE meets quarterly with nurse managers from both sites. These meetings are forums for information sharing and brainstorming around professional issues, labor issues, and mandatory compliance concerns. Labor management meetings take place monthly. The membership consists of the directors of nursing and union association delegates.

The governance model supports the institutional strategy of moving toward a total managed care environment. The concept of caring for patients across the lifespan and providing primary care services to reduce unnecessary overutilization of expensive healthcare interventions is a basic tenet of managed care. The shared governance model allows for coordination and integration of nursing services from every sector of care delivery, whether they are in the acute care hospital, school-based clinic, or primary care sites. This model aligns the organization with managed care principles.

CARE DELIVERY MODEL

At MMC, coordinated care management (CCM) is the professional interdisciplinary model of care delivery. This model ensures that each patient's written care plan is implemented and evaluated by the interdisciplinary team. Nurses are point-of-care providers. They coordinate each patient's care plan with his or her physician. Professional nurses integrate, coordinate, and facilitate the delivery of healthcare. The CCM model promotes the proper utilization of resources and reduced length of stay. An interdisciplinary care team conducts rounds every day. The team consists of the nurse caring for the patient, a social worker, a clinical care coordinator (CCC), a physician, and other care team members as necessary. The bedside nurse is responsible for coordinating the patient's direct care needs and initiating consultation with other healthcare providers. The nurse caring for the patient is responsible for initiating the discharge plan. The CCC, when involved in the case, facilitates the care for complex cases. The CCC also helps the patient's nurse ensure that the plan of care is followed and that the patient and family have a safe and appropriate discharge. Due to budget cuts and downsizing of the number of CCCs, the staff manage the direct patient care, whereas the CCCs perform utilization management. In the ED, the nurses, in collaboration with physicians, ensure that all admissions to the acute care hospital are appropriate.

Nursing's Contribution to this Strategy

With the direct responsibility of the care delivery model, the CNE oversees both quality patient care and resource utilization. The CCM model of care delivery places the nurse as the coordinator of care responsible for discharge planning as soon as the patient is admitted to the hospital. Each professional nurse has a caseload of patients to manage. For the complex cases with multiple discharge needs, there are CCCs who facilitate the discharge process. There are daily rounds on each unit in which the nurses present their patients to the team. The team consists of a CCC, a social worker, physicians, and other professionals. With an ever-growing number of patients under a global risk contract, it is essential to manage their care to ensure that the length of stay is appropriate. The team meetings identify problems and issues that delay appropriate care.

The driving forces that provided the impetus to change MMC's care delivery model were excess length of stay for patients, delays in service delivery, interdisciplinary duplication of work, lack of an outcome focus, and discharge planning inefficiencies. The CCM model ensures that each patient has a collaboratively developed plan of care, which is implemented and evaluated by an interdisciplinary team. Professional nurses integrate, coordinate, and facilitate the delivery of cost-effective healthcare. This model provides a clinical infrastructure, which supports interdisciplinary clinical practices and processes in a managed care environment. The nurse is the point-of-care provider and coordinates the patient's plan of care with the physician. As a patient advocate, the nurse ensures that care is appropriate and that the potential problems are identified and corrected, thereby improving the quality of care delivered to the patient.

In redesigning the clinical nursing infrastructure, there was a focus on being outcome driven. The leadership team was challenged to use data to measure successes. This data included measures of length of stay reductions, denial by insurance companies, patient satisfaction scores, access to care, wait times for patients, and cost per case reductions.

In the MMC model, the care center leaders, the vice president, and the directors of nursing are accountable for the nursing services provided within each center. The CNE at MMC retains the governance responsibility for monitoring the quality, safety, and competency of professional nursing practice.

Utilization Management

The director of CCM also oversees utilization management. The need for more accurate documentation was identified by the leadership team as the denials of payment by insurance companies increased. Out of this need, the clinical documentation program was developed. A team of nurses reviews the medical records of hospitalized patients, seeks out the interdisciplinary team members as appropriate to improve documentation on medical records to reflect severity of illness, and helps resident house staff, physicians, and other disciplines understand appropriate diagnosis assignments. This program improves the quality of diagnostic-related group (DRG)-related documentation and improves medical center reimbursement for actual services and care rendered.

BALANCED SCORECARD

To determine if MMC's strategy is working and if MMC as a large institution is in alignment with its strategy, it is necessary to measure this company's goals, which need outcome measures. The methodology selected by the institution as a measurement tool is the balanced scorecard (ANA, 1995b; Kaplan and Norton, 1996, 2001). In the future, MMC will be able to determine if it operationalized the strategic plan effectively. The balanced scorecard allows the institution to measure integrated balanced performance measures against targets, and it assigns accountability for performance.

The measurements of the balanced scorecard are divided into four categories: (1) innovation and growth, (2) internal processes, (3) financial performance, and (4) customer's view. Innovation and growth focuses on looking forward. Internal processes include measures that look down, from the inside out. Financial performance allows us to look back. The customer's view is looking down from the outside inward.

For the care centers, innovation and growth measures include market share, equipment actual age versus useful life, percentage of new programs, referring physicians, and patients per referring physician.

Internal process measures include length of stay, appropriate bed usage, case length, actual versus planned utilization, ancillary tests per discharge, readmission rate, denial rate, percentage of patients on plan of care, patient satisfaction with the environment, aggregate wait times, aggregate procedure times, and patient outcomes.

Financial measures are cost per unit of service, revenue per unit of service, and overall units of service.

The customer view includes patient satisfaction scores, point of service surveys, complaints and compliments, and time to first appointment.

Each care center selected measures based on the balanced performance categories, which prevented conflicts that might have been reinforced by separate and sometimes opposing performance measures and reward systems. Small cuts in one area can sometimes result in significant increased expenses or reduction in service in other areas. Each care center and service line developed indicators using the balanced scorecard framework. The management team agreed on a set of indicators that would track the individual and the collective performance of their areas of control. Working with the care center leadership, the management team set specific improvement targets for each of their performance measures. Each care center then tracks and reports its progress to the rest of the management team.

Nursing's Balanced Scorecard

The vice president of clinical services/CNE has the authority and responsibility to provide a methodological framework for promoting continuous improvement in the quality of nursing services through the conduct of quality measurement, clinical and functional performance, and outcomes management. The goal of the CNE is to ensure the provision of quality nursing care services to patients and families, deploy resources effectively, and facilitate response to patient care issues in a timely manner to achieve continuous improvement in nursing care services and patient outcomes.

The nursing quality plan is an integrated component of the overall MMC quality management program. All nursing personnel are involved in the planned, systematic, ongoing performance improvement program designed to objectively and systematically monitor and evaluate the quality and appropriateness of nursing care services, pursue opportunities to improve patient care, and resolve identified problems. The plan is customer focused, interdisciplinary, data-driven, outcome-oriented, and proactive.

Although each care center measures many nursing indicators, it is essential to analyze these indicators and quality measures in the aggregate, which is accomplished by using the balanced scorecard methodology. Data are collected, analyzed, and presented using this format. Under innovation and growth, or looking ahead, nursing measures the number of visits to MMC's nursing Website. The Website, which can be accessed through the Montefiore Website, is a comprehensive view of professional nursing practice at MMC. As part of innovation and growth, nursing measures the number of nurses who have received their certification in their specialty. Another innovation and growth measure is the number of nursing research projects, as well as publications in professional journals by the nursing staff.

To assess MMC's operations or internal processes, nursing is measuring the percent of patients with an activated plan of care, and the number of referrals to the New York Organ Donor Network, a regulatory requirement. As a proxy for staff satisfaction, MMC is measuring mandatory overtime and protests of assignment. These two measures provide MMC with data that do not directly measure staff satisfaction but provide an ongoing measure that allows the medical center to make assumptions about staff morale.

Financial performance, or looking back, is measured by the number of patient stay and patient day denials and MMC's success in appealing denied days. Variances from coordinated care management are measured, which provides a view of variances by type. The types of variances include system variances, family variances, interdisciplinary team variances, community variances, physician variances, and patient or physiological variances. The variances are tracked by looking at days at risk, as well as financial impact. These measures allow MMC to determine how well its coordinated care model of patient care delivery is working from a fiscal perspective.

Another financial measure that MMC looks at in the aggregate is sick time use and overtime uses. MMC also measures and assesses nursing care hours. For this measure, it uses both internal and external benchmarks. Internally, MMC compares similar nursing care units, and externally, it compares itself with other institutions. This measure is an important one, since managed care drives the length of stay down and the patient acuity up.

Nursing measures that provide the customer's view are specific indicators in MMC's patient satisfaction survey, the number of hospital-acquired pressure ulcers, the appropriate use of restraints, and patient falls. Medication errors are measured as part of a collaborative effort with pharmacy, medicine, and nursing to identify and analyze prescriptive, dispensing, and administration errors.

Nursing's integrated balanced performance measures are presented to the NEC each quarter. They are presented at the MQC and at the Medical Committee of the Board of Trustees. In addition, they are presented at multiple nursing forums to ensure that the information reaches all staff nurses and nursing personnel.

OPPORTUNITIES FOR NURSING

The CNE remains central to the success of the organization and is responsible for maintaining professional nursing practice through quality of care, competency, knowledge-based practice, and support of new nursing knowledge. Managed care has provided many opportunities for nursing to provide leadership in MMC. With the responsibility of resource utilization and quality patient care, nursing has been a major player in promoting the mission of this institution.

REFERENCES

American Nurses Association: *Nursing's social policy statement*, Washington, DC, 1995a, American Nurses Publishing.

American Nurses Association: *Nursing care report card for acute care*, Washington, DC, 1995b, American Nurses Publishing.

Kaplan RS, Norton DP: *The balanced scorecard*, Boston, 1996, Harvard Business School Press.

Kaplan RS, Norton DP: *The balanced scorecard*, ed 2, Boston, 2001, Harvard Business School Press.

Person and Community: Coauthors of Health and Care

Sandra Schmidt Bunkers

KEY LESSONS IN THIS CHAPTER

- Serious access to care issues and delivery gaps have led to the need for innovative community nursing practice models.
- Community nursing practice models provide a framework to help people, families, and the community achieve their own health promotion, goals, hopes, and dreams.
- Honoring the community's voice is a challenge for nursing and requires courage in today's economically focused healthcare climate.
- Implementing a program requires not only vision but an ability to operationalize that vision.
- It may be necessary to seek funding at local, state, and national levels to support the creation of new and innovative practice models.

The complexity of healthcare for persons and communities continues to challenge both providers and consumers. The defining role nursing can take to address this challenge arises from the knowledge base of the discipline and the ability of nursing to respond to public concern. This chapter focuses on the components and processes involved in developing science-based community nursing practice models, which can respond to continuum of care issues. The Health Action Model for Partnership in Community (HAMPIC) (Bunkers et al, 1999) is used as an example of a community nursing model based on Parse's theory of human becoming in nursing. HAMPIC responds to the needs of those disconnected from health and social services and those underserved by the healthcare community. Healthcare management issues are framed within the perspective that the person-community is the expert in knowing their own way (Parse, 1998). The challenge of nursing is to help the person-community actualize their plans and goals for changing health patterns.

THE CALL TO COMMUNITY

The meaning of community, from a human becoming perspective, is framed within the idea of community as process (Bunkers, Michaels, and Ethridge, 1997; Parse, 1999). Parse writes concerning community:

The prefix *com* means *with* and the term *unity* means *oneness*. Community then means *oneness* . . . From a human becoming perspective, the human and universe are in mutual process co-creating what is, thus co-creating community . . . A community, then, is co-constituted with all the personal histories of the individuals who are present. What arises as the distinctiveness of a community reflects the diverse meanings of the individuals, and although the evolution of community over time has recognizable patterns of constancy, the ever-changing process incarnates diverse patterns . . . Whether the community is an individual, a city, a group, or whatever, the constituents continuously change, co-creating diverse patterns. Thus community is an ever-changing process, not a static geographical location (Parse, 1999, p 119).

The call for innovative community nursing practice models has never been clearer than it is today. The present healthcare delivery system is developing serious access to care issues along with various gaps in needed services. New community nursing practice models are emerging as the discipline attempts to respond to the health needs of society. Such models include parish nursing programs, nursing centers in inner city neighborhoods, and education-service models originating in nursing schools that link community care with the acute care setting. The management of care, or *case management,* across a continuum of health services is a critical part of these various community nursing practice models.

Many disciplines, including nursing, have been vying for the role of case manager in these various community health models. In this author's opinion, the most appropriate person to be a case manager of a health situation is the person living that health situation. Future community nursing practice models can be developed guided by this belief. Cody initiates this notion when he writes, "The role of *case manager,* if the term is taken literally, seems to this author to fit only one person per 'case'—and that is *the person* whose 'case' is at issue" (Cody, 1994, p 181). Cody further states:

Increasingly, individuals are asserting control over their own healthcare, insisting on making their own choices, and choosing alternative modes of healing or choosing no intervention at all, based on information they have acquired on their own and evaluated in light of their own relationships, beliefs, and values . . . It is possible, even likely, that nursing as a discipline would progress further, faster, by recognizing the *person* as case manager rather than claiming that role for the nurse (Cody, 1994, pp 181-182).

Community nursing practice models, based on the belief that the person is the most qualified to make decisions about his or her life and health, can help individuals, families,

---

BOX 11-1
Core Belief Components for Nursing Practice Model Building

Person: patterns of relating
Community: patterns of interconnectedness
Health: patterns of human becoming
Nursing: patterns of presence

---

and communities find new and unique ways to address health concerns of the twenty-first century. Shaping such new and innovative care delivery systems involves intentional reflection on the underlying beliefs and values guiding nursing practice. There are four core components that serve as cornerstones in creating a theory-based nursing practice model: (1) beliefs about the person, (2) beliefs about the community, (3) beliefs about health, and (4) beliefs about nursing (Box 11-1).

When creating a theory-based community nursing practice model, the core components must be defined from a particular nursing theoretical framework. For example, these core components are taken from the perspective of Parse's theory of human becoming. Other frameworks within nursing also can be the basis for the defining characteristics of these core components.

CORE COMPONENTS FOR CREATING A THEORY-BASED NURSING PRACTICE MODEL

Person: Patterns of Relating

The person, from the human becoming perspective, is a unitary being different from the sum of his or her parts and is recognized through ways of relating that "distinguish one human being from another" (Parse, 1998, p 22). The individual's pattern of relating is "illuminated through speech, words, symbols, silence, gesture, movement, gaze, posture, and touch" (Parse, 1998, p 22). Also, the person is free to choose within situations. Thus individuals choose how they will relate to others and to the universe. Nursing practice based on the belief that persons are unitary beings who are free to choose within situations focuses on the meaning that lived experiences hold for individuals, groups, families, or communities and on the quality of life they want to choose. Individuals and communities freely choose meanings, which create their reality of health. From this perspective, a nursing practice model would be designed with the idea in mind that the person-community will coshape with professionals the healthcare process in multiple complex interrelationships. A nursing practice model will continuously evolve as the nurse-person and nurse-community process unfolds.

An example of such a nursing practice model exists at Augustana College in Sioux Falls, South Dakota, where the Department of Nursing has developed a community nursing practice model, HAMPIC. The graphic model in Figure 11-1 depicts important concepts of Parse's

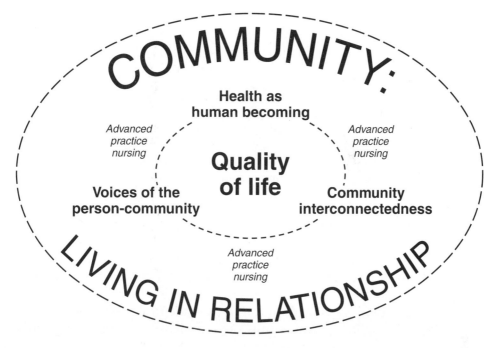

Figure 11-1   The Health Action Model for Partnership in Community. (From the HAMPIC model, Augustana College Department of Nursing, Sioux Falls, South Dakota, Copyright 1997.)

theory of human becoming, such as health as human becoming, the nursing focus of quality of life from the person-community's perspective, and community as a relational process. Bunkers et al write concerning this model:

This model is based on Parse's human becoming school of thought and focuses on the primacy of the nurse's presence with others . . . This advanced practice nursing model is an alternative to the present-day customs of healthcare experts diagnosing, prescribing, and providing what *they see* as needed services to those disadvantaged in a community. HAMPIC is grounded in the formation of collaborative relationships with persons, families, and groups who are living the experience of marginalization and disenfranchisement. The purpose of the model is to respond in a new way to nursing's social mandate to care for the health of society by gaining an understanding of what is wanted from those living these health experiences (Bunkers et al, 1999, p 94).

The person as a unitary pattern of relating underscores the importance of focusing on such patterns of relating in developing nursing practice models. The quality of the relationships between the nurse, persons receiving care, other healthcare providers, and the larger social and economic structure of the community must be one of the guiding components in developing and evaluating the practice model.

Community: Patterns of Interconnectedness

HAMPIC is an example of an advanced community nursing practice model, which focuses on community as process. Bunkers et al suggest that the process of community interconnectedness

involves the interrelationship of persons, ideas, places, and events . . . The interconnectedness of community involves relationship that transcends separating differences . . . Nurses practicing in this model understand that community as process entails a moving together in seeking mutual understanding while holding as important the unique perspectives presented by individuals and groups in complex health situations. Moving together in seeking mutual understanding calls for a type of listening to one another in which both nurse and person-community engage in contributing to expanding choices for living health (Bunkers et al, 1999, p 95).

In HAMPIC, listening occurs in many ways in the nurse-person-community process. One of these ways involves a Steering Committee, in which over 32 persons formally come together four times a year to discuss health concerns of the community, as well as ongoing program operations. The Steering Committee consists of representatives of healthcare delivery systems in the Sioux Falls area, as well as "individuals who are experiencing economic marginalization and homelessness and who are active in the Health Action Model" (Bunkers et al, 1999, p 97). Individuals and groups present ideas to address health concerns. Community as patterns of interconnectedness is lived out with the Steering Committee and the staff of HAMPIC.

Community as patterns of interconnectedness allow a community nursing practice model to address a wide range of human health experiences. Nurses practicing from this belief about community work with individuals, groups, families, and communities. The nurse, in listening intently to these various voices of the community, will move with the meanings of health situations as they emerge to understand what healthcare is wanted and needed.

Health: Patterns of Becoming

Health, from the human becoming perspective, is a process. Health is a personal commitment to a lived value system; it is the process of human becoming (Parse, 1990). Persons live health by choosing what is important to their quality of life. Thus health is defined by the person and not the nurse or any other healthcare provider, and quality of life is "not what those outside the life looking in think it is, but rather it is what the person *there* living the life say [sic] it is" (Parse, 1994, p 17). Parse writes concerning health:

Health is how I live my life—my own personal commitment to being the who that I am becoming . . . Listen to me nurse, when I tell you how I am, and what I will do—since that is how I am going to be me (Parse, 1990, p 140).

A nurse practicing with the belief that health is a process of living one's own chosen way will focus on what the person, family, and community desire in relation to changing or not changing patterns of health. A nursing practice model guided by these beliefs about health focuses on patterns of choosing how to live, since health is the pattern of choosing human becoming. For example, in HAMPIC, the nurse talks with individuals and communities about what life is like for them now, what hopes and dreams they have, what goals they would like to work on for their quality of life, and how the nurse can work with them to meet these goals (Bunkers et al, 1999). HAMPIC is an example of a nursing practice model focusing on patterns of individuals and communities in choosing how to live:

The intent . . . is to connect in true presence with persons and communities and to understand their health experiences . . . Advanced practice nurses in the model work with individuals, families, and "site" communities in creating personal health descriptions and health action plans . . . It is in this process of identifying a health action plan that the nurse explores how she or he can work with the person-community in changing patterns of health (Bunkers et al, 1999, p 96).

The belief that health is a pattern of human becoming provides possibilities for a future nursing practice model to address a variety of lived experiences for individuals, families, and communities. In one neighborhood health project within HAMPIC, bicycle safety and wearing helmets is addressed, and the local Optimist club helps the nurses fix and repair children's bicycles while the children also learn about bicycle safety. Another community group donates bicycle helmets to this project. Nursing practice focusing on patterns of human becoming can help persons and communities create unique opportunities for health and quality of life.

Nursing: Patterns of Presence

From a human becoming perspective, nursing practice involves the process of being with people in true presence and bearing witness to others' health patterns. Parse writes concerning true presence:

The nurse in true presence joins the reality of the person at all realms of the universe and is open to him or her without judging or labeling. The person at all realms of his or her universe experiences the intent of the nurse, which is to bear witness to changing health patterns. The intent of the nurse is languaged in his or her whole being, in the subtle knowings of messages given and taken at all realms of the universe, so words are not necessary to live true presence in the nurse-person process (Parse, 1997, p 35).

In true presence, which is an interpersonal art grounded in the beliefs and value system of Parse's human becoming theory, the nurse moves with the person-community as they illuminate the meaning of their health experiences. The nurse responds to the rhythms of the person-community as they live paradoxical patterns of relating such as revealing-concealing and connecting-separating with self and others. The nurse explores with the person-community ways of working together on health issues as the person-community make choices about moving on with new and valued ways of living health. Patterns of presence emerge as the nurse engages others in community. Although the notion of "caring for" others is inconsistent with the human becoming perspective, care as "being with" others and honoring their chosen way is lived in the nurse-person-community process.

The notion of care as being present for others arises out of the works of such philosophers as Heidegger (1962) and Helminski (1992). Heidegger writes in *Being and Time* that the essence of being human (Dasein) is care, and that care "is always concern and solicitude" (Heidegger, 1962, p 238). Concern involves an interest in the possibilities of others. Solicitude is a moving toward others and engaging "entities in the world" (Heidegger, 1962, p 239). Helminski posits, "Presence is the way in which we occupy space, as well as how we flow and move . . . Presence determines our degree of alertness and openness and warmth" (Helminski, 1992, pp viii, ix). Presence is "a receptivity to the energies of possibility" (Helminski, 1992, p 32).

Bearing witness and honoring the voices of community is a challenge for nursing and requires courage in today's economically focused healthcare climate. A community nursing practice model based on nursing as patterns of presence focuses on the interpersonal art of being truly present to others and participating in an ongoing dialogue in exploring the endless possibilities for changing patterns of health.

PROCESSES OF THEORY-BASED NURSING MODEL DEVELOPMENT

Developing community nursing practice models based on nursing theory involves ongoing processes of co-creation and collaboration. The processes presented here are not numbered in any particular order to emphasize the notion that they are not linear but are ongoing mutual processes of envisioning what can be. Box 11-2 lists these processes.

Imaging the Vision

The key to establishing a theory-based community nursing practice model is to imagine that it can and will be. This imaging of the vision must be linked to a desire to respond to healthcare concerns of particular individuals or groups in society. From the human becoming perspective, the focus of a community nursing practice model is "for the betterment of humankind" (Parse, 1998, p 95). For example, HAMPIC was conceptualized as a nursing practice model that would work with persons and groups who struggled with a lack of economic, social, and interpersonal resources and access to healthcare issues (Bunkers et al, 1999). The model seeks to create connections between persons and agencies and to create services where none exist.

BOX 11-2
Processes for Creating a Theory-Based Community Nursing Practice Model

Imaging the vision	Participating in teaching-learning processes
Engaging the community	Obtaining funding
Developing a conceptual framework	Conducting research
Naming operational components	Publishing the prototype
Creating a documentation system	

Once the conceptualization of the model occurs, others must capture the vision of the model. The inventor(s) need a clarity of purpose and a passion for the work, which is expressed to others in inviting ways. From a human becoming perspective, imaging involves the construction of personal knowledge (Parse, 1998). By imaging the vision, one can begin to create a new reality. Nevertheless, there are obstacles to making the vision a reality. In *The Company of Strangers,* Palmer (1997) suggests that we live in a culture of fragmentation where individualism and autonomy are more compelling than visions of unity. The historian Harding writes:

> . . . a truly pluralistic and humane society must be undergirded and overarched by a common vision of the public good . . . For without that capacity to see ourselves ultimately as a community, without that common basis on which community must be built, we are in danger of disintegrating into hundreds of private, warring, special interests (who will not, for instance, pay taxes to support the well-being of the whole; who will, for instance—at astonishingly young ages—physically attack helpless elderly citizens to grab the pittances of their social security and welfare money; who will, for instance, pour life-destroying industrial wastes into rivers, or produce essentially poisonous products for profit alone). Where there is not vision the people perish (Harding, 1978, pp 350-351).

Thus imaging the vision needs to be coupled with an appreciation for community interconnectedness. Key persons within site communities need to capture the vision. Imaging the vision then becomes an ongoing process of creation as project staff and site communities work together continuously to reshape the emerging nursing practice model.

Engaging the Community

A site community consists of collaborating agencies, programs, and individual groups that become partners with the community nursing practice model to deliver and create health services. Identifying site communities requires intimate knowledge of the community in which the project is to be developed. For example, in HAMPIC, site communities are critical in co-creating connections for underserved populations in the Sioux Falls area: "Representing different disciplines and areas of interest and expertise (public and private entities, healthcare and social action, and education), all are committed to the creation and implementation of the model" (Bunkers et al, 1999, p 98). From a human becoming perspective, "the nurse knows quality of life is different for everyone and s/he does not expect people to live a certain set of norms to achieve it" (Parse, 1997, p 172). Thus each site community will voice different expectations concerning their quality of life and how they want to live their health. Nursing practice in the site communities that addresses quality of life issues is guided by the model's conceptual framework.

Developing a Conceptual Framework

Nursing theories and conceptual frameworks provide a nursing science foundation for practice models in community. The unique contributions of the discipline of nursing can be derived from this nursing science base. Those imaging the vision for a community nursing practice model identify the nursing theory whose values and beliefs they choose to guide the nursing practice. Once a nursing theory is selected, drawing the conceptual framework for the model is helpful to articulate the values, beliefs, and focus for nursing practice. For example, HAMPIC is based on Parse's theory of human becoming (Bunkers et al, 1999). Parse writes concerning the human becoming theory as a guide to practice:

With Parse's human becoming theory as a guide to practice, the nurse's major focus is on the meaning the person or family give [sic] to the situation. The nurse is with individuals and families as they describe their meanings and move with their choices of hopes and dreams. The nurse in true presence is *there with* the other as the other discovers new meanings along his or her own way of life. The nurse does not try to force persons to do things that they find upsetting; the person is respected as the guide to choosing personal patterns of health (Parse, 1996, p 58).

Developing a conceptual framework based on nursing theory to guide practice "contributes to fortifying nursing's identity as a scientific discipline, the practice of which is unique in the health care system" (Parse, 1996, p 55). With nursing theory-based practice focused on co-creating with communities, a nursing practice model can evolve where "the main concern is the person's perspective of health" (Parse, 1996, p 55).

Naming Operational Components

In the development of a community nursing practice model, it is important to identify the essential components that operationalize the work of the model. These model components must be developed thoughtfully, with ongoing consultation with the community. For example, HAMPIC "consists of three simultaneous integrating components—advanced practice nursing, the steering committee, and site communities" (Bunkers et al, 1999, p 96). Each of these components is clearly developed with designated roles and responsibilities. At the same time, however, there is openness to modifications as healthcare issues surface in the site communities. In fact, modifications have been made in all three components of HAMPIC since its inception. In the advanced practice nursing component, staff have been added due to the increasing demand for the services of HAMPIC; the Steering Committee has expanded with several new members joining from community sites; and two new site community projects have been added that include working with youth in neighborhoods and with elders in a day care and community dining site. The components of a community nursing practice model can continuously evolve and expand as long as they have been clearly identified and developed. The model components form the operational structure of the healthcare delivery model.

Creating a Documentation System

A documentation system for a new community nursing practice model must respond to the overarching objectives of the model and be consistent with the nursing theoretical framework guiding the model. Such a documentation system includes forms for ongoing monitoring of individual or community health plans and ongoing evaluation processes. For example, in HAMPIC, booklets were created for individuals or communities to use to describe their personal health descriptions (Bunkers et al, 1999). The personal health descriptions, consistent with the theory of human becoming, are written in the words of the person, family, or community. The personal health descriptions include: "What life is like for me now; My health concerns are . . . ; What is most important for me now . . . ; My hopes for the future are . . . ; My plans for the future are . . . ; How I can carry out my plans . . . ; My specific health action plan is . . ." (Bunkers et al, 1999, p 97). A variety of additional documentation forms have been created to facilitate the work of the model. A conceptually consistent documentation system is the foundation for the development of meaningful and concise evaluations that report the effectiveness of the practice model to the larger community.

Participating in Teaching-Learning Processes

To create theory-based community nursing practice models, nursing professionals and others involved must participate in ongoing teaching-learning processes. The nursing theory guiding the model must be studied and discussed with all involved. It is essential to seek the involvement of nursing scholars with expertise in the nursing theory used to guide the practice. The depth and degree of study of the theory will depend on the person(s)' level of involvement in the practice model. For example, Parse identifies the following four essentials to successfully integrate the human becoming theory as a basis for nursing practice:

Willing learners who have freely chosen a commitment to learning and living the theory; consistent administrative support evidenced in attitude and allocation of time and resources; an on-site master's-prepared nurse who is knowledgeable about the theory in practice and whose job description includes teaching the theory; regular consultation with theory-in-practice experts, both on-site and through telecommunications (Parse, 1996, p 59).

Thus all participants in the community practice model must make a considerable commitment to theory-based practice. Ongoing discussions and teaching-learning processes can be woven throughout the components of the model. For example, in HAMPIC, an aspect of the human becoming theory is presented at each Steering Committee meeting (Bunkers et al, 1999). In one clinic location, a staff meeting was held where the physicians and other allied health personnel were introduced to the human becoming perspective.

Obtaining Funding

One of the most challenging aspects of creating new and innovative practice models is to search for and obtain sources of funding that will ensure long-term success of the model. Funding that includes local, state, and national resources should be explored, as well as both private and public sources of funding. Again, the purpose and objectives of the model must be communicated clearly and concisely to potential funders. To expand one's resource base, the community nursing practice model must link with community organizations that affirm the model's vision. The original funding for HAMPIC involved local private and public sources, including Augustana College, Sioux Valley Health System Community Fund, Sioux Falls Area Foundation, Sioux Falls School District Head Start Program, and the Sioux Empire United Way.

In *Building Partnerships,* Richards writes, *"The new linking organization itself must have a vision.* Organizations must continually seek to define a vision—one that all participants recognize and affirm—to sustain long-term efforts" (Richards, 1996, p 189). An example of this organizational linking exists within HAMPIC (Bunkers et al, 1999). Sioux River Valley Community Health Center in Sioux Falls, one of the original site communities for the model, decided it wanted to develop the advanced practice nursing role of HAMPIC into its ongoing operations, thus contracting for the time of one advanced practice nurse in the model. This contractual agreement creates an ongoing funding source. Having research and evaluation processes in place, which can help demonstrate the effectiveness of the community nursing practice model, is essential to obtain ongoing funding.

Conducting Research

Research, whether qualitative or quantitative, basic or applied, needs a primary place of importance within a community nursing practice model. The nursing theory and conceptual framework guiding the practice model will determine much of the focus for research. For example, Parse's theory of human becoming encompasses two types of research studies: basic research that focuses on uncovering the structure of lived experiences of health and applied research, "the goal of which is to evaluate human becoming as a guide to practice" (Parse, 1996, p 61).

In HAMPIC, the project director is presently conducting a study on "The Lived Experience of Feeling Cared For" with women who are struggling to become economically and socially self-sufficient (Bunkers et al, 1999). Parse's basic phenomenological-hermeneutical research methodology is guiding the study. The research will add to the understanding of human experiences and will expand the knowledge base of the human becoming theory, thus informing nursing practice. Persons involved with HAMPIC will be presented with the findings of this study.

Publishing the Prototype

The importance of publishing the work of co-creating theory-based community nursing models must be underscored. Publishing new prototypes for practice informs the members of the discipline of nursing, other healthcare disciplines, and the public on what is possible; it keeps the agenda for healthcare reform and change in health policy alive. Individual stories, documentation of program operations, conceptual framework, and model development efforts are all important for publication. Imaging the vision and sharing the vision in publications contribute to the ongoing development of the discipline of nursing, as well as to the "betterment of humankind" (Parse, 1998, p 95).

Persons and communities are the coauthors of health and care. This coauthorship involves a complex interconnectedness of person and community. Theory-based community nursing practice models that trust in the possibilities of this interconnectedness can create new and uncharted places. These uncharted places hold the promise of tomorrow.

REFERENCES

Bunkers SS, Michaels C, Ethridge P: Advanced practice nursing in community: nursing's opportunity, *Adv Pract Nurs* Q 2(4):79-84, 1997.

Bunkers SS, Nelson M, Leuning C, et al: The health action model: academia's partnership with the community. In Cohen E, De Back V, editors: *The outcomes mandate: case management in healthcare today*, St Louis, 1999, Mosby.

Cody W: Radical health-care reform: the person as case manager, *Nurs Sci Q* 7:180-182, 1994.

Harding V: Out of the cauldron of struggle: black religion and the search for a new America, *Soundings* 61(3): 350-351, 1978.

Heidegger M: *Being and time*, New York, 1962, Harper & Row.

Helminski K: *Living presence: a Sufi way to mindfulness and the essential self*, New York, 1992, Putnam.

Palmer P: *The company of strangers*, New York, 1997, Crossroad.

Parse RR: Health: a personal commitment, *Nurs Sci Q* 3:136-140, 1990.

Parse RR: Quality of life: sciencing and living the art of human becoming, *Nurs Sci Q* 7:16-21, 1994.

Parse RR: The human becoming theory: challenges in practice and research, *Nurs Sci Q* 9:55-60, Copyright 1996 by Sage Inc. Quotes reprinted by permission of Sage Publications.

Parse RR: The human becoming theory: the was, is, and will be, *Nurs Sci Q* 10:32-38, 1997.

Parse RR: *The human becoming school of thought*, Thousand Oaks, Calif, 1998, Sage.

Parse RR: Community: an alternative view, *Nurs Sci Q* 12:119-121, 1999.

Richards R: *Building partnerships: educating health professionals for the communities they serve*, San Francisco, 1996, Jossey-Bass.

12

Nurse/Physician Partnerships: Essential to Care Management?

Ruth A. Hanson

KEY LESSONS IN THIS CHAPTER

- Physicians, partnered with seasoned nurse managers, can be effective change agents in improving the quality and efficiency of patient care delivery systems.
- Financial viability should not be the only compelling incentive driving healthcare organizations.
- Excellent care management is a blend of both quality and cost-effectiveness.
- Nurses and physicians are the two constant players needed to design, deliver, and manage patient care.
- Virtually all organizations must learn that political, social, and economic partnerships are necessary building blocks for their sustainable future.

What differentiates managed care from care management? What is the relationship between managing patient care and nurse/physician partnerships? How can infrastructure facilitate these partnerships? What are the outcomes of nurses, physicians, and others working in collaboration to design and deliver patient care? MeritCare Health System, based in Fargo, North Dakota, is nearly 2 years into a bold new company design that features formal partnerships among nurses and physicians in leadership positions. The hypothesis driving the design was this: physicians, in accountable, decision-making roles, partnered with seasoned nurse managers, would be effective change agents and would better position the company to improve the quality and efficiency of patient care delivered throughout the system.

IN THE BEGINNING

Once there was a tertiary care hospital physically attached to a multispecialty clinic. They shared patients but remained quite separate in most ways, including ownership, governance, personnel, resources, and culture. Both were founded in the early 1900s and coexisted for the most part like toddlers in parallel play. Along came diagnosis-related groups (DRGs), health maintenance organizations (HMOs), and other rude awakenings as managed care entered the healthcare horizon. Compete or collaborate? became the question for these two successful but separate healthcare organizations who boasted a number of duplicative services. Merger talks commenced. After several intense months, negotiations were suspended for 18 months. Talks were reopened, and today these two entities comprise MeritCare Health System (MCHS), which is a not-for-profit integrated physician-hospital health system, created in 1993 with the merger of the former Fargo Clinic and St. Luke's Hospitals in Fargo, North Dakota. (For specific demographics, see Appendix 12-1, Who Is MeritCare Health System? at the end of this chapter, or take a virtual tour on MeritCare's Website at http://www. meritcare.com.) The merger was a significant milestone in the transformation of MCHS into a company designed as a collaborative matrix, with formal nurse and physician partnerships leading all clinical services.

Role of Nurses and Physicians

Nurses and physicians are constant players in nearly every patient care experience. Depending on the individual patient and his or her family, many other disciplines are essential to complement medical and nursing care. Research has demonstrated that nurse/physician collaboration results in better patient outcomes (decreased mortality and morbidity) (Knaus et al, 1986). If one believes what Wheatley says, "None of us exists independent of our relationships with others," it makes good sense to intentionally focus on building relationships among nurses, physicians, and other colleagues (Wheatley, 1999, p 35). Building relationships is what MCHS did when it created its new organizational design, which is described in a later section.

Physicians are facing many transitions: from independent loners to interdependent team members, from competing with hospitals and other providers to partnering and collaborating, from avoiding financial risk to sharing risk. Physicians were not taught to be partners; they were taught to be sole decision makers. Porter-O'Grady, Hawkins, and Parker observe:

MDs have been acculturated to share power with no one, not even their own peers. Physicians are no longer customers in the health system. They are instead partners, creating a whole new set of relationships. The independent and unilateral practice of medicine in America is now dead. The physician of the future will exemplify a partner approach to practice in a much stronger team orientation (Porter-O'Grady, Hawkins, and Parker, 1997, pp 192-195).

As pivotal players on both sides of the cost/revenue balance sheet, physicians are also critical stakeholders in effective care management and practice redesign. When MCHS envisioned what the ideal nurse/physician partnerships could accomplish, several assumptions were made. Physician partners in formal leadership roles will do the following:

1. Address physician culture and behavioral issues
2. Facilitate standardization of clinical practice
3. Maintain their clinical practices, balanced with administrative hours
4. Build "ownership" and accountability for MCHS's performance among physician colleagues
5. Acquire new skills and management competencies
6. Challenge the paradigm that physicians are "superior" partners
7. Eliminate the need for a separate physician management structure

ORGANIZATION DESIGN PROCESS AND CRITERIA

Taking a proactive stance in 1996, Dr. Roger Gilbertson, MCHS's chief executive officer (CEO), began to lead the company through its own creative design process, guided by these mutually established expectations. The new company will do the following:

1. Integrate physicians into accountable decision-making roles
2. Facilitate physician/nonphysician partnerships
3. Facilitate cohesive connections across settings of care and among service areas
4. Instill ownership in associates across the system
5. Facilitate alignment of cultures
6. Enable prioritization, coordination, and tracking of systemwide projects
7. Enable standardization and implementation of appropriate processes
8. Promote consciousness of systems (systems thinking) and minimize internal competition
9. Balance line responsibilities with system requirements
10. Clarify accountabilities
11. Facilitate allocation of resources
12. Facilitate decision making
13. Facilitate communication

When Gilbertson introduced the new design, he emphasized, "The way we do our work (culture) is as important to customer satisfaction, bottom line, etc., [sic] as the work we do. MeritCare's new organizational design addresses the way we do our work." The structure facilitates interaction among clinical and support services across the health system. All clinical services, both inpatient and ambulatory, are led by two senior executives, a physician and a nurse. The senior executive who leads support services (e.g., human resources, material services, financial services) also serves as the chief financial officer (CFO). A chief information officer (CIO) and in-house general legal counsel complete the senior executive team.

During the design phase, the two major components of the matrix model were nicknamed *Clinical* and *Everything Else*. The entire MeritCare company is organized into intersecting clinical and support services, called *aggregates* (Figure 12-1). All clinical aggregates (e.g., heart services, oncology services) are co-led by two executive partners (EPs), a physician

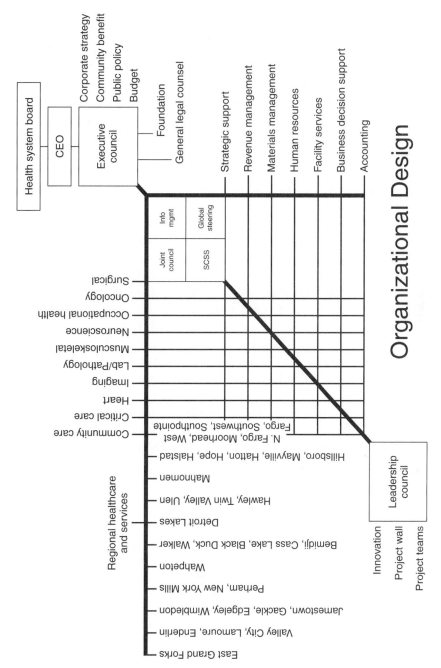

Figure 12-1　MeritCare Health System's organizational matrix design. (From MeritCare Health System, Fargo, North Dakota.)

and a nurse or other clinician. This physician/nonphysician partnership model is replicated within each clinical aggregate at the point of service. (At this level, the physician leaders are called *managing physician partners* [MPPs], and their counterparts, usually nurses, are managing partners.) All formal physician leaders share accountability for business, as well as clinical performance outcomes. Support service aggregates, such as human resources and material services, are led by one nonphysician EP. In the clinical arena, a unique aggregate, system and clinical support services, provides focus and staff support for education and development, research, quality improvement projects, and development of practice guidelines and clinical pathways. The physician leader of this group is also the assistant dean of the local campus of the University of North Dakota School of Medicine and Health Sciences and oversees the clinical practice experience of all medical students and residents.

MANAGED CARE: A SUBSET OF CARE MANAGEMENT

Managed care is defined by Reinhardt as the "external monitoring and co-managing of an ongoing physician-patient relationship, to ensure that the provider delivers *only* appropriate care" (Reinhardt, 1994, p 277). Managed care is intended to control costs while maintaining quality and access to appropriate care. To be successful under managed care contracts, healthcare providers must be good managers of care and conscientious stewards of the resources they use to provide care. Financial viability should not be the only compelling incentive to improve patient care management. Dr. Bruce Pitts, MCHS's physician leader of quality management, has repeatedly emphasized, "Ethically, our care must not differ among patients covered by different health plans; rather, we must learn to manage care consistently well for all patients." He defines quality care as care that adds value instead of cost.

The phrase *care management* evokes many images, including coordination, integration, standardization, timing, sequencing, streamlining, patient advocacy, holistic assessment, and tailoring to address individual needs. Ideal care management has three cardinal aims: patient/family satisfaction, clinical quality, and fiscally sound utilization of resources. Cohen and Michaels provide this insightful description:

Care management is a way for clinicians to link their disciplinary efforts, programs, and services across the continuum of care for the benefit of patients in like situations. To be effective, care management needs to be cycled across the continuum—at a minimum from the hospital to home, and across primary or specialty care settings. The necessary clinical mindset for care management is to consider one's patient care unit as the entire continuum of care, not just a single point on that continuum, like a medical-surgical unit or home health. As such, no patient is ever discharged, but moves along the continuum of care matched to self-care or whatever services are needed to support health and well-being. Then, by developing clinical guidelines and linkages to weave together disciplinary efforts within the multiple points across the continuum of care, the therapeutic relationship between interdisciplinary providers and patients is supported rather than 'taken over,' as is the case with many clinical protocols and mandates (Cohen and Michaels, 2001, p 33).

CARE MANAGEMENT AND NURSE/PHYSICIAN PARTNERSHIPS AT MERITCARE HEALTH SYSTEM

Although North Dakota lags behind Minnesota in managed care penetration, care coordination and management is an ongoing MCHS strategic priority. Current goals include the following:

- Reducing variation in chronic disease assessment and care management practices across settings
- Improving care coordination among multiple providers who manage patients with chronic health conditions through the designation of a primary care provider
- Redefining provider roles

The development and implementation of interdisciplinary clinical pathways in the early 1990s ushered in a more disciplined partnership approach to care management at MCHS. By 1995, over 3000 patients had been managed on pathways, length of stay was decreased by 4700 days, direct costs were decreased more than $4 million, and the level of patient satisfaction was maintained or increased. Several clinical practice guidelines have also been developed to standardize and streamline care. Tools such as pathways and guidelines, however, are relevant only if developed in partnership with all care providers. From the very beginning, MCHS engaged physicians and other discipline members in the development of pathways, and today, new physicians are hired with the understanding and expectation that they will adopt existing pathways. At MCHS, all orthopedic surgeons follow the same pathway (and use the same hip and knee prostheses), and all cardiovascular surgeons follow the same pathway for open heart surgery and other procedures. Since being named EPs, the nurse and physician leaders of surgical services have successfully implemented standardized procedure packs versus "designer packs" for individual surgeons, which is a major breakthrough.

PROPERTIES AND PRINCIPLES OF PARTNERSHIP

"Partnership is an unnatural act between two nonconsenting adults. Partnership, while intuitive, is not done naturally" (Troseth, 1999). This witty definition offered by Troseth, who researched nurse/physician partnerships for her master's thesis, implies that partnership requires intentional investment. Porter-O'Grady and Krueger Wilson concur: "Partnership does not occur without effort; rather, partnerships must be created. They demand a mutual value that drives the players into the relationship and requires work to define the essential characteristics of the partnership" (Porter-O'Grady and Krueger Wilson, 1998, p 13). Partnership is a work in progress requiring continual renegotiation, dialogue, and renewal. MCHS's approach to partnership has been shaped by three experts who share synchronous views. Peter Block, Tim Porter-O'Grady, and Bonnie Wesorick all have served as on-site consultants to MCHS leaders.

Bonnie Wesorick, president and founder of the Clinical Practice Model Resource Center, author, and mentor, has taught MCHS much about partnership. Partnership within a systems thinking framework is the essence of her professional practice model. Wesorick (1995) describes partnership as a mental model for relationships that nourish others. She has discovered that although many people can describe a positive working relationship, they do not know how to make it happen. Wesorick (1995) describes partnership as a conscious decision or a choice to go beyond the superficial, the robotic, and the physical domain. Partners dare to be different and to take risks and can address conflict without intimidation. Through her research, Wesorick (1995) has distilled the following six principles underlying partnership:

1. *Intention:* a personal choice to connect with another at a deeper level of humanness
2. *Mission:* a call to live out something that matters or is meaningful
3. *Equal accountability:* a relationship driven by ownership of mission, not power or fear
4. *Potential:* an inherent capacity within oneself and others to continuously learn, grow, and create
5. *Balance:* a harmony of relationships with self and others necessary to achieve one's mission
6. *Trust:* a sense of synchrony on important issues or things that matter.

In his book *Stewardship: Choosing Service over Self-Interest,* Block (1993) outlines the following four requirements of partnership:

1. Exchange of purpose
2. Right to say no (partnership does not mean you always get what you want)
3. Joint accountability; each person is responsible for the outcomes and the current situation. (There is no else to blame.)
4. Absolute honesty.

Partnership demands that there be a sense of equality between the players. Each person contributes something of value to the relationship and needs to be honored for that contribution. Also, each partner's expectations include the right to receive full value from the relationship. Each member must give fully to the work of the partnership to advance the partnership and ensure it produces desired outcomes (Porter-O'Grady and Krueger Wilson, 1998, p 15).

Partnership also requires clarity and honesty of interaction so that each member is able and free to bring up issues and concerns regarding the character of the partnership. When he met with MCHS leaders, Porter-O'Grady illustrated the following properties of partnership:

- Role expectations are negotiated.
- Equality exists between the players.
- Relationships are founded on shared risk.
- Expectations and contributions of each person are clear.
- Solid measures of contribution to outcomes are established.
- Horizontal links are well defined.

SO WHERE ARE WE, REALLY? ACTUALIZED VISION, FAIRY TALE, OR SOMEWHERE IN BETWEEN?

To find out where we really were, this author interviewed nurse/physician partners. (Their responses are presented in the next section of this chapter.) They were asked to define partnership and care management and to talk about how they have been affected by the new design. A physician partner shared this metaphor, "Like a three-legged race, partners need common goals, or they trip over one another and get nowhere." Another observed that "partnership takes practice, communication, commitment, and collaboration." One of the nurse partners explained his partnership this way: "We think completely differently, but we think about the same things. Having different approaches is the beauty of a partnership because one may work better than the other. Both of us know our destination, and there are lots of ways to get 'there.'" A different nurse partner stressed this advantage: "Partnership allows you to examine issues from a broader perspective. Decisions are more sound and long lasting, because together partners see a more complete picture. It's like creating an orchestra . . . who plays what and when. It doesn't happen overnight." Another nurse partner observed, "Having a physician partner is absolutely phenomenal. Their clinical expertise is critical for managing accurate coding and understanding denials of payment."

Common Partnership Views

Many common themes were expressed in the nurses' and physicians' responses, which are highlighted as follows:

Partnership is:
- Having a common vision and goals but different approaches
- Synergistic; being more effective as a team than either could be individually
- Stimulating us to learn new things
- Having the best of two worlds because two can see more of the universe
- Sharing responsibility and accountability for the work
- Standing together on tough decisions
- Complementing each other's talents

Partnership is not:
- Hierarchical (one partner considered "superior")
- Judgmental
- Controlling (power over another)

Successful partnerships are built on:
- Trust, honesty, and the ability to speak freely
- Collaboration versus competition
- Sense of equity among the partners
- Listening actively to understand, not just reacting
- Equal commitment to making it work
- Mutual mission, vision, and values
- Mutual successes and crises
- Appreciation for the other's unique skill sets

Advantages of a Nurse/Physician Partnership

Nurses and physicians share a common heritage, namely, patient care. Having a physician partner gives the nurse the "whole" picture. It strengthens the capacity of the team to work with all physicians and to address medical issues of care delivery. Because physicians respect and respond more readily to peers, physician leaders are able to facilitate practice changes by "walking the talk" and role modeling the desired change. Physicians need to be key players in quality improvement. Now they are participating; they bring good ideas and are developing an appreciation for the need to standardize. They are developing a sense of ownership in MCHS and are realizing that if MCHS does not do well, neither will they. This attitude also leads to wiser use of resources.

What Are the Components of Care Management?

The goals of care management are optimal patient outcomes (including a peaceful death), timeliness, and cost-effectiveness. Care management requires an interdisciplinary and holistic (body/mind/spirit/financial) approach to patient care that deals with all aspects related to care. Failure to address financial issues can result in family stress and lack of coordination of patient care. Forming partnerships with patients can help manage their care and their cost of care.

Excellent care management is a blend of both quality and cost-effectiveness. Financial stewardship is *not* in conflict with quality patient care; it is using resources wisely, providing the right care, moving the patient effectively through the system, and moving beyond the walls to tackle hot spots "upstream" in the community.

What Does Ideal Patient Care Management Look Like?

When asked, "What would ideal patient care management look like?" the nurse/physician partners responded with the following characteristics:
1. Processes of care are designed by all players who contribute to patient care (e.g., continuum pathways).
2. Every player ensures personal accountability for his or her aspect of care and works with team members to monitor quality and reduce variation.
3. Everyone owns the outcomes, whether good or bad; no one service takes credit or blame.
4. Patient experience is seamless.
5. Communication is open, and there is a feeling of trust.
6. Data is readily accessible in a timely manner.

What Impact Has the New Design Had?

A third question posed in every interview, "What impact do you think the new organizational design is having on partnership and care management?" evoked several observations, which are listed as follows:
- Patients expect and deserve consistency and collaboration across providers and fast, flexible service. The integrated organization of MCHS is an advantage because acute care and ambulatory care can be connected under one system with the same infrastructure.
- The merger and new design facilitate standardization of care and conservation of resources. When physicians are not part of the system, they do not necessarily share nurses' vision or goals. It is much easier to implement changes when physicians are employees of the system.

- Accountability is shared without blame or finger pointing. Energy is focused in a positive way.
- It is now much smoother to convert 350 physicians to new systems.
- Physician partners who are active members of operations become better able to share information and rationales with peer physicians.
- "Class distinction" and privilege are evening out, and there is a blurring of roles. Physicians will soon be paid on market value just like everyone else.
- Care management is facilitated by the new aggregate structures. The services required for the entire patient care continuum are in one group and one team, so they have a better view of the whole picture and the flow of care across settings. Programs that take the whole picture into account are being developed. Care teams have a broader systematic view and are better connected to essential support services such as finance and information systems.
- Selection versus election for physician leadership roles has changed the playing field. Competency and commitment are the new criteria versus the "old boys' club" politics.
- The broker concept of aligning consistent business experts with clinical aggregates has forged new relationships between clinicians and financial analysts.

*V*IGNETTES: Interviews with Nurse/Physician Partners

■ **Jeff Hoss, RN, and Rich Wacksman, MD**
Executive Partners of Critical Care Services (emergency center, walk-in clinic, medical surgical intensive care unit and acute inpatient units, air ambulance service, renal transplant program)
Jeff: Managers are seeing a more systemic view and are willing to help each other. This didn't used to happen. They have voluntarily put things on hold in one area so another service can proceed with something more pressing.
Rich: The new design fosters relationships among nurses and physicians at all levels. They don't clash any more. They have common goals. In the past, the traditional physician role was very different. For example, the medical director of the [emergency room] ER was often in conflict with the nurse manager. Now people are willing to help across services; RNs and MDs are working closer together to solve common problems.
Jeff: A huge positive has been the change from a medical director to a managing physician partner (MPP) position. Medical directors were basically knighted, with no clear expectations of their role. The MPP is selected and has a defined job description. The MPPs in our aggregate are very committed and function as partners with the nurse managers. They attend every meeting; they listen. Our walk-in clinic had never met its budget contribution. In one quarter, the MPP has turned that around. He takes resource management very seriously; he looks into all issues. Because of his leadership, the physician culture is changing. The old culture was characterized by physicians asking, "What is MeritCare going to do for me?" The new cultural message is changing to, "My job is patient care, and MeritCare provides the resources I need to deliver that care."

■ **Kathy Hanish, RN, and John Leitch, MD**
Executive Partners of Oncology Services
(Roger Maris Cancer Center, inpatient oncology, radiology oncology)
Kathy: Non-MD managers couldn't begin to influence physician practice in the same way that peer MDs can. A good example was when we started using the templates for dictation. It means much more coming from

John, because he lives and works with the same changes they have to. Clinical improvements can't happen without physician partners; their expert knowledge is a must. For example, they know which patient can safely be treated with generic drugs. They also can identify new ways of using existing modalities in more cost-effective ways. Nonphysicians don't have the clinical knowledge, nor do they have the same influence. Physicians are now partnering with our doctorate-prepared pharmacists who have bioequivalence data to better manage drug choice. Sometimes the choices may vary in cost from $2 to $200! And in the past, MDs didn't necessarily have this information.

Physician EPs have some development needs. They need to learn the art and science of management. But they have validity, by virtue of being a physician, to lead change among other physicians. If they have always been a part of a big clinic, they don't know the business side of healthcare and haven't had management training or experience. Stellar clinical expertise is not enough. If you have poor business skills, you will repeatedly go out of business. You have to bill correctly, dictate correctly, and meet requirements for reimbursement. Just because you work hard doesn't mean you will get paid. Physicians who have never had their own business don't understand this. They have been insulated. Other team members need to support the physicians so they can do their work to achieve the best outcomes. If the physician doesn't get paid, we won't either.

John: I value Kathy's experience in administration and her ability to manage various personnel issues, be they managerial, nursing, physician, etc. in a fair and straightforward manner. She has the ability to prioritize aggregate projects and work on many simultaneously. She works hard and takes pride in her work and, most importantly, the achievements of the people she leads. I depend on Kathy for feedback, criticism, information, and help with administrative issues about which I have little knowledge. I enjoy the challenges and exchange of information and ideas that our joint administrative responsibilities generate.

Kathy: Physicians are learning that they can't be a part of a group and function like they are in solo practice. As we focus on access problems, collect the data, and report on it, physicians are beginning to see why they need to think as a group. Some want the advantage of group practice and none of the responsibility. That's been one of the biggest frustrations.

John: We are making progress. There is a greater understanding that standardization, outcomes measurement, and [plan-do-check-act] PDCA cycles need the "joint" effort of everyone involved and are the keys to improving healthcare.

Kathy: John and I may disagree on approaches but *not* on our messages. I may move quicker than John. He is learning to be more firm, and I am learning to be more polished.

John: We are in the midst of a revolution in healthcare. Legislation may catalyze even more rapid change. The new design places us in the best position to adapt to change.

■ Evelyn Quigley, RN, and Bruce Pitts, MD
Senior Executive Partners of System and Clinical Support Services

Bruce: We all have arranged marriages. These can and do work in Eastern culture, but they work because of support and nurturing from both families who brought them together, strong cultural traditions, and clear rules and objectives. In business terms, parallels for developing healthy partnerships might be clear roles and expectations, culture that values the relationships, and clear objectives.

Evelyn: From a global perspective, partnership was introduced around our mission, values, and core beliefs for MCHS. Partnerships exist at all levels, but it is the RN/MD partners at the point of service who will be our movers and shakers, depending on the organizational support they have. The opportunities for creativity at point of service are remarkable! Bruce and I are very clear on the ultimate goal of moving the partnership to the bedside/point-of-service. We have a formal partnership now, but we also had a strong relationship prior to being named [executive partners] EPs. It was driven by skill set and interests related to quality improvement.

Bruce: One disturbing caveat occurs to me. Care management is not just dependent on RN/physician partnerships. Nurses and doctors don't have all the skills they need to manage patient care. They need others.

Any project undertaken to change the way care is delivered, such as development of guidelines, pathways, and work redesign, are all facilitated by partnerships among RNs, physicians, financial experts, and others. The essential ingredient is getting the people together who have some insight into the process (who do the work) and allowing them to change it. That invariably involves doctors and nurses. The RN and physician are constants, but many other partners, such as facilitators, analysts, educators, and receptionists, are also necessary.

The role of discipline/professional specific affiliations also comes into play. The goal in care management is to bring better value to patients. To accomplish this we need to blur boundaries across disciplines, renegotiate roles, and blur hierarchy among RNs and physicians to provide better value at a lower cost to the family. The partnerships we are building are challenging the traditional relationships that have existed among physicians and RNs. When it comes to patient care, the boundaries should become meaningless.

Evelyn: Effecting change requires partnership and creative leadership. It takes creativity to make guidelines and pathways work in different sites with different teams. That's part of managing change.

Bruce: For example, to implement diabetes guidelines, the minimum specifications of the redesign are stated, and then it becomes the accountability of the clinicians to work out implementation. We expect implementation approaches to vary across sites, but all must achieve better diabetes care. Every detail of how is not scripted. This has proved uncomfortable for the RN educator who wants more detail before she begins. The nurse becomes the teacher, and the doctor becomes the student. This role reversal is a radical paradigm shift, even though as residents, we all learned a great deal from nurses. It requires that the nurse renegotiate his or her roles with the physician, who may have a hard time accepting the change.

Evelyn: This is a major challenge for nurses, who have historically been highly controlled and regulated.

Bruce: My vision of the future is that highly skilled nurses, partnered with physicians, will transform care to a higher quality by becoming protectors of the guidelines and outcomes. Ingredients for success will include:

- RNs who are confident enough to renegotiate roles with physicians
- Relationship-building skills
- Tools such as practice guidelines, evaluation criteria, and processes
- Minimum specifications
- A dose of creativity and freedom to shape practice and approaches to fit each setting

■ Joan Justesen, RN, and Greg Post, MD
Senior Executives for all Clinical Services
(All clinical executive partners report to Joan and Greg.)

Joan: Partnership means equal/mutual accountability. It requires trust and being intentional. You have to talk about the relationship. You don't instantly become partners. It's a becoming process. Each partner has personal strengths and needs to build on them. I can't walk in the shoes of a physician, but Greg can.

Greg: Partners need to intentionally communicate on a daily basis. Our communication needs to be a mirror image to foster credibility. It shouldn't matter which of us is at a meeting. Our message would be the same.

Joan: You need to be loyal; don't talk about one another behind his or her back . . . Be very deliberate about not saying anything disrespectful or that could be construed as condescending about each other or other senior executives. Partners need to focus on what, not who. The new design is good. Our partnership works well, and so should the EP's and MPP's manager partnerships. If the model works well at our level, it should work well at other levels.

Greg: Nurse/physician relationships have to be cultivated and taken to the point of service. In my department of urology, we hold weekly meetings with nurses. I have always treated nurses as equals and have dealt with patient issues and behavioral issues openly and honestly. When the urology joint practice council was formed, we included the inpatient nurses and other staff to look at the whole continuum. It's really a "no-brainer" to consider nurses as partners in care.

Joan: Partnerships require that you put egos and competition spirit aside. You can't always have the upper hand or the last word. Some of the reasons we struggle with building teams in healthcare can be linked directly back to how physicians are trained to stand alone and be the best. They need to learn new skills to partner effectively.

Greg: In some cases, we've forced partnerships. For example, the EPs were paired, and the MPPs were paired with managers. New relationships are developing at the point of service through aggregate planning meetings.

Joan: The new design has helped us look more broadly at the continuum. Ideally the patient is in the center. We learn the patient's story and tailor their care to them. More caregivers are paying attention to patient flow and not leaving out or forgetting key players. For example, home health is integrated.

Greg: The building blocks of care management are common mission and vision, electronic connections, and stakeholder involvement. MCHS has all of these in place now. It's very exciting to see it coming together. From a patient standpoint, their data flows readily across the system from primary care to specialty [care] and back, and it's all within one system because all elements are connected.

Greg: Communication across aggregates is heightened. More people are starting to think about the domino effect (i.e., what they do has an effect on others). Before, with our strategic planning, it was separate from budget process. Now they are connected.

Joan: The budgeting process in the last 2 years has brought more people into the loop. Patient care is the driving force. For example, patient safety was the number-one priority used to evaluate new technology. Will it improve patient care is always a consideration. Having financial brokers assigned to each aggregate is facilitating business decisions. It also connects clinical and support services as partners. Business and clinical concerns are intertwined. We have to work together in the new design. Clinicians weren't trained in finance, so this connection is necessary. Compliance and coding is another example of a partnership between clinicians and business experts.

Greg: Implementing compliance requirements is challenging. Having MD leaders has made this easier. With partnerships, you gain credibility among stakeholders. For example, all the changes moving us closer to the electronic patient record (EPR) have been facilitated by them.

Joan: Partnership between managers and managing physician partners is critical to EPR progress. We are learning that the formal partnerships are much more effective in leading change than appointed coleaders of a task force.

Greg: The expected behaviors, principles, values, ethics, and ground rules spelled out for the new company all support partnerships.

Joan: You can't hide a poor fit anymore. If you lack a good fit, a change is made. Staff are relieved to see this.

Joan: I feel really good about how we have connected the rural community clinics with the main campus. We chose a good leader, and Greg and I have made many trips to the regional sites. We now are able to recruit much more readily for the regional clinics.

Greg: Clinical pathways, our work in defining best practices, and standardizing care are all making positive impacts on care management. And we have done this without sacrificing customer satisfaction. Our market share has increased. The new hospitalist service is improving patient care by ensuring expert medical care 24 hours/day. Hospitalists have no interruptions from office practice, and there are only two, so nurses have far fewer physicians to team with, which makes their work easier. We also now have job descriptions for managing physician partners, as well as the doctor on call, and we have a code of conduct for on-call physicians.

■ Carla Hansen, RN, and Craig Kouba, MD
Executive Partners of Heart Services

Craig: In 1986, cardiology began a pooled practice that was the beginning of a shift away from independent private practice. Up to this time, physicians all worked individually and covered everything for our patients. We all did things a little differently. The goal of our pooled practice was to manage the process (of seeing patients in the clinic and hospital) and improve work life for nurses and doctors. We began to see some advantage to uniformity, which laid the groundwork for pathway development. Pathway work led to greater respect for nurses' time and talent. Outcomes improved, and fewer variations and mistakes were made. It became clear to physicians that if the process was standardized, the outcomes got better, things happened quicker. They began to see value in working with nurses and others to design processes of care.

Carla: Early on, Craig and I identified values that we share and promise to hold consistently. They are:

- Quality care (have to be able to demonstrate it, monitor it, define it, and talk about it)
- Value of the team (recognizing that it takes people to provide quality care and that everyone's contributions are recognized as valuable)
- Viewing ourselves as members of the team with an administrative role, not as detached leaders.

MD/RN partnerships have been the key to bringing together the formerly very separate, strong hospital and clinic entities. Our aggregate is a microcosm of the hospital clinic merger. Premerger, we were a service line. I didn't have the accountability for the medical group practice. They were "over there," separate from the hospital. Now we have integrated the business; all inpatient and ambulatory departments are accountable for the success of the whole. We have a common bottom line.

Craig: I describe my role as a facilitator. I try to translate the importance of team behavior, which is in sharp contrast to the old guard, "lone wolf" mentality. I reinforce why changes are needed. As an MD partner, I can speak "doctor" to other MDs. Because I maintain a full clinical practice, work at the same level, and take the same call, when we have a meeting, my voice is just as authentic as anyone else's. This is a key piece. If I decreased my clinical time considerably, I think I would be viewed with skepticism by my MD colleagues. This requires my partner to share disproportionately in the work load. The bulk of the work detail has to reside with the non-MD partner. Carla does 95% of managing the business, yet decisions are joint. If decisions come across as single partner decisions, they are not viewed as favorably by the team as decisions that have clearly been made jointly. In the case of unpopular decisions, we stand together. Weekly leadership team meetings provide me with direct connections to leaders and leaders to other MDs. This keeps me current on issues, pitfalls, etc. and so when I hear conversation in the clinic (e.g., about hospital census issues), I know the situation firsthand and can be supportive.

Carla: The MD perspective broadens the team's thinking and can help identify early, potential hot spots or "Be careful"s and avoid some "I told you so"s.

Craig: Managing physician partners are also being paired with nurses, and they meet together with Carla and I. This is in the development phase now. The next evolution will see more operational management coming from these partners. Physicians are seeing the value of partnerships with nurses in several of our ambulatory programs, like the lipid clinic, congestive heart failure clinic, and cardiac rehabilitation/secondary prevention clinic. Interdisciplinary teams are more successful if the physician member is an active participant. When all the players come together, things happen, and they happen quickly. Things don't get left out. But if the physician is not an active member, it slows the progress. There is not much tolerance for that anymore. Replacements are quickly sought; "not playing" is no longer acceptable.

Carla: The new design has created many new partnerships across aggregates. We now have shared system-wide goals, values, and strategic and operational priorities that create greater collaboration and interdependency.

Craig: The physician EP leader position became accountable and thus has more effect on other physicians. (I felt like a figurehead when I was named service line medical director in 1992.) In the past, physicians would listen but not act. Change was slow. If you don't have the power to effect change, it didn't happen. "The gun is now loaded."

We are now able to deal with long overdue behavioral issues that cross aggregates. Issue resolution has required intense collaboration with other EPs because the players played in more than one playground, and singly, the behavior was not enough, but collectively, when the patterns were put together, the need to change became very clear. In the past, offenders could run to the other group and bargain; "divide and conquer." This was a sentinel moment; associates feel supported in bringing out tough issues. The expectation bar is higher.

Carla: Collaboration among physicians and nurses has increased and so has the team's ability to continuously monitor and improve quality. Changes in practice are ongoing and research-based. For example, revisions to our postprocedure care and assessment for cardiac catheterization has safely decreased the amount of bed rest and observation time needed, and pacemakers are now inserted in the cardiac catheterization laboratory.

Summary

DePree's partnership insights summarize what MCHS's nurse/physician partners are learning:

We need to be able to count on the other person's special competence. When we think about the people with whom we work, people on whom we depend, we can see that without each individual, we are not going to go very far as a group. By ourselves we suffer serious limitations. Together we can be something wonderful (DePree, 1989, p 50).

Nurses and physicians are the two constant players, with many other partners needed to design, deliver, and manage patient care. Having doctors at the table from the beginning is a huge asset. It provides a more complete picture and facilitates sound financial and medical decisions that are more timely. The historic "we/they" paradigm is being replaced with a "we are one and the same; if MCHS does not do well, neither will we" paradigm. Formal physician leaders can influence and change behavior and practice. They know the work, they do the work, they "walk the talk," and when they speak, peer physicians listen.

Partnership is essential to building relationships and is the foundation for constructing the future of organizations (Porter-O'Grady and Krueger Wilson, 1995). It is a work in progress, requiring ongoing dialogue, renegotiation, and renewal.

Partners bring different skill sets to the relationship; when differences are valued, each learns from the other; together they see a more complete picture, and they make more sound decisions.

FUTURE DIRECTIONS

The concept of partnership is driving changes at every level of the social order. Virtually all organizations will learn that political, social, and economic partnerships are necessary building blocks for their sustainable future.

By combining services into logical groups based on the customers served and bringing physicians into accountable leadership roles, MCHS has improved its decision-making and communication capabilities and its capacity to manage change. As an integrated system, MCHS is better equipped to address the health needs of the individuals, businesses, and communities it serves.

In terms of managed care, the physician will always be the main player, with the nurse a close second. As lines blur, managed care will influence future curricula in medicine, nursing, and other fields. New approaches will increase awareness and knowledge about the skill sets and contributions of others to patient care, and they will also challenge regulatory boundaries. We need to ask, What are the implications for nursing faculty? How will we increase collaboration between nurse administrators and deans of nursing and medicine?

MCHS is currently exploring the option of a formal partnership with Bonnie Wesorick and her resource center. MCHS leaders believe that implementation of her model is a logical next step to strengthen partnerships centered around managing patient care at the point of service.

The delivery of healthcare, which is affected by countless internal and external variables, is increasing in complexity at astonishing rates. The next skill that must be developed is how to manage complexity. As this new science becomes better understood, it may help MCHS leaders better manage nonlinear change, keeping the patient in the center of all their decisions.

REFERENCES

Block P: *Stewardship: choosing service over self-interest*, San Francisco, 1993, Berrett-Koehler.

Cohen EL, Michaels C: Two strategies for managing care: care management and case management. In Cohen EL, Cesta TG, editors: *Nursing case management: from essentials to advanced practice applications*, St Louis, 2001, Mosby.

DePree M: *Leadership is an art*, New York, 1989, Dell.

Knaus WA, Draper EA, Wagner DP, et al: An evaluation of outcomes from intensive care in major medical centers, *Ann Intern Med* 104:410-418, 1986.

Porter-O'Grady T, Hawkins M, Parker M: *Whole-systems shared governance: architecture for integration*, Gaithersburg, Md, 1997, Aspen.

Porter-O'Grady T, Krueger Wilson C: *The leadership revolution in healthcare: altering systems, changing behaviors*, Gaithersburg, Md, 1995, Aspen.

Porter-O'Grady T, Krueger Wilson C: *The healthcare team book*, St Louis, 1998, Mosby.

Reinhardt UE: Providing access to healthcare and controlling costs. In Lee P, Estes C, editors: *The nation's health*, ed 4, Boston, 1994, Jones & Bartlett.

Troseth MR: Physicians and you: the power is in partnering with each other, Panel presentation at the Clinical Practice Model International Conference, Fort Worth, Tex, Oct 7, 1999.

Wesorick B: *The closing and opening of a millennium: a journey from old to new thinking*, Grand Rapids, Mich, 1995, Practice Field.

Wheatley M: *Leadership and the new science: discovering order in a chaotic world*, San Francisco, 1999, Berrett-Koehler.

APPENDIX 12-1
Who is MeritCare Health System?

MeritCare Health System (MCHS) includes a 404-bed tertiary care hospital, a 330+ physician medical group, and 33 primary care clinics located throughout eastern North Dakota and western Minnesota. A telemedicine network connects 12 rural clinics with MCHS's main facility in Fargo, North Dakota. Other major components include the Roger Maris Cancer Center, and a Children's Hospital. Serving a population of 795,000 people in a predominantly rural environment, MCHS spans two states, North Dakota and Minnesota, and 50,000 square miles. MCHS offers a full line of heart, cancer, maternal child, surgical, orthopedic, and business health services, with care coordination provided between inpatient and outpatient settings. A 24-bed transitional care unit and home healthcare services complement acute care services, ensuring continuity of care between hospital and home. MCHS's commitment to education is evidenced in its active participation in over 75 student internship/clinical experience programs, including the University of North Dakota School of Medicine and Health Sciences. For more detailed information about MCHS or to take a virtual tour, access the MeritCare Website at http://www.meritcare.com.

13

Integrating Concepts of Managed Care and Nursing Case Management into Academic Curricula

Patricia A. Chin and Judith L. Papenhausen

KEY LESSONS IN THIS CHAPTER

- As case management has transcended from a mere trend to a common practice in nursing, nurse educators have recognized the need to incorporate managed care and case management into nursing curricula.
- The American Nurses Association, in a 1992 position statement on nursing case management, recommended a baccalaureate degree in nursing as the minimum preparation for assuming a nurse case manager position.
- Content and competencies for effective case management include foundational threads of healthcare finance and reimbursement and clinical and systems issues.
- Currently, it is not clear whether nursing case management will evolve into a unique new advanced practice role or whether the nursing case management process and strategies will be incorporated into other roles.
- As long as managed care and case management continue to evolve in the practice arena, it will be difficult to provide specific answers about the most effective ways to prepare professional nurses for the managed care environment.

Periodically, nursing practice is challenged by shifts in healthcare delivery and reimbursement of services. Since the mid-1980s, the phenomenon labeled *managed care* has been the driving force modifying and reshaping American healthcare. Some newly pervasive concepts do not enjoy widespread acceptance in practice or cannot withstand the rigors of research and eventually fade away, but that has not been the case with managed care.

Managed care concepts, including nursing case management strategies and interventions, have gained wide implementation in the American healthcare delivery system. This implementation has been due primarily to the potential financial gains and benefits to the system. Research regarding the fiscal advantages of these models and strategies can be found in healthcare delivery and nursing literature. Studies that examine the impact of case management strategies on the cost and quality of care delivery in general and on specific high-risk and vulnerable populations have emerged.

In response to the shifting managed care environment, several noticeable consequences for nursing education have occurred. Specific nursing case management models have been developed and adopted by major healthcare institutions. Population outcomes are being tracked and documented. Literature on managed care concepts and nursing case management has rapidly developed and has emanated beyond periodical literature into mainstream textbooks. These benchmarks indicate that nursing case management strategies have transcended the "nouveau trend" stage and have entered the nursing lexicon. Case management has become a viable choice as an effective, efficient nursing care strategy. Nurse educators have considered these events to be signals of the necessity to incorporate managed care and case management concepts into nursing curricula.

As is often the case when a new, innovative approach is introduced into practice, the academic community is initially interested yet cautious regarding inclusion into the mainstream content. Once models of managed care and case management have been forged in practice and tested and refined by research, however, they ultimately will be recognized as essential content by faculty of educational institutions for incorporation into the curriculum. Although this integration has already begun, the essential managed care concepts and the breadth and depth of coverage at the various levels of nursing education have yet to be universally established. Even the definition of managed care and case management remain ambiguous and are subject to regional influences.

There are considerable differences of opinion regarding which healthcare providers are best prepared to assume the role and responsibilities necessary for managing client care. Both nurses and nonnursing personnel have been assigned to case management positions. Agencies vary in the level of education and the type of preparation required for performing case management functions. Nurse educators and the healthcare industry also debate the educational preparation needed for functioning effectively in the position of nurse case manager. Some agencies use nurses prepared at the associate degree level, many agencies require preparation at the baccalaureate level, whereas others will hire only nurses prepared at the master's level (Koerner et al, 1989).

Ethridge and Lamb (1989) concluded that a minimum of a baccalaureate education is needed for competent nursing case management. Zander (1990) suggested that the baccalaureate degree be the minimum level of educational preparation unless the individual demonstrated highly developed skills in use of the nursing process, disease and system management, communication, and decision making. The American Nurses Association's (ANA) (1992) position statement on nursing case management also recommended a baccalaureate degree in nursing as the minimum preparation for assuming a nurse case manager position. As nursing case management has evolved over time, other authors have suggested that the development of the required capabilities and skills necessary for nursing case management are only possible through educational preparation at the advanced practice level (Hamric, 1992; Glettler and Leen, 1996; Mahn and Spross, 1996). With the current growth and expansion of managed care and case management and the demand for nurse case managers, however, it may not be practical to expect an educational preparation standard at the master's level (Conger, 1999).

Nurses must be familiar with managed care concepts and case management even if their practice areas are not directly identified as managed care systems. This chapter examines the integration of managed care and nursing case management skills and strategies into academic nursing curricula. The perspective offered regarding the integration of these concepts into academic nursing curricula is grounded by the authors' decade-long experience with case management in the progressive managed care environment of southern California. The discussion includes implications for associate degree, baccalaureate degree, and graduate degree programs. Suggestions for curriculum content, competencies, and student activities are provided to level academic curricula across the continuum. Components of sample syllabi of a baccalaureate theory course and a baccalaureate clinical course focusing on case management with high-risk clients are provided in Appendices 13-1 and 13-2 at the end of the chapter.

LITERATURE REVIEW

The challenge to nursing education is to prepare a healthcare provider who can function effectively in an integrated healthcare system. A review of current literature offers those interested in curriculum design and development limited insight for integration of content in the area of case management. Regional differences in the specifics of implementation of managed care and case management and the significant variations in the conceptualization of the term *nursing case management* across institutions also contribute to the uncertainty and challenge regarding curricular integration. Mundt (1996) identified several key elements for consideration for educational and curricular reform. Those elements included a client-centered approach, coordination of care and services across healthcare settings, an outcome orientation to planning and implementation of care, resource efficiency, and collaborative and cooperative team approaches to care. She proposed that the curriculum itself become the vehicle for teaching case management instead of merely interjecting case management concepts into traditional curriculum courses and unrelated independent student experiences. The latter method is an antiquated approach that results in fragmentation. Her discussion was general, however, and did not identify the specific content, capabilities, or activities to be used to drive educational case management curricula.

Much of the literature found in nursing education, nursing administration, and clinical nursing journals provides little beyond anecdotal reflections on personal experiences in the role of case manager (Cesta, 1993; Daleiden, 1993; Tidwell, 1995; Nolan et al, 1998). In a quantitative study, Nolan et al (1998) asked 20 acute care case managers to identify skills and knowledge of value to nurses involved in case management. Acute care case managers identified the top educational needs. There was a difference in the topics identified as the most valuable for educational preparation. Baccalaureate-prepared case managers focused on clinical issues, identifying family coping, patient education, quality of life, and social support as valuable, whereas master's-prepared case managers focused on systems-related issues. Knowledge about community resources, discharge planning, and third-party reimbursement were identified as the top three educational needs for all case managers.

The literature does provide information regarding the variety of preparatory programs available to those assuming case management positions. The range of those programs includes the following (AACN, 1996; Cesta, Tahan, and Fink, 1998):

- Noncertificate programs offered by institutions as part of training or orientation
- Certification programs offered by independent agencies and healthcare institutions
- Multiple credit certification courses offered by colleges and universities
- Postbaccalaureate certificate programs
- Master's level case management degree programs

The review of literature on managed care, case management, nursing case management, and the review of information on certification programs, degree programs, and certification examinations assisted in the identification of the following seven basic themes:

1. Healthcare and nursing organizations and systems
2. Coordination and service delivery
3. Physical and psychosocial factors
4. Budget concepts
5. Benefit systems and cost/benefit analysis
6. Case management concepts
7. Community resources

CURRICULUM DEVELOPMENT AND DESIGN

Several factors influence the following discussion regarding the integration of managed care and nursing case management concepts into academic curricula:

- A review of current professional literature
- A definition of managed care
- A definition of case management
- A perceived case manager role
- A perception of differentiated nursing practice

Operational Definitions

Managed care is viewed as the generalized structure and focus for managing the use of resources and personnel to accomplish established client outcomes and enhance the quality of care. Managed care links the client to provider services (Cesta, Tahan, and Fink, 1998).

Case management is a client care delivery system under the organizing framework of managed care. It is both a process and an outcome model of care. The system focuses on managing costs and quality and achieving positive client outcomes. Case management is a collaborative interdisciplinary approach that covers the entire continuum of care and crosses all healthcare settings in which the client receives care, from admission to discharge (Cesta, Tahan, and Fink, 1998).

The *case manager* is the individual responsible for coordinating the care delivered to an assigned population of clients based on diagnosis or need. The case manager focuses on complex needs of high-risk patients, families, and populations along a continuum of care (Sinnen and Schifalaqua, 1996). Case manager functions include but are not limited to care coordination, client education, client advocacy, and discharge planning, and a major role of the case manager is to remove barriers to the efficient delivery of care within the hospital.

Currently, most nurse case managers function in an unstructured environment. They must be extremely flexible and must be comfortable with ambiguity, uncertainty, and change (Fralic, 1992). There is an increasing emphasis on accountability for both cost and quality outcomes (Conger, 1999), and nurse case managers must have an understanding of both quality management techniques and risk management principles. The nurse case manager must be familiar with a variety of financial reimbursement systems and strategies and managed care arrangements and must be able to evaluate client care alternatives and options from a financial basis. Autonomy is required to carry out this role successfully.

Differentiated nursing practice can be conceptualized as a structure or framework of nursing roles based on education, experience, and competency (AACN-AONE Task Force, 1995). Such a framework provides shared values for levels of nursing practice, shared sets of competencies for those levels, and a time (shift versus life span), space (unit versus community), and motion (capacity to integrate) orientation for practice roles. This framework also recognizes that the ability to handle variations of client and situational complexity is gained through education and practice. Differentiated nursing practice transcends all clinical settings (CSPCN, 1999).

The authors of this chapter offer their composite view of appropriate leveling of managed care and nursing case management concepts in Table 13-1, which includes varying levels of these concepts in the associate degree or diploma, baccalaureate, and graduate level nursing curricula. These curricula are discussed in the following sections.

ASSOCIATE DEGREE CURRICULUM

The curriculum for the associate-degree nurse (ADN) prepares an individual to provide direct care to individuals and families with usual, uncomplicated, and well-defined diagnoses with predictable illness and care trajectories. The knowledge base of the associate degree program emphasizes facts, concepts, principles, demonstrated relationships, and verified observations. In addition to nursing courses, the curriculum includes general education courses and natural and behavioral science courses that support the nursing curriculum. ADN graduates function in structured healthcare settings where policies, procedures, and protocols for the provision of care are clearly established. An ADN possesses

TABLE 13-1
Leveling of Managed Care and Case Management Concepts for Curriculum Integration

Category	Associate Degree/Diploma	Baccalaureate	Graduate	Doctorate
Healthcare delivery systems/models	Introduction to basic concepts	Examination of concepts Implementation of selected models	Application of models to specific client populations Modification of models based on need	Evaluation of existing models Development of new models
Hospital/community-based tools	Introduction to established care maps, clinical pathways, and other tools	Utilization of care maps and clinical pathways Monitoring of client progress	Application of developed tools for specific population and participation in development of clinical pathways and care maps	Development and evaluation of intervention tools and strategies and evaluation of effectiveness of case management tools
Implementation of nursing case management and symptom/disease management strategies and competencies to enhance self-care capabilities	Exposure to basic interventions, strategies, and competencies	Implementation of fundamental strategies in acute care and home settings with individuals and families	Advanced case management strategies for specific populations across care continuum	Design of innovative case management and symptom/disease strategies Evaluation of efficacy of case management strategies Evaluation of fiscal and quality care outcomes with specific populations
Financing and reimbursement	Basic elements of healthcare financing	Introduction to third-party payer reimbursement systems System costs Introduction to risk management concepts Basic "gatekeeper" role	Examination of cost/benefit ratio Brokering/negotiation with third-party payer reimbursement systems System costs Risk management analysis	Evaluation of cost/benefit ratio of selected reimbursement methods Advocate for healthcare accessibility and equality of care

Continued

TABLE 13-1
Leveling of Managed Care and Case Management Concepts for Curriculum Integration—cont'd

Category	Associate Degree/Diploma	Baccalaureate	Graduate	Doctorate
Educational strategies and clinical settings	Clinical observations with case manager in acute care settings with uncomplicated, predictable, reoccurring clinical scenarios	Preceptor field work in acute and home care settings with complex, unpredictable clinical scenarios using strategies of journaling, case logs, case studies, and clinical seminars	Advanced field work managing case load of high-risk vulnerable individuals and/or populations in acute, home, and community-based settings Utilizing seminars and case presentation	Advanced field work residency with practitioner focusing on specific high-risk population in variety of settings Seminars, case presentation, and publications
Research	Introduction to research	Consumer of research	Consumer of research Participant in collaborative studies, assists others in utilization of research findings in practice settings	Participant and designer of independent studies Research consultant Contributor to theory and research literature
Client advocacy	Introduction to concept of advocacy	Promotion of climate for client empowerment and autonomy Participation in multidisciplinary efforts to identify healthcare options targeting client specific needs	Participation in advocacy programs for high-risk individuals and populations to improve healthcare outcomes for clients in variety of settings	Modification, design, and/or implementation of consumer standards, policies, or procedures Synthesis and/or management of research and dissemination of findings related to client advocacy

foundational knowledge of biological, social, and psychological science that facilitates decision making about the care of clients by applying tested criteria and norms. ADN nurses work with a time frame that is based in the present (Koerner, 1992). The setting provides them with appropriate resources for assistance and support from the full breadth of nursing expertise.

ADNs provide direct care by doing the following:

- Collecting data using established assessment tools
- Organizing health pattern data from an established list of diagnoses
- Establishing goals for a specified work period that are consistent with an overall comprehensive plan of care
- Implementing established protocols
- Coordinating and overseeing care for a limited number of patients of minimal complexity
- Documenting and communicating data concerning clients to other members of the healthcare team
- Using basic communication skills and established communication channels to participate as a member of an integrated healthcare team

The role of the ADN in nursing case management is to participate as an active member of an interdisciplinary care team. The ADN case management functions include the following:

- Providing hands-on direct client care using a plan of care established by the case manager or the interdisciplinary team
- Patient teaching using established teaching plans
- Identifying clients who may benefit from case management
- Referring clients to the nurse case manager or other appropriate personnel responsible for the implementation of case management

Educational preparation to develop the competencies to carry out these functions includes an introduction to basic concepts of managed care and case management and the role of the case manager. The curriculum should include a basic understanding of financing healthcare as it relates to individual clients. Clinical experiences should include clinical observations with case managers when available as a part of the traditional client care experiences. Experienced nurses with an associate degree will need to have additional educational experiences to become effective in case management positions.

BACCALAUREATE DEGREE CURRICULUM

The curriculum for the baccalaureate degree program prepares an individual to provide direct care to individuals and families with complex complicated diagnoses and unpredictable illness and care trajectories. The educational program includes a liberal arts education and nursing education components. Graduates of a baccalaureate program possess a greater understanding and appreciation of the various disciplines involved in client care and a broader perspective on client care. There is an emphasis on thinking and analyzing critically, making inferences, and communicating effectively. The bachelor of science nurse

(BSN) functions in both structured and unstructured healthcare settings. The setting may or may not have established policies, procedures, and protocols. There is potential for variations in client situations requiring independent nursing decisions.

Baccalaureate-prepared nurses provide both direct and indirect care by doing the following:

- Expanding the collection of data to identify complex healthcare needs
- Organizing and analyzing complex health pattern data to develop nursing
- Establishing goals with clients to develop a comprehensive plan of care from admission to discharge
- Developing and implementing a comprehensive plan of care
- Interpreting the medical plan of care into nursing activities to formulate a plan of care
- Evaluating the nursing care delivery system
- Promoting goal-directed change to meet individualized client needs
- Facilitating outcomes by being an interdisciplinary team leader

The extent of the responsibilities of the BSN in case management is often dictated by the conceptualization of case management, the case management model used, and the job description of the employer institution. Implementation of the role will be affected by the type of organization, the placement of the case manager in the organization, the power embedded in the role, the management model implemented, the specific nursing goals, and the area of practice or care setting (Cesta, Tahan, and Fink, 1998). The role of the BSN in nursing case management may include but is not limited to the following:

- Clinical expertise in symptom and disease management
- Consultant or counselor
- Coordinator and facilitator of client care
- Manager of client care
- Educator
- Negotiator or broker
- Client advocate
- Outcomes manager
- Quality manager
- Risk manager
- Change agent
- Ethics

Content and competencies for effective case management include the following threads: (1) foundational concepts, (2) healthcare financial and reimbursement concepts and issues, and (3) clinical and system issues.

Foundational Concepts

Nursing students need to understand the nature of the healthcare environment that they will experience when they gain entry into practice (Conger, 1999). Nurses employed in a managed care environment and engaged in case management must be able to respond to the quality, cost, and access imperatives of the system. The baccalaureate-prepared nurse must be able to focus on clients and families with complex issues in a dynamic healthcare delivery environment. An introduction to the following foundational concepts will help the nurse develop an appreciation of the breadth and scope of managed care and case management. These concepts provide an understanding of managed care's historical, political, and social contexts and provide a basis for working as an effective and efficient member of an integrated delivery system:

- Managed care terminology
- Historical, political, and social perspective on healthcare reform
- Historical, political, and social perspective on managed care
- Benefits and limitations of managed care
- Systems theory
- Change theory
- Integrated delivery system
- Case management process
- Case management models
  - Inside the walls
  - Beyond the walls
  - Continuum of care

Healthcare Financial and Reimbursement Concepts and Issues

Two content areas that historically have not been well addressed in nursing education are healthcare costs and healthcare financing. Many nurses have a limited understanding of the financial realities of healthcare delivery or of the maze of third-party payers and managed care organizations. Containing the cost of services and resources while maintaining quality of care is a goal for the case manager. To accomplish this goal, an understanding of fundamental concepts of healthcare financing and fiscal outcomes is necessary. This understanding is also necessary if the case manager is to help clients and families navigate capitation and fee-for-service healthcare systems. Key concepts should include the following:

- Driving forces behind managed care and cost containment
  - Medicare/Medicaid
  - Fee-for-service
  - Health management organizations
- Provider organizations
- Cost containment
- Financial risk, risk analysis, and risk management
- Market forces

Clinical and System Issues

The case management process helps promote a client-centered approach to care, which requires a broad knowledge base and clinical reasoning skills. It also involves developing competencies in negotiating, coordinating, and procuring services and resources needed to provide cost-appropriate quality care. The case manager must also have the skills necessary to develop multiple interdisciplinary relationships. Key concepts should include the following:

- Participating as an active member or leader of an interdisciplinary care team
- Case finding and screening
- Assessing client needs
- Identifying actual and potential problems
- Facilitating interdisciplinary care planning
- Serving as an organizational gatekeeper

To further develop skills in this area, the content can be more concretely identified into categories of clinical and systems issues as follows:

- Clinical issues
  - Competencies:
    - Assessment
    - Communication skills
    - Collaboration
    - Negotiation
    - Delegation
    - Conflict management
  - Role of the case manager across settings
  - Referrals
  - Care outcomes
  - Case management tools
  - Discharge planning
  - Patient education
  - Client and family coping strategies and social support
- System issues
  - Community resources
  - Leadership
  - Informatics
  - Utilization review
  - Continuous quality improvement monitoring and evaluation
  - Patient mix
  - Staff education
  - Legal issues
  - Ethical issues
  - Consumer rights
  - Healthcare policy and legislation
  - Professional practice legislation

Educational Experiences

For the past several years, educators at all levels have identified the need for more active learning in education. This need is especially true of the educational experiences for nurses entering the managed care environment, who need to incorporate active teaching methods. The managed care environment and case management approaches require critical thinking, reflection on practice, a comprehensive view of the client and client care, and a set of skills for working effectively as an member of an integrated healthcare team. Active teaching strategies involve hands-on learning techniques. Students need to develop skills for analysis and evaluation and need to explore their own attitudes and values, as well as those of other healthcare providers. Activities facilitating active teaching include questioning, cooperative learning groups, debates, role-playing simulations, and problem-based learning.

Distinct differences exist between the learning experiences of generic baccalaureate nursing students and RN-BSN students. These authors have observed that at California State University–Los Angeles, the clinical experiences are structured to address these differences. Courses are scheduled so that only generic or RN-BSN students are in a specific section to match skill level and provide a more homogenous student profile.

Generic nursing students were more comfortable in the acute care setting. Most of the generic students lacked the experience with patients and the understanding of symptom and disease management to work outside the direct supervision of preceptors. These students were more apt to focus on procedural clinical situations as ordered and regulated. These are characteristics described by Benner, Tanner, and Chesla (1996) as being consistent with those entering the nursing field as advanced beginners. Very few of the students had an awareness of or an interest in healthcare financing issues or the need for cost containment. Generic nursing students had a more difficult time understanding the concept of benchmarking and developing a care plan that did not focus on direct patient care.

RN-BSN students possessing clinical experience (i.e., those with 4 or more years in a clinical setting) were more responsive to case management strategies. The experience and clinical expertise of RN-BSN students enabled them to take a more holistic approach to planning for the client's current and future healthcare needs. They were more aware of tertiary aspects of client care than were generic students. RN-BSN students possessed the broader knowledge base necessary to engage in case management. They were comfortable in both acute care settings and home healthcare settings and required less direct supervision from their clinical preceptors. These students were more aware of the need for comprehensive discharge planning and the need to work with clients and families to ensure adherence to treatment regimes after hospitalization. They were more comfortable working on complex client problems, networking with other healthcare providers, and making necessary referrals. At evaluation, RN-BSN students who had taken the course expressed an appreciation of the degree of autonomy associated with the case management approach and the development of a keener sense of professional accountability.

RN-BSN students demonstrated pattern recognition, pattern differentiation, and salience, described by Benner, Tanner, and Chesla (1996) as characteristics of competent and proficient nurses. They also demonstrated a greater understanding of the life experiences of clients, patients, and families. This understanding facilitated their problem solving, decision making, and relationship building with clients, patients, and families.

Both generic and RN-BSN students expressed frustration with the system and with trying to deal with insurance providers. It was often difficult for them to come to terms with the various ways in which case management is operationalized in the "real world." A great deal of seminar time was spent initially discussing what case management meant at the various institutions used for clinical placements. Sample baccalaureate-level course syllabi for both the theory course and the companion clinical course are provided in Appendices 13-1 and 13-2 at the end of this chapter.

MASTER'S DEGREE CURRICULUM

Most graduate level curricula prepare nurses for advanced roles in nursing, such as nurse educator, nurse administrator, clinical nurse specialist (CNS), nurse practitioner (NP), nurse anesthetist, or nurse midwife. Of the present advanced practice options, the roles of CNS and NP are most closely associated with the concepts embedded in the process of nursing case management. It is not clear whether nursing case management will evolve into a unique new advanced practice role or whether the nursing case management process and strategies will be incorporated into other roles.

Changes in the healthcare delivery system driven by the implementation of financial tactics imposed by managed care often impact the evolution or expansion of advanced practice roles in nursing. The degree of that impact may be regional and related to the degree to which the managed care market has penetrated a specific area of the country. In southern California, the resultant fiscal gains of managed care have been a significant force in the healthcare market and have influenced current nursing practice.

In southern California, the number of CNSs employed in the acute care setting has declined significantly over the past 5 years. This decline has transpired largely as a result of cost-savings measures by healthcare institutions. The role of the CNS traditionally includes staff development, education, and clinical consultative functions. These CNS activities deeply impact the overall quality of nursing care in an institution, but in times of fiscal crisis, they can be viewed as indirect service functions and can be deemed expendable and subject to elimination as a short-term and short-sighted cost-savings measure. Therefore in southern California, the CNS position has become vulnerable and is subject to downsizing efforts that result in reduced demand for nurses prepared for those positions. This reduction of available CNS positions drives the declining enrollments seen in CNS programs. Two other factors have been associated with declining enrollment in acute care CNS programs, namely, the subtle yet progressive shift in care delivery from acute care to community-based settings and the marked increase in graduate level NP programs.

The popularity of the NP advanced practice option has created a proliferation of NP programs at the graduate level, creating concern in some regions of the country that supply will soon exceed demand. Others (Elder and Bullough, 1990; Forbes et al, 1990; Hixon, 1996) have concluded that although the CNS and the NP have different practice domains, there is considerable overlap in the core curricula found in graduate programs. This overlap suggests a possible role evolution and a blending of these roles. This is particularly true of the acute care CNS and the acute care NP, whose clinical roles, arenas of practice, and population focus may be indistinguishable.

The NP employed in a primary ambulatory care setting may also use strategies associated with case management. The extents to which those strategies are implemented in such settings are directly linked to the type of client seen and whether the healthcare problems of the population are episodic or chronic. Many NPs work in practice settings where they care for essentially healthy persons, monitor health status on a fixed routine, and treat episodic health problems. These practitioners see many clients a day for a limited time. Other NPs focus on a population of clients whose health conditions are chronic and recurrent, requiring frequent intensive monitoring and adjustment to their therapeutic regimens and education related to self-care strategies to stabilize their health problems. It is with this type of population-focused practice that the overlap of NP skills and competencies with case management techniques is most pronounced.

Benoit suggests that case management is "a systematic process of mobilizing, monitoring, and controlling resources that a patient uses over the course of an illness" (Benoit, 1996, p 108). She further suggests that superb communication skills, clinical expertise, the ability to collaborate with members of a multidisciplinary team, and critical thinking ability are essential to successful case management. This combination of characteristics is more likely to be found in nurses prepared at the advanced practice (graduate) level. Also, case management strategies are most effective when specific high-risk, vulnerable populations are closely followed by a healthcare professional who frequently monitors and adjusts the therapeutic regimen, explores alternatives to care, and educates the client about self-care monitoring and symptom management strategies (Rogers, Riordan, and Swindle, 1991; Weyant, 1991; Gibson, 1996; Papenhausen, 1996). Many graduate programs now include courses in advanced assessment, pathophysiology, and pharmacology, as well as specific clinical courses, as core requirements of their advanced practice graduates.

The graduate-prepared nurse possesses the clinical competencies to function in unstructured settings, such as the community and the home, in autonomous but collaborative practice with clients with highly complicated and interrelated health problems. It is still unclear whether a separate advanced practice role, that of the nurse case manager, will evolve or whether case management is a process, strategy, or set of interventions to be practiced by advanced practice nurses such as CNSs, NPs and others.

Advanced practice nurses provide direct care by doing the following:

- Applying advanced assessment skills to identify and monitor complex healthcare needs in selected client populations in acute and community settings
- Providing expert clinical interventions to facilitate symptom management of a specific vulnerable client population
- Establishing disease management goals with clients to develop a comprehensive plan of care from admission to discharge

- Providing continuity of care from the acute care to the home setting, depending on the practice setting
- Managing a caseload of specific vulnerable clients in collaborative practice arrangements with other healthcare providers
- Evaluating and modifying the nursing care delivery system

The functions of the advanced practice nurse in nursing case management may include the following:

- Clinical expertise in symptom and disease management
- Expert consultation to specific clients in acute care or community settings
- Resource and outcomes management for individuals or a client population
- Client and family education and advocacy
- Primary healthcare provision for specific vulnerable client population
- Coordination and evaluation of cost and quality of care in acute care and other managed care settings

How the graduate curriculum is modified to prepare these advanced practice nurses remains unclear. A search of Web-based university catalogs was conducted to determine recurrent content themes and phrases reflective of nursing case management and managed care in various graduate curricula. A regional convenience sample of Web-based catalogs was obtained by accessing Websites listing graduate programs in nursing from the western United States. The catalog descriptions of graduate curricula were scrutinized for courses or course descriptions that indicated inclusion of nursing case management content and for advanced practice options that used this content. The descriptions of the functions or characteristics of the various advanced practice graduates were examined for the use of the word *case manager*. Instances of the use of advanced practice nurses with special populations were considered, as well as specific nursing case management strategies, such as symptom/disease management, symptom/disease monitoring, resource/service brokering, and interdisciplinary collaboration. The setting of nursing case management practice was noted if it could be determined. Although this survey of case management content in graduate curricula of western universities is not comprehensive, nor does it purport to represent all university graduate programs, the preliminary trends and program designs are noteworthy. These trends and program designs are summarized in Table 13-2. These trends were considered as a factor in the construction of the graduate level content in Table 13-1.

What does appear clear is that graduate education that prepares advanced practice nurses for the managed care environment needs to include advanced knowledge and experience in organization theory and nursing systems. Advanced practice nurses need to possess practical knowledge of financing, budgeting, risk management, and marketing in healthcare. Broad clinical specialty preparation needs to focus on care coordination, including clinical management, continuity of care, and the means to procure and deliver healthcare services. The content of graduate programs needs to be augmented with skills of collaboration, brokering, negotiation, referral making, conflict resolution, networking, and resources. Research strategies that focus on analysis of the broad context of models or systems, the benefits of

TABLE 13-2
Selected Advanced Practice Graduate Programs in the Western United States

Universities		CONTENT/THEMES			
	Advanced Practice Roles/Incorporates NCM Concepts	Focus of NCM Clientele	Description of Role/ Function of Advanced Practice Nurse	Focus of NCM Strategies or Interventions	Location of Practice Site
University of Washington, Seattle	Blended CNS and NP role Advanced practice home care NP	Population-based, focus on acute and chronic illnesses	Clinical nurse manager, CNS, clinical expert, nurse manager and educator	Dx and management of illness and complications Symptom management and client education	Community-based settings and home healthcare
University of San Francisco	Multiple CNS specialties in gerontology, CV, and home and acute care adult and gerontological NP	ACANPs focus on complex acutely ill CNSs focus on older adult and acute and/or chronic illness	ACANPs case manage in collaboration with medical team Home health CNSs and gerontological NPs provide clinical management	ACANPs coordinate care, perform PEs and therapeutic procedures, and order Dx tests and medication CNSs provide management in Dx and Tx of responses to complex responses to illness	ACANPs in acute care settings Home health CNSs and gerontological NPs in community and home settings
University of Arizona, Tucson	NCM option at graduate level	NCM option for either population-based or system-based practice	NCM practicing management and coordination within care delivery systems NCM of individual and/or specific population groups	Systems-based focus on data management and evaluation of home care delivery systems Population-based focus on management and coordination of chronic illness across continuum	Systems-based NCM in acute care or other managed care settings Population-based CNS in community-based settings and home

ACANP, Acute care advanced nurse practitioner; *CNS,* clinical nurse specialist; *CV,* cardiovascular; *Dx,* diagnosis; *NCM,* nurse case manager; *NP,* nurse practitioner; *PEs,* physical examinations; *Tx,* treatments.

Continued

TABLE 13-2
Selected Advanced Practice Graduate Programs in the Western United States—cont'd

| Universities | Advanced Practice Roles/Incorporates NCM Concepts | CONTENT/THEMES | | | |
		Focus of NCM Clientele	Description of Role/ Function of Advanced Practice Nurse	Focus of NCM Strategies or Interventions	Location of Practice Site
Oregon Health Science University, Portland	Adult health and illness CNS and gerontological population health management specialist	Individual, family, and groups and focus on long-term recovery, chronic illness, or end of life issues	CM, program coordinator, and independent CNS	Dx and management of symptoms, functional problems, and risk behaviors	Community nursing centers, clinics, home healthcare
Samuel Merritt College, Oakland, Calif	CM specialist	CMs prepared in systems-based theories, epidemiology, and quality assurance	CM as coordinator of care, monitoring of care quality and provision for continuity of care	Management of quality of care from cost-sensitive perspective	Acute care and managed care settings Prepared to practice in payer/insurance industry
California State University, Los Angeles	NCM	NCMs prepared for system-based practice and for high-risk, population-based practice	NCM within acute care settings as monitor of cost and quality and in community with specific high-risk population groups	Focus on quality assurance in acute care settings and with high-risk individual for disease/symptom management in community setting	Acute care and/or community settings Population- or system-based practice

CM, Case manager; *CNS,* clinical nurse specialist; *Dx,* diagnosis; *NCM,* nurse case manager.

case management on client outcomes and client satisfaction, and managed care's influence on issues and trends in healthcare need to be stressed.

DOCTORAL LEVEL CURRICULUM

The inclusion of managed care and case management concepts in doctoral level education is a necessity for all programs. The clinical content included should be similar to that of the previously mentioned advanced practice level content. Doctoral level content differs in that these students also do the following:

- Evaluate the effectiveness of existing models
- Develop new models
- Develop and evaluate case management tools to monitor quality and costs
- Design innovative case management strategies for symptom/disease management
- Evaluate the cost/benefit ratio for selected reimbursement models
- Evaluate fiscal and quality care outcomes with specific populations
- Advocate for healthcare accessibility and equality of healthcare

QUESTIONS

Many questions remain unanswered. How can educators create and modify academic curricula to prepare for and promote case management? What are the implications of preparing nurse case managers for the preferred model of managed care? What are the benefits for clients, patients, families and the system of nursing case management? How can we facilitate nursing case management and collaborative practice and reduce interdisciplinary conflicts and biases in managed care competition? The answers to these questions can only come from practice and research.

SUMMARY

Curriculum can be described as a design for formal education for limited purposes. Often the development of curricula for fields of practice are influenced by the social perspective of practice and the purposes related to that perspective (Taylor, 1985). This influence is true for managed care and case management at this phase of evolution. The preceding discussion undoubtedly raises more questions than it provides answers or insights into the integration of managed care and case management content into the academic curriculum. The level at which content related to managed care and case management is taught will be determined by several factors, primarily the philosophy of the nursing program, the expected outcome of the program, and the degree to which managed care influences regional medical and nursing practice. It is possible to educate nurses for managed care and case management from both concrete applied and abstract theoretical perspectives. How the organization of those concepts, capabilities, and skills of case management are incorporated in the curriculum will vary greatly. As long as managed care and case management continue to evolve in the practice arena, it will be difficult to provide specific answers for educators on the most effective way to prepare professional nurses and advanced practice nurses for the managed care environment. Until there is greater agreement and standardization of the evolving models of case management and the role of the nurse in managed care, especially in case management, it will be difficult to determine the educational preparation for nurses. The profession itself may need to take a proactive position and establish the acceptable educational preparation for professional nurse case managers.

REFERENCES

American Association of Colleges of Nursing: *Master's education via interdisciplinary links, case management, and nursing informatics*, Washington, DC, 1996, The Association.

American Association of Colleges of Nursing, American Organization of Nurse Executives, and National Organization of Associate Degree Nursing Task Force: *A model for differentiated nursing practice*, Washington, DC, 1995, The Association.

American Nurses Association: *Case management by nurses*, Washington, DC, 1992, The Association.

Benner P, Tanner CA, Chesla C: *Expertise in nursing practice: caring, clinical judgment, and ethics*, New York, 1996, Springer.

Benoit CB: Case management and advanced practice nurses. In Hickey JL, Ouimette R, Venegoni S, editors: *Advanced practice nursing*, Philadelphia, 1996, Lippincott.

California Strategic Planning Committee for Nursing: *Model for differentiated practice*, Sacramento, Calif, 1999, The Committee/Colleagues in Caring Education/Industry Interface Task Force.

Cesta TG: The link between continuous quality improvement and case management, *J Nurs Admin* 23(6): 55-61, 1993.

Cesta TG, Tahan HA, Fink LF: *The case manager's survival guide: winning strategies for clinical practice*, St Louis, 1998, Mosby.

Conger MM: *Managed care: practice strategies for nursing*, Thousand Oaks, Calif, 1999, Sage.

Daleiden A: The CSN as trauma case manager: a new frontier, *Clin Nurse Spec* 7:295-298, 1993.

Elder RC, Bullough B: Nurse practitioners and clinical nurse specialists: are the roles merging? *Clin Nurs Spec* 4(2):78-84, 1990.

Ethridge P, Lamb G: Professional nursing case management improves quality, access, and cost, *Nurs Manage* 20(3):30-35, 1989.

Forbes KE, Rafson C, Spross J, et al: Clinical nurse specialist and nurse practitioner core curricula survey results, *Nurse Pract* 15(43):20-23, 1990.

Fralic M: The nurse case manager: focus, selection, preparation, and measurement, *J Nurs Admin* 22(11):13-14, 46, 1992.

Gibson SJ: Differentiated practice within and beyond the hospital walls. In Cohen EL, editor: *Nursing case management in the 21st century*, St Louis, 1996, Mosby.

Glettler E, Leen MG: The advanced practice nurse as case manager, *J Case Manag* 5(3)121-126, 1996.

Hixon ME: Professional development: socialization in advanced practice nursing. In Hickey J, Ouimette R, Venegoni S, editors: *Advanced practice nursing*, Philadelphia, 1996, Lippincott.

Koerner JG: Integrating differentiated practice into shared governance. In Porter-O'Grady T, editor: *Implementing shared governance*, St Louis, 1992, Mosby.

Koerner JG, Bunkers LB, Nelson B, et al: Implementing differentiated practice: the Sioux Valley Hospital experience, *J Nurs Admin* 19(20):13-20, 1989.

Mahn VA, Spross JA: Nursing case management as an advanced practice role. In Hamric AB, Spross JA, Hanson CM, editors: *Advanced nursing practice: an integrative approach*, Philadelphia, 1996, WB Saunders.

Mundt MH: Key elements of nursing case management curricula. In Cohen EL, editor: *Nursing case management in the 21st century*, St Louis, 1996, Mosby.

Nolan M, Harris A, Kufta A, et al: Preparing nurses for the acute care case manager role: educational needs identified by existing case managers, *J Contin Educ Nurs* 29(3):130-134, 1998.

Papenhausen J: Discovering and achieving client outcomes. In Cohen EL, editor: *Nursing case management in the 21st century*, St Louis, 1996, Mosby.

Rogers M, Riordan J, Swindle D: Community-based nursing case management pays off, *Nurs Manage* 22(3):30-34, 1991.

Sinnen M, Schifalaqua M: The education of nurses: nurse case manager's view. In Cohen EL, editor: *Nursing case management in the 21st century*, St Louis, 1996, Mosby.

Taylor SG: Curriculum development for preservice programs using Orem's theory of nursing. In Riehl-Sisca J, editor: *The science and art of self-care*, Norwalk, Conn, 1985, Appleton-Century-Crofts.

Tidwell S: The role of the critical care case manager CNS in case management, *Am J Nurs* 95:163-166, 1995.

Weyant J: St. Joseph's Medical Center in Wichita. Community-based nurse case management department report. Paper presented at a meeting of nurse case managers, Tucson, Feb 1991.

Zander K: Managed care and nursing case management. In Mayer GG, Madden MJ, Lawrenz E, editors: *Patient care delivery models,* Gaithersburg, Md, 1990, Aspen.

APPENDIX **13-1**
Sample Baccalaureate Theory Course Syllabus

California State University–Los Angeles
Nursing 496, Nursing Case Management for Vulnerable Populations

Units: 3 units of didactic lecture/discussion
Prerequisites: Completion of all lower division nursing courses
Corequisite: Nursing 497, Nursing Case Management for Vulnerable Populations

Course Description: Introduction to the emerging collaborative professional role that nurses perform through managed care and case management strategies for high-risk client populations. Focus is on needs assessment, brokerage and monitoring of healthcare services and resources, comprehensive care coordination and discharge planning, client advocacy, and the provision of nursing interventions. These interventions include educative, supportive, and counseling strategies to increase self-care abilities and symptom management of chronic illness.

Course Objectives: At the completion of the course, students will be able to do the following:

1. Define specific high-risk client populations appropriate for case management strategies and identify issues related to access and utilization of the healthcare system for these populations.
2. Discuss current trends for financing healthcare.
3. Differentiate between types of managed care organizations.
4. State the goals of managed care and case management.
5. Describe and discuss prospective payment system and the application of diagnosis-related groups (DRGs).
6. Describe and discuss current healthcare trends driving managed care and case management.
7. Describe the current healthcare trends driving the evolution of cost-effective, quality intensive nursing care modalities for high-risk client populations.
8. Discuss and distinguish the roles of the various interdisciplinary team members who might participate in case management.
9. Describe and compare the current case management models and the respective role functions of the case manager.
10. Define and discuss the role of the nurse in developing and coordinating collaborative plans of care using "within-the-walls" and "beyond-the-walls" case management models.
11. Discuss the key elements for establishing a case manager/client/family relationship.
12. Define quality assurance and continuous quality improvement and relate to managed care and case management.
13. Define and discuss risk management.
14. Discuss research findings to support the financial and quality benefits of case management, specifically nursing case management.
15. Demonstrate the use of the Internet to locate national, regional, and local resources for nursing case management.

Content Outline:
Vulnerable populations
   Definition of vulnerability
   Identification of vulnerable populations
   Chronic illness
   Care access
   Ethical implication of managed care and case management
Financial and reimbursement issues
   Historical overview of healthcare financing and reimbursement
   Prospective payment systems
   The managed care marketplace

Cost-effective care

Monitoring of costs

Development of managed care and case management models

Origins of managed care and case management

Managed care terminology

Goals and objectives of managed care

Goals and objectives of case management

Differentiation of managed care, case management, disease management, and nursing case management

Differentiation of case management, quality improvement, and discharge planning

Hospital-based ("within-the-walls") case management

Models of case management

Appropriate clients for case management

Collaborative practice arrangements

Interdisciplinary team approach

Hospital-based management tools and case management strategies

Care multidisciplinary action plans (MAPS)

Clinical pathways

Benchmarks

Computer-generated decision trees

Outcomes-specific care planning

Monitoring of outcomes

Systems assessment

Employee education

Case manager characteristics and functions

"Beyond-the-walls" case management

Models of case management

Appropriate clients for case management

Development of a nurse/client relationship

Case manager preparation, characteristics, functions, and strategies

Outcomes-specific care planning

Monitoring of outcomes

Interdisciplinary team approach

Development of a referral network

Documentation of quality of care

Definition of quality

Quality care outcomes

The continuous quality improvement (CQI) process

Physician and institution quality "report cards"

Cost containment methods

Population demographics affecting healthcare cost

Relationship of cost to length of stay

Risk analysis process and methods

Research

Summary of research studies documenting fiscal impacts of managed care

Summary of outcomes and case management productivity research

Internet resources for nursing case management

Nurse case managers on the World Wide Web

Local, regional, and national resources

Legislative Websites

(Developed by Patricia A. Chin, Judith L. Papenhausen, and Jane Hook, School of Nursing, California State University–Los Angeles, 2000.)

APPENDIX 13-2
Sample Baccalaureate Clinical Course Syllabus

California State University–Los Angeles
Nursing 497, Nursing Case Management for Vulnerable Populations Laboratory

Units: 3 units or 7 clinical hours/week and 2-seminar hours/week

Prerequisites: Completion of all lower division nursing courses

Corequisite: Nursing 496, Nursing Case Management for Vulnerable Populations

Course Description: Clinical nursing case management laboratory for high-risk clients who have complex healthcare problems due to an acute physiological or psychological dysfunction or acute exacerbation of a chronic health problem. Focus is on comprehen-

sive care coordination, brokerage, monitoring, discharge planning, client/family advocacy, and nursing interventions.

Clinical Outcomes: A specific clinical agency for the Nursing 497 experience *will vary* in terms of the case management model used or the conceptualization of case management. This will result in variability in the nature and extent of the clinical experience. The exact clinical objectives will need to be negotiated by the student, clinical instructor, and preceptor.

The following clinical goals *are not applicable* in every setting due to variation in agency, instructor, and/or preceptor focus:

1. Identify and manage a minimum caseload of three to six high-risk clients per week. Exact

caseload will be determined in collaboration with the preceptor, depending on variables of complexity and preceptor caseloads.

2. Professional clinical nursing interventions under the direction of a clinical faculty member and clinical preceptor will include, but not be limited to the following:

    2.1. Participate in collaborative interdisciplinary goal setting, focusing on quality and cost containment.

    2.2. Assessment of client/family self-care capabilities and deficits.

    2.3. Development of a comprehensive plan of care, including discharge planning and education.

    2.4. Nursing case management and monitoring of critical client objectives during the hospitalization.

    2.5. Participation in accessing and coordination of healthcare services beyond the hospital stay.

    2.6. Establishing a partnership with the client/family by doing the following:

        2.6.1. Assessing health status and potential for self-care

        2.6.2. Creating mutual client/family goals

        2.6.3. Assessing, brokering, and coordinating healthcare and supportive services

        2.6.4. Providing professional nursing case management interventions related to educational, supportive, and counseling strategies to increase self-care agency and symptom management.

        2.6.5. Monitoring and evaluating care plan outcomes and quality of care.

3. Extension of the nurse/client relationship beyond the acute hospital stay with selected clients in selected settings. It is preferred that each student be able to make a home visit to client(s).

4. Participate in the agency's quality of care assessment and/or cost containment protocols. The level of permitted participation will vary.

Student Clinical Objectives: The exact clinical objectives may vary across agencies and will be determined at the beginning of the course by the student, the clinical instructor, and the preceptor. The student will create four objectives in correct format and give a copy to the clinical instructor and the preceptor. Refer to the guidelines provided in the syllabus.

Course Requirements: Clinical performance is evaluated on the basis of successfully completing the negotiated clinical objectives based on the judgment of the clinical instructor and preceptor. Written guidelines are provided for each of the assignments.

Competition of clinical hours and activities	Credit/No credit
Student negotiated objectives	Credit/No credit
Clinical journal assignments	Credit/No credit
Clinical case logs and seminar presentations	20%
Written midterm case study	30%
Written final case study	30%
Oral case study presentation	20%
Total	100%

Settings: A clinical setting that provides traditional acute care, transitional or extended care facilities and/or community-based healthcare services, community outpatient clinic, and hospice-based case management services may be used with the approval of the instructor and may include: cardiac/stroke rehabilitation settings, diabetic education programs, community/hospital-based support groups/education programs, and community health clinic settings.

Appropriate Populations:

The elderly who need coordinated healthcare services and case management

Other patients who require coordination of potentially high-cost healthcare services

Chronically ill and disabled children and adults across the life span

Persons with AIDS across the age span

Mothers and infants identified as high-risk patients

Persons with repeated hospitalizations for chronic physical or mental illness

Homeless individuals and families who need care and services

(Developed by Patricia A. Chin, Judith L. Papenhausen, and Jane Hook, School of Nursing, California State University–Los Angeles, 2000.)

Legal and Ethical Issues

14

Legal Issues in Managed Care

Barbara A. Ryan and Tina H. Sernick

KEY LESSONS IN THIS CHAPTER

- The three primary legal issues that surface as consequences of cost containment are professional liability exposure, licensing issues, and risk management. They exemplify the conflict between cost containment and quality of care.
- Each state is responsible for regulating its own quality of care.
- Nurses should maintain a working knowledge of current federal and state legislation as it relates to healthcare, such as ERISA, HIPAA, and others.
- A lack of information has been cited by consumers as an impediment to making informed choices about health plans.
- Health providers must abide by the rules of their profession, regardless of payment or reimbursement issues.

UNDERLYING PRINCIPLES

To fully appreciate the legal issues that nurses face in this "new" healthcare environment, a basic understanding of the concept of managed care is necessary. As a principle, managed care is an insurance concept that combines the idea of healthcare financing and delivery into one entity. Typically, this is accomplished through the establishment of a single corporate entity that delivers healthcare through arrangements with selective healthcare providers. There are as many definitions of managed care as there are managed care policies (Huntington, 1997). Managed care has been around, at least in a limited role, for decades. The initial push for the widespread implementation of managed care began with a national healthcare reform movement in the late 1980s. Nevertheless, in 1994 when the government-driven healthcare reform proposals failed, private industry, namely insurance carriers and corporate entities, fostered market-driven change with full force. Consequently, we now see healthcare that is driven by traditional economic forces, supply, demand, fierce competition, and a complicated regulatory framework.

The overall impact of the managed care invasion has been basic restructuring as new models of healthcare are delivered. This restructuring affects every aspect of healthcare from physician practices to outpatient care to hospital care. Budget tightening on both the state and federal levels has resulted in a dramatic increase in financial stress on both for-profit and not-for-profit hospitals. For-profit care is frequently criticized for being driven by financial forces. These providers must decrease costs so they can be fiscally responsible to their shareholders. This profit motive is in sharp contrast to the motive of charitable institutions, which focus on survival while fulfilling their mission to deliver patient care. This new marketplace has resulted in an unprecedented amount of politicizing and competition, particularly since government regulators allow market forces to shape new models of healthcare delivery—rather than a system of rate-setting. For example, the New York Healthcare Reform Act of 1996 supplemented previously enacted measures that set hospital rates prospectively. Compounding the stress on hospitals are cuts in government aid, increased numbers of uninsured patients, and the expansion of managed care (*New York Times*, 1999).

To survive in this volatile market, healthcare providers, whether they are hospitals or outpatient practices, have had to adapt in various ways. Hospitals frequently focus on achieving the needed savings by reducing labor costs through work redesign and substitution of lower-paid unlicensed assistant personnel. This approach frequently results in job reductions, including nurse positions, causing a ripple effect of increasing the workload for the nurses who remain on the job (Huntington, 1997). This new healthcare environment leaves almost every healthcare worker, nurses included, at risk for liability exposure due to increased demands. Such stress has caused many to complain about a conflict of interest between professional responsibility and the need to meet the company's bottom line; there is also a potential violation of state and federal laws that regulate the delivery of healthcare for professionals who must also bear the brunt of patient complaints.

Managed care is not all negative, however. The principle behind managed care—linking the financing of healthcare to the delivery of services—theoretically should provide a coordinated set of services that emphasizes prevention and primary care (Huntington, 1997). In 1992 the American Nurses Association (ANA), along with various specialty nursing organizations, developed and endorsed a healthcare policy statement called the *Nursing Agenda for Health Care Reform*. This agenda states that the managed care system should provide universal access to a defined standard package of essential health and treatment services, encompassing a balance between treatment of disease, health promotion, and illness prevention (ANA, 1992). Unfortunately, this model of healthcare delivery may still be a rarity.

The rapid and continued growth of managed care resulted in predictions that nearly 80% of the U.S. population would receive some form of managed healthcare by the year 2000 (Ladden and Steinberg, 1996). This prediction has largely become a reality. Nearly every nurse practicing in the next 10 years will be affected by the concept of managed care. Nurses therefore must have an understanding of the principles behind the managed care environment in which they are employed and must dictate their practice in a legally acceptable and ethical way within the bounds of their employment. Although both federal and state governments have introduced nearly 1000 bills nationwide that affect healthcare, relatively few bills have passed. The overall goal of the statutory schemes has been to control managed care so that the profit motive of these companies is not a priority over access to care, delivery of quality care, and distribution of services.

LEGAL ISSUES

In principle, managed care seeks not only cost containment but improvement in the *quality of care.* Most managed care entities have a definitive *quality assurance cost containment program.* Nevertheless, cost containment initiatives can leave RNs at odds with their legal and ethical obligation to provide quality care.

The three primary legal issues that surface as a result of cost containment are professional liability exposure, licensing issues, and risk management. All three essentially exemplify the potential conflict between cost containment and quality of care.

Professional Liability

Nurses face a difficult task when trying to render competent, responsible care and fulfill their advocacy responsibilities in an environment of extreme cost containment. As professional healthcare providers, nurses are held accountable for providing care that meets the prevailing standard of care in the nursing community. Frequently, managed care plans have strict guidelines and administrative procedures that control the delivery of healthcare, whether it is in a hospital setting (such as in an emergency room) or an outpatient center. Regardless of the setting in which nurses practice, however, they will be held accountable for malpractice for failure to provide the appropriate level of nursing care that meets the standards of nursing practice within the community in which they work, even if the managed care plan dictates nursing practice. *Medical malpractice* is a term used to describe a form of professional negligence. In the context of nursing, it is failure to do what a reasonable nurse would do under the same or similar circumstances. Generally, each state is responsible for the regulation of the quality of healthcare. Thus each state regulates who may be sued under the theory of malpractice and how long a person who is perceived to have been injured as a result of improper treatment has a right to bring a lawsuit.*

There are four universal elements to a claim for medical malpractice: (1) duty, (2) breach of duty, (3) causation, and (4) injury.

For the nurse to be held accountable to a patient who is claiming malpractice, the person suing, or the *plaintiff,* has to be able to establish that there was some sort of professional relationship between the nurse and the plaintiff and that the nurse had a duty or responsibility to provide a certain level of care. A typical example of this in the managed care setting occurs when nurses manage patient screening telephone lines at health maintenance organization (HMO) centers. A patient or an HMO member may call the HMO with a complaint and be put in contact with a nurse who screens the call and makes a recommendation as to whether the patient should be seen at an urgent care center or for a routine visit. The nurse in that setting arguably has a duty to the patient who has called, even though that nurse may not have met that patient or even had an opportunity to examine the caller. The patient then might act in reliance on the nurse recommendations. The nurse in this case has a *duty* to the patient to render sound advice.

There must also be a departure from the accepted standards of nursing practice for the plaintiff to have a right to bring a medical malpractice action against a nurse. When there is a breach of the standard of care rendered by the nurse, that is called a *departure.* The standard against which the nurse is measured can vary from state to state. In New York State, for example, the nurse's standard of care is measured against that of other nurses in his or her community. Thus if the nurse's action fails to meet the standard of care within the community in which he or she practices, that would be deemed a *breach of duty* or a departure from the accepted standards of nursing care.

The third essential element is known as *causation.* Causation is best described as the event or circumstances that happened as a consequence of the nurse's departure, resulting in injury. Causation can be direct or indirect. An example of direct causation is if a nurse administers an intramuscular injection in such a way as to cause an intravenous administration of the medication that was intended only for intramuscular injection. Any untoward effects that occur would be a direct result of the nurse's improper administration of the injection. An example

---

*For example, in New York State, the Civil Practice Laws and Rules (CPLR) regulate that generally, medical malpractice actions for adults must be brought within 2½ years of the date of the alleged medical malpractice.

CPLR §214(a) states: "Action for medical, dental, or podiatric malpractice to be commenced within two years and six months; exceptions.

An action for medical, dental or podiatric malpractice must be commenced within two years and six months of the act, omission or failure complained of or at last treatment where there is continuous treatment for the same illness, injury, or condition which gave rise to the said act, omission or failure; provided, however, that where the action is based upon the discovery of a foreign object in the body of the patient, the action may be commenced within one year of the date of such discovery or of the date of discovery of facts which would reasonably lead to such discovery, whichever is earlier. For the purpose of this section the term 'continuous treatment' shall not include examinations undertaken at the request of the patient for the sole purpose of ascertaining the state of the patient's condition. For the purpose of this section the term 'foreign object' shall not include a chemical compound, fixation device or prosthetic aid or device" NY CPLR §214(a) (McKinney Suppl, 2001, p 261).

of indirect *proximate cause* is as follows: A nurse finds a patient in respiratory distress but attempts to administer oxygen instead of calling a code. There is a clear delay in calling the code, and as a result, the code team does not arrive into the patient's room until 10 minutes after the respiratory distress was detected. Unfortunately, the patient dies. At the time the patient was suffering from respiratory distress, however, she or he was suffering from a massive pulmonary embolism that could not be treated. The patient would have died even if a code was called immediately. In this scenario, the nurse's failure to call a code in a timely manner was not the absolute proximate cause of this patient's death—but as a substantial contributing factor, a jury might still find the element of causation and award monetary damages.

The fourth essential element is that the plaintiff must have actual or real injuries as a consequence of the treatment or breach of duty. In legal jargon, the injury is also termed *damages,* which is an essential element of a malpractice claim. Even if a nurse clearly departed from the accepted standards of medical practice, if no harm has resulted, that patient does not have the right to sue for compensation for *malpractice.* An example is a situation in which a nurse administers the wrong medication to a patient, and fortunately, the patient suffers no untoward or ill effects as a consequence of that error. Without damages, a plaintiff does not have a right to be compensated. In medical malpractice cases such as these, the compensation can include damages for pain, suffering, and economic losses that occurred as a consequence of the departure.

Various statutory schemes under state and federal law result in the exemption of various managed care entities from being held responsible under the rubric of medical malpractice. For example, in New York State, there is a specific statute that exempts all HMOs from malpractice liability, although it does not protect the professional staff in this manner.* Additionally, the federal Employee Retirement Income Security Act (ERISA) shields employee benefits plans from state malpractice actions.†

The concept of managed care and cost containment has resulted in the emergence of clinical practice tools such as clinical practice and case management guidelines, which are directed at limiting or containing the length of hospital stay. These guidelines may result in the use of "canned" nursing care plans. Nurses must recognize, however, that nothing can replace the art and skill of nursing. A nurse's greatest tool is his or her assessment ability. Yet this environment may place constant pressure on the nurse to provide more for less, at the risk of sacrificing quality of care.

Reorganization of staffing is another common phenomenon. Reengineering of healthcare frequently results in decreased staffing, even if downsizing is not the primary goal. Increasing an RN's workload may compete with the nurse's ability to provide appropriate and skilled care. The result is a divided loyalty to duty of care versus economics and cost containment.

---

*Public Health Law §4410.
†ERISA preempts state law claims "relating to" employee benefit plans. Thus, many managed care plans are exempt from state malpractice claims. However, this statute, at least in New York State, does not insulate individual physicians who are employees of the plans from claims of failing to timely refer patients (*Nealy v. Yung, New York Law Journal,* 1999, p 26).

Decreased time with each patient has the impact of increasing the risk for mistakes and decreasing a nurse's ability to develop relationships with patients. A patient's subjective impression of the type of care provided by the nursing staff may directly impact his or her decision of whether to sue for malpractice.

Expanding nurse practice roles also leave nurses at a higher risk for malpractice suits. In outpatient settings, nurses are asked to perform tasks previously reserved only for physicians. The motivation generally is cost control. A nurse who practices in this arena will be held to the appropriate standard of care for a nurse practitioner in this arena. Nurses who function in this environment and are not qualified cannot hide behind the mask of ignorance. They have a legal and ethical responsibility to practice within their clinical skill level.

Nursing departments have input in clinical practice guidelines, case management orders, and nursing practice guidelines. The role of nurses in the reengineering of healthcare provides an unprecedented opportunity to have a positive impact on the delivery of healthcare. Risk management, sensitivity to health costs, quality improvement, and interdisciplinary collaboration are just some of the curricula being taught in baccalaureate nursing programs throughout the United States. Nurses also have a responsibility to "keep up with the times," hone their administrative and computer skills, and keep up to date with standards of medical practices.

Licensure

With reengineering, there has been a redistribution of various tasks, from skilled nurses to unlicensed assistant personnel. Hospitals are increasingly substituting unlicensed assistant personnel for nurses as a cost-saving strategy. Many state boards of nursing and state legislatures are considering methods to regulate these unlicensed providers. This concept is a new one, however, and legislatures are often slow to act. The ANA has proposed a comprehensive position on the regulation of unlicensed assistant personnel. Frequently, the existing state laws that regulate nursing practice use broad-based language, making it difficult to pinpoint when a line has been crossed by unlicensed personnel.* Furthermore, the unlicensed personnel generally work under the "supervision" of a nurse. The use of unlicensed personnel to perform duties and tasks previously reserved for nurses leave the nurses supervising the unlicensed personnel open to potential liability. The nurse is still responsible for patient care and making sure that the care is delivered.

One of the most significant challenges facing the nursing profession is the licensure issue. A movement to eliminate *individual professional licensure* is underway. Over the years, the nursing profession has been able to preserve the concept of individual professional licensure and thereby protect the scope of nursing practice despite strong challenges to the contrary.

---

*New York State's Nurse Practice Act, Education Law §6902(1) states:
"The practice of the profession of nursing as a registered professional nurse is defined as diagnosing and treating human responses to actual or potential health problems through such services as case finding, health teaching, health counseling, and provision of care supportive to or restorative of life and well-being, and executing medical regimens prescribed by a licensed physician, dentist or other licensed health care provider legally authorized under this title and in accordance with the commissioner's regulations. A nursing regimen shall be consistent with and shall not vary any existing medical regimen" NY Ed. L. §6902(1) (McKinney, 2001, p 504).

Recently the American Hospital Association affiliates have been advocating the expansion of the institution's authority to determine the scope of nursing practice, giving the hospitals the authority to determine what tasks nurses and assistant personnel may perform. The ANA, on the other hand, supports a move toward national licensure laws but not institutional licensure. The advantage of national licensure is that it preserves individual accountability of the practitioner to the patient (Huntington, 1997).

Risk Management

Institutions laboring under the concept of managed care are motivated to cap and limit the length of hospital stay. This model dates back to the 1980s, when Medicare switched to a prospective payment model (diagnosis-related groups [DRGs]). With the advent of the managed care revolution, however, there has been a strong movement to limit length of stay beyond what was deemed acceptable 10 years ago. This movement often results in a backlash, which causes a demand for remedial legislation. One example is the backlash that occurred as a result of the practice of insurance carriers enforcing a 24-hour stay for uncomplicated obstetrical deliveries. Ultimately this backlash led to successful efforts to require a minimum of 48 hours coverage for normal childbirth, with passage of legislation by the 104th Congress to prevent premature discharge policies (Huntington, 1997). In cases of early discharge, the nurse's best intervention was to ensure that the appropriate follow-up care in the home was made available on discharge and to ensure that the environment to which the patient was going was a safe one. Today there are still many early discharge issues arising, with outpatient mastectomies and 3-day cardiac surgery stays. Nurses must identify the potential for difficulties with early discharge. To provide nursing care within the acceptable standards of care, the nurse must ensure that the appropriate services are available once the patient is discharged.

   State law may dictate that managed care programs have a definitive quality assurance (QA) program. A potential problem arises, however, when the managed care system's cost containment policy is also part of the QA program (Friedberg, 1997). Although as a concept QA's primary goal is promoting quality of care, when cost containment becomes the primary function of a QA program, problems arise. Strict cost containment measures have a disparate impact on those most vulnerable, including the chronically ill, the physically disabled, and the unemployed. The 106th Congress (1999) addressed the issue of utilization review (UR) and QA by pushing for legislation that called for national standards, such as a "minimum uniform data set" (CRS Report for Congress, 1999, p 24). Nevertheless, these types of QA programs sometimes conflict with nursing judgment. To avoid this problem, it is imperative that nurses follow up with management in the development of sound nursing practice guidelines.

STATUTORY SCHEMES

The criticism has been made that incentives exist under managed care to underutilize necessary services. In contrast, financial incentives existed under traditional fee-for-service insurance arrangements, which led to wasteful and perhaps even harmful excesses in the provision of care. While Congress was busy from 1998 to 1999 tending to the unfortunate business of impeachment, some of the laudable initiatives of the 105th Congress remained in committee. The 106th Congress also did not accomplish much in terms of managed care legislation. Such bills responded to the consumer and healthcare provider concerns about managed care by proposing federal standards that regulated certain aspects of managed care products and establishing federal standards to reflect initiatives on the state level, as well as incorporating recommendations from the President's Advisory Commission's Consumer Bill of Rights. There was a flurry of legislative activity on both state and federal levels under the rubric of consumer protection, in response to the perceived ills of managed care. Congress is still trying to decide on a Patients' Bill of Rights package. In the wake of the terrorist attacks of September 11, 2001, however, Congress has not yet revisited this legislation at the time of this publication.

Central to the effort to protect consumers in the age of managed care is the attempt to hold payers accountable for negligent medical decision making. Individual patients who have been aggrieved by what they perceive as negligent medical care are frustrated in their attempt at finding a legal remedy against a managed care plan. ERISA* is largely to blame, since this federal law (enacted to standardize pension and welfare benefit plans throughout the country) preempts state tort law claims† as they relate to employee benefit plans. A patient who suffers harm as a result of negligent medical decision making by a managed care intermediary generally has limited remedies if the coverage in issue is provided pursuant to an employee benefit plan. Since many people receive health insurance as part of an employee benefit plan, ERISA has served to frustrate many litigants.

Employers may elect to self-insure their health plans (known as *self-funded plans*), in which the employer bears all or part of the risk (in terms of payment) in covering applicable services. ERISA preempts state regulation of employee health plans, which means that a self-insured plan is subject to ERISA but not to state regulations. If an employer arranges for a fully-insured benefit policy from an *insurer* (i.e., an HMO), however, then the policy would be regulated by state law with respect to the HMO issues (and the employer [plan sponsor] would still have to abide by ERISA). (For an example of a state HMO law, see NY Pub. HL, article 44 [McKinney, 1993].)

Although there have been a number of proposed bills in Congress over the past few years, the most prominent stem from two major initiatives introduced by the Republicans and one major bill introduced by the Democrats, which have some common features (CRS Report for Congress, 1999). Banning "gag clauses," which prevent physicians from openly recommending care; improving access to specialists in emergency treatment; increasing information available to consumers and expanding "point of service options," as well as requiring internal and external appeal procedures, are the major highlights. Unlike the

---

*Employee Retirement Income Security Act of 1974, 29 USC §1001 et seq.

†Medical malpractice is a type of "tort," which describes a legal cause of action brought by an injured person who has suffered harm because the "tortfeasor" breached the standard of care. In the context of medical malpractice, this means that the medical care rendered fell below the prevailing standard of care in the medical community.

Republican proposals, the Democrat bill sought to allow self-insured plans to be sued in certain cases, answering in damages for negligent medical decision making (CRS Report for Congress, 1999). This imposition of liability (as contemplated by the bill prominent in the 105th and 106th Congress) would require an amendment to ERISA to remove the impediments resulting from a long line of case law permitting preemption of state tort law claims. The Republican bills originally did not provide for additional causes of action against health plans; however, they sought to expand penalties for plans that do not comply with external review decisions. It remains to be seen if any Patients' Bill of Rights legislation will pass. Still, on the state level, efforts have been made to redress problems with managed care.

Regulating insurance is traditionally the role of state government. Congress can regulate in the area of healthcare, however, since the healthcare economy is part of interstate commerce, and hospitals, as recipients of federal and Medicare funds, are necessarily responsive to federal requirements. One of the last great examples of Congress flexing its strength in the area of insurance regulation is the Health Insurance Portability and Accountability Act of 1996 (HIPAA), effective January 1, 1997 (Ryan, 1997). One of the main provisions is to ensure portability of health insurance for individuals as they change jobs and move their homes. HIPAA imposes such requirements even on insurance plans, as well as ERISA plans. Only certain aspects of eligibility and coverage are addressed. It does not regulate the choice of providers, grievance procedures, or QA.

The opposition to the federal regulation of managed care plans argues that the marketplace should be free from federal interference so that market forces can respond to consumer demands, particularly for affordable quality care. Furthermore, regulation increases the cost of health insurance, which also increases the number of uninsured workers. The opposition also believes that national standards create inflexibility and interfere with cost-effective measures in the design of health plans.

The argument that information and choice are the hallmarks of a free market assumes that consumers are properly informed and that purchasers will choose among competing products to get the best value. If cost and quality data are available, this may in fact be sound logic. A lack of information has been cited by consumers as an impediment to making informed choices about health plans, however. Congress responded by proposing a requirement in various bills that information be disclosed about benefits, providers, medical decision making, and quality of healthcare (CRS Report for Congress, 1999). Benefit information that includes the type of existing coverage (e.g., services, emergency care, experimental treatment, drug formularies) and the responsibility of the policyholder for cost sharing was written into some of the proposals under consideration by Congress. Most importantly, the type of financial incentives used in provider contracts (as well as contract exclusions) were also part of the consumer-oriented proposals.

One of the bills introduced in the House of Representatives in April 1997 (HR 1415, known as *PARCA*, with 232 cosponsors) required disclosure of UR criteria and computer algorithms to health providers on request. Other bills required a general description of a UR program directly to the enrollees. The concept of value-based purchasing arguably requires the disclosure of quality data. Measures of enrollee satisfaction, health outcomes, voluntary disenrollment rates, and utilization data illustrate a plan's performance. The consumer-oriented bills under consideration generally agreed that such information should be accessible. Without national standards for a *core data set* to evaluate quality data in a plan, it would be extremely difficult to compare data across various plans.

Further compounding the debate is how to determine who would receive such information. The legislative proposals in Congress generally required that information go directly to the enrollees—or even to potential enrollees. State and federal authorities and plan sponsors would be permitted access as well. One approach under consideration was to avoid informing enrollees directly of UR procedures and to disclose the information to an accreditation body instead (or to a state agency or other regulator with oversight responsibility).

Congress has not gone so far as to become the nation's benefit manager. Once a benefit plan is available, however, the government has defined its role in providing procedural safeguards for enrollees. ERISA (and many state HMO plans) have a mechanism for hearing grievances and appeals by enrollees deprived of certain benefits. The criticism is that the appeals are generally within the plan (rather than before a disinterested third party) and that the damage done by negligent decisions or delays in treatment are never fully redressed, as they would be in a medical malpractice action. For example, an aggrieved individual can appeal to the ERISA plan to obtain a benefit previously denied and can even bring such an action in federal court; however, under ERISA, only contractual damages would be available (i.e., the cost of the service denied). This result should be contrasted with the *consequential damages* typically seen in a medical malpractice action involving lost wages, pain, and suffering. Thus consumer-driven remedies typically involve the proposal to impose tort liability on managed care payers (under ERISA plans or otherwise) who engage in negligent medical decision making.

Medical decisions made by unlicensed personnel (as opposed to physicians and nurses acting as case managers or UR agents) might enjoy greater insulation, depending on the case law precedent in a given state. On a case-by-case basis, attorneys have tried to carve out managed care liability on various theories, including negligent UR. A more compelling argument can be made for negligent medical decision making when the decision is made by a licensed health professional as opposed to an insurance manager. It is arguably within the mandate of state licensure boards to take issue with negligent medical decisions by a plan's medical director. Still, without an affirmative piece of legislation to provide a cause of action directly against a managed care plan, the change in accountability may unfold slowly. As such, case precedents may be most solid when premised on liability against licensed health professionals functioning as case managers, since they arguably have a duty of care commensurate with their professional experience.

Health professionals must also be careful when producing clinical practice guidelines (CPGs), which must be flexible enough to permit individualized application to avoid the "cookbook approach" to patient care (although such guidelines can enhance patient care). The federal Department of Health and Human Services has approved such initiatives, facilitating a Website for CPGs. The danger of reflexive application must be appreciated. For example, applying one CPG (e.g., treatment of pneumonia in an adult) may not necessarily encourage the analysis of comorbid factors in complicated cases. In other words, multiple CPGs may be necessary in any given case, and their use may cause inflexibility in the way care is delivered. Also, the criticism has been made that "teachers teach to the test," meaning that nursing and medical educators will stay within the confines of CPGs without appreciating the subtleties of disease presentation and medical and nursing management.

Nurses and other health professionals who establish CPGs must consider the need (and likelihood) of cases involving comorbidities. Enhancing medical decision making by providing multiple CPGs in complicated cases is not only important for the patient but is essential from a risk management point of view, since the lack of a comprehensive approach, from the standpoint of CPGs, poses significant liability. Since the role of a plaintiff's attorney (who brings an action on behalf of a patient suffering harm) is to prove that there was a breach in the duty of care that caused damages, the CPGs will be "center stage." The CPG will be evidence in the trial court, and a breach of the guideline will provide compelling evidence to a jury that the patient was cared for negligently. Making matters worse, if multiple CPGs are necessary (and only a few make their way to the medical record), the inference drawn by the jury may be that the patient was neglected.

CPGs therefore should be drafted with great care and should include a statement reminding the practitioners to evaluate each case on an individual basis. Furthermore, if such guidelines are drafted as part of the QA process, there may be less likelihood that they will be subject to disclosure during a malpractice case, depending on the laws in a given jurisdiction.*

SUMMARY

The dramatic shift in the way healthcare is delivered, which involves payers in medical decision making, has created an unprecedented strain on nurses and medical providers in general. The impact may not have been readily apparent to consumers, who generally are not familiar with the complexities of the healthcare delivery system. Accordingly, remedial legislation, state and federal regulations, and case precedents (from malpractice cases) come slowly to the aid of aggrieved consumers. The move to redress some of the substandard practices associated with managed care is in many respects just beginning, and where it equilibrates remains to be seen. Congress may ultimately pass consumer-oriented legislation in response to widespread complaints about managed care. The alliance of medical associations and consumers is a formidable one and is a force that lawmakers cannot ignore. On the other side, the insurance industry has made compelling arguments to keep tort liability restricted so that overall costs of healthcare delivery do not skyrocket. It is against this backdrop that traditional legal principles (such as tort liability) interact with the dynamic changes in the health industry. When the dust settles (perhaps several decades from now), there may be clearer legal guidelines for nursing practice—assuming it survives in its currently regulated form. In the interim,

---

*In New York, quality assurance materials and peer review proceedings are protected from disclosure in a medical malpractice action, subject to very narrow exceptions. NY Pub. HL §2805 m (McKinney, 1993, p 493); NY Ed. L. §6527 (McKinney Suppl, 2001, p 290).

nurses should be careful to abide by the standard of care notwithstanding economic forces that may antagonize traditional nursing principles. The fact that coverage for certain health-care may not be available does not permit an alternate level of care. A healthcare provider must abide by the rules of the profession, leaving the issue of payment and reimbursement for the insured. Simply stated, the standards should not be tuned to what care is likely to be paid for. The rules of nursing (dictated on a state-by-state basis) are not likely to become more relaxed in response to economic forces. The continuation of such professional mandates gives the professional nurse little choice but to maintain professional standards.

REFERENCES

American Nurses Association: *Nursing's agenda for health-care reform,* Washington, DC, 1992, American Nurses Publishing.

Congressional Research Service (CRS) Report for Congress: *Side-by-side comparison of selected patient protection bills: HR 358/5.6, HR 448 and 5.1344,* Washington, DC, July 26, 1999, Congressional Research Service, Library of Congress.

Friedberg R: Accountability and managed care, *Radiology* 205(2):833a-885a, 1997.

Huntington JA: Healthcare in chaos: will we ever see real managed care, *Online J Issues Nurs* 2(1), 1997.

Ladden MT, Steinberg S: *Managed care implications for nursing,* Boston, 1996, Harvard Community Health Plan.

McKinney's consolidated laws of New York annotated, 2001-2002 Interim Supplementary Pamphlet, Eagan, Minn, 2002, West Group.

McKinney's consolidated laws of New York annotated, Eagan, Minn, 2001, West Group.

Nealy v. Yung, New York Law Journal, p 26, Mar 26, 1999.

Ryan B: Health law promises access, portability, *New York Law Journal,* p 85, Feb 10, 1997.

U.S. tells Albany to aid failing hospital, *The New York Times,* pp 3-5, April 10, 1999.

15

Managed Care and the Nurse: Legal Issues

Margaret Davino

KEY LESSONS IN THIS CHAPTER

- Although the number of malpractice lawsuits has increased over the past several years, it does not seem to be caused by the increasing number of managed care health insurance plans in the population.
- From a legal perspective, the nurse's primary responsibility is to the patient and not to the managed care company.
- All members of the healthcare team should act in the best interest of the patient. The law does not require healthcare professionals to render care without compensation, however, except when a patient seeks emergency care.
- Legally, patients should not be discharged simply because the payer refuses to pay for continued days in the hospital if the discharge poses a danger to the patient's life or health.
- Although nurses may encounter a number of legal issues pertaining to managed care in their practice, these issues should not impose any additional liability on them.

Managed care has become increasingly prevalent as employers and others have become concerned about the cost of healthcare and look for ways to decrease healthcare insurance premiums. Nurses may become involved in managed care arrangements in the following ways:

- As providers of nursing care to patients whose insurance is through a managed care organization (MCO)
- As case managers attempting to control the utilization of resources provided to a patient insured by a managed care plan
- As discharge planners locating appropriate posthospital care for a patient insured by a managed care plan
- As patients whose MCO may or may not authorize the care desired

A number of legal issues relate to managed care arrangements in which nurses may become involved. MCOs, when defending themselves against allegations of liability, will emphasize that the MCO is only the payer of care provided, and not the decision-maker as to what care will be rendered. In reality, given the cost of healthcare today, payment is often equated with care itself and directly influences (if not directs) whether a patient will seek care.

PAYMENT METHODS

There are several different methods by which MCOs pay providers, including capitation, fee-for-service, discounted fee-for-service, globally (payment includes both the hospital and the physician), case rates (payment is made to all the providers involved in a case such as a cardiac bypass), or other payment mechanisms in which the provider is put "at-risk" (withholding part of the payment until a later time to see how efficiently the provider managed the patient's care). The method (and amount) of payment will be negotiated between the managed care payer and the providers of care, which may include the hospital, employed physicians, unemployed (attending) physicians, nursing staff, and other staff employed by the hospital.

Payers establish certain methods of payment both to control the amount paid and to attempt to influence providers to provide more cost-efficient care. In capitated arrangements, a provider (usually a primary care physician such as an internist or a pediatrician) is paid a flat amount per month for a patient (called a *per-member-per-month* payment), regardless of whether the patient is seen by the physician every day for an acute problem or is not seen at all. In the ideal world, capitation emphasizes that the physician should maintain the patient in a healthy state, promotes preventive care, and decreases the frequency with which the patient needs to see the physician.

In the case of capitated arrangements involving legal disputes, a lawyer may allege that the physician did not provide care needed by the patient because the physician would not be paid anything extra for providing that care. The same allegations may be made if the provider is paid through any type of a "risk" arrangement: that the physician did not provide the care needed by the patient because the physician was going to make more money by *not* providing care and was influenced by these monetary incentives.

Regardless of the payment arrangement, most managed care payers implement mechanisms to manage specialty care, hospitalization, or other care provided under their various contractual arrangements. Management can occur through a requirement that patients must have the approval of their primary care physician before they see a specialist, or the MCO may require that an admission to a hospital be "preapproved" or "precertified" by the managed care payer. They may authorize payment only for a certain number of days in the hospital, or for a certain number of days or hours of outpatient treatment or home care. Other examples of management include denial of payment for procedures that MCOs do not consider to be "medically necessary." They may not pay for certain hospital care because that same care can be provided in an outpatient setting, or they may not pay for certain procedures because they are considered "experimental" (e.g., bone marrow transplant for breast cancer).

RECEIVING NONREIMBURSED CARE

Although managed care payers argue that they are not denying *care delivery* but are only denying *payment* for care, the effect of this nonpayment is usually the same. Most people are unable or unwilling to pay for treatment that may be extremely expensive if their insurance company says it is not "medically necessary." Therefore they may not ultimately receive the care they were seeking. If a patient suffers injury due to lack of treatment, the allegations in a lawsuit are that the insurance company should have paid for treatment, that the patient's primary care physician should have appealed the payer's denial of payment for care, and/or that the hospital, home care agency, nurse, or other provider should have continued to provide care or given the patient more education about what could happen after discharge or if certain care was not continued.

The Role of the Nurse

The underlying role of the nurse should be to provide care to the patient without regard for the patient's payer status. Hospitals, by virtue of their agreements outlined within their managed care contracts, are required to implement mechanisms to comply with managed care payers' requirements (e.g., precertification, approval for continued stay, and review of whether services will be considered to be "medically necessary").

The nurse's employer, or the case manager or discharge planner, may be influenced to retain, discharge, or provide certain care to a patient based on whether the patient's payer has authorized payment for that care. Although most hospitals are not-for-profit, they will not remain financially viable for long without payment for the services they provide. Therefore hospitals are essentially required to provide care not only effectively but efficiently, with "efficient" viewed from both an operational and a cost perspective.

Patient Care Issues

When operationalized, these mechanisms may result in moving patients out of acute care settings earlier than in the past. If a lawsuit results from this earlier patient transition to a lower level of care, the patient's lawyer may allege that care needed by the patient was not provided because of the hospital's financial incentives.

The nurse may get involved in a lawsuit involving allegations that managed care requirements and payments improperly influenced the care of a patient. Although the role of the nurse is usually as a witness, nurses sometimes are included as defendants in such suits.

FREQUENTLY ASKED QUESTIONS ABOUT LEGAL ISSUES IN MANAGED CARE

This section focuses on some areas in which legalities may be involved in patients with managed care arrangements. The remainder of this chapter is presented in a question-and-answer format to address questions frequently asked by nurses about these areas.

Question

Does managed care cause more malpractice suits that the nurse may get involved in?

Answer

Managed care influences care provided to patients in the following three ways:
1. An MCO may pay *providers* (e.g., nurses, physicians, hospitals) in ways that may influence the amount of care provided.
2. An MCO may impose certain requirements before care will be paid for. One example is if the patient or the hospital is required to obtain "preapproval" before the payer will pay for hospital care.
3. An MCO may refuse to pay for continued care or other care recommended by the patient's physician. If a patient is denied payment for care and does not receive that care, the patient may sue, alleging that he or she suffered injury because appropriate care was not received. Sometimes these suits are brought solely against the MCO; sometimes they also include the physicians and nurses involved in the patient's care.

There has been no real study as to whether managed care patients sue more frequently for medical malpractice than do other patients. The number of malpractice lawsuits has been increasing over the past several years, but this is probably due more to society's increasing propensity to sue than to the increasing percentage of the population's health insurance that is through a managed care arrangement.

Question

What is my responsibility as a nurse to a managed care patient?

Answer

The nurse's responsibility to any patient, regardless of whether that patient pays or how that patient pays, is the same. The nurse is responsible for providing good, reasonable care as should be provided by a reasonably prudent nurse acting within the scope of ethical guidelines, the law, and his or her employer's policies.

A nurse who is not involved in case management or discharge planning may never need to know what type of payment arrangements exist for a patient or the identity of a patient's health insurer.

A staff nurse's duty to a patient may at some time be affected, however, because a managed care payer questions the care being rendered or has refused to approve payment for continued hospitalization. In such cases, the physician and hospital will need to decide whether to appeal the payer's denial of continued payment. The nurse may become involved in this decision either directly or indirectly. The staff nurse may be directly involved by participating in an interdisciplinary case conference where the need for continued hospitalization for the patient is reviewed. The staff nurse may be indirectly involved, since the hospital's and payer's case manager may review the nurse's notes to determine whether continued hospitalization is medically necessary. A nurse's note stating that a patient's wound is still draining purulent fluid, that a patient has pain requiring injectable pain medication, or that a patient is unable to ambulate independently may cause a managed care payer to approve payment for continued hospitalization that would otherwise be denied or questioned.

Question

Do I have any additional malpractice liability to a managed care patient?

Answer

As stated earlier, the nurse's duty to a patient does not depend on the specifics of reimbursement. A patient who brings a negligence suit against a healthcare provider must show the following four things:

1. That the provider had a duty of care towards that person
2. That the provider breached his or her duty and failed to act like a reasonably prudent person under the same or similar circumstances
3. That the patient suffered some actual injury or harm
4. That what the provider did (or failed to do) caused the patient's injury or harm

Patients who bring negligence suits involving MCOs often allege that the payer refused to pay for services the patient claims were medically necessary. If the nurse is included as a defendant in such a suit, the plaintiff's attorney will look for the following things that are always reviewed in assessing the nurse's liability:

- Did the nurse act reasonably prudent when assessing the patient and providing patient care?
- Did the nurse provide appropriate discharge instructions to a patient being discharged from the hospital?
- Did the nurse communicate any problems to the responsible physician(s)?
- Did the nurse's documentation reflect his or her actions and the justification for taking or not taking actions?

As with any malpractice case, the nurse's documentation will be essential in defending his or her actions.

Question

Do I as the nurse have any responsibility or liability to the MCO?

Answer

No. The responsibility of the nurse is to the patient. In addition, the nurse is responsible to his or her employer and should follow the employer's policies and procedures in providing care to patients and in documenting that care.

Question

If an MCO denies payment for care ordered by a patient's physician, what is my responsibility as a nurse?

Answer

The nurse's responsibility is to act in the best interests of the patient at all times. Nevertheless, the nurse's actions need to conform with his or her employer's policies and the law, which states in the Nursing Practice Act that the nurse generally works under the direction of a licensed physician.

A nurse may be involved in caring for a patient whose MCO denies payment for either continued inpatient care, outpatient care, home care (entirely or at the level recommended by the physician), or a specialized procedure. Unless the patient is willing and able to pay for private care, a number of factors will be involved in deciding how the patient's care will proceed. These factors include whether the denial of continued payment is appealed and what alternatives for care exist. If a hospitalized patient's MCO refuses to authorize continued hospitalization but will pay for home care, the nurse's duty is to educate the patient and family about their responsibilities in managing the patient's care in the home, such as the signs and symptoms to watch for that should be brought to a healthcare professional's attention and tasks that will have to be performed in the home (e.g., toileting, feeding).

Question

Are there other members of the care team (e.g., the physician or hospital) that may have liability if an MCO refuses to authorize continued care for a patient?

Answer

Like the nurse, all members of the care team should always act with the best interests of the patient in mind. The law does not require healthcare professionals to render care without compensation, however, except when a patient seeks emergency care from a hospital with an emergency room. The general concept that a hospital or physician cannot be forced to provide care to a patient who cannot or does not wish to pay for that care must be balanced against the malpractice liability that may result from refusal of care.

As stated earlier, a patient suing a hospital, physician, or other healthcare provider must show the following four things to prove that the provider was negligent and guilty of malpractice:

1. That the provider owed the patient a duty of care
2. That the provider breached his or her duty of care and failed to act like a reasonably prudent healthcare professional under those circumstances
3. That the patient suffered some injury or harm
4. That what the healthcare provider did (or failed to do) caused the patient's injury or harm

With very few exceptions (for example, in an emergency room), a healthcare provider has no duty to someone with whom there has been no previous relationship. For example, a physician or nurse practitioner in a private setting cannot be forced to accept a patient for an appointment who has not previously been seen as a patient of that practice. Similarly, a home care agency that does not wish to accept a patient because the managed care company authorized fewer hours than the home care agency feels is appropriate is generally not required to accept that patient.

When a healthcare professional is already in a provider-patient relationship, however, the provider can be liable if she or he terminates that relationship without making sufficient efforts to ensure that the patient will not suffer harm. In addition to malpractice liability, many state licensing agencies may take action against the license of a healthcare professional or a hospital who "abandons" a patient. Therefore if a patient's payer is refusing to pay for continued care, the provider must decide whether it is medically appropriate and legally defensible to discharge the person from care or whether the patient's care should be continued, either without payment or seeking payment directly from the patient.

If a patient is currently hospitalized and the payer refuses to pay for additional hospitalization, an assessment must occur as to whether the patient is truly ready for discharge. Legally the patient should not be discharged simply because his or her payer refused to pay for continued days of hospitalization if the discharge will pose danger to the patient's life or health. In cases alleging premature discharge, documentation is essential. A plaintiff's attorney often will review the medical record to look at what the various caregivers' notes said about the patient's condition in the days before discharge and whether the nurses' notes are consistent with the physician's notes.

For example, in the case *John Bell v. NYCHHC,* 90 AD 2d 270 (1982), a patient who attempted suicide by setting himself on fire 1 week after he was discharged from a psychiatric unit claimed that the caregivers had discharged him prematurely, without a proper medical examination. In its finding in favor of the patient, the court emphasized that the nurse's note the day before discharge read that the patient was delusional and became physically resistant when attempts were made to medicate him, requiring that the patient be placed in restraints. The court added up the amount of Thorazine documented as given by the nurses and noted that the patient required more Thorazine the day and night before discharge than any other day. Later that day, however, the attending physician determined that the patient could be released.

When the patient is ready for discharge, a safe discharge plan is required. The court in the Bell case noted that the hospital record was silent about discharge planning and that the patient's wife testified that she was not informed that her husband was being discharged. To protect against claims that the hospital failed to explain the discharge plan or that the patient did not understand it, the nurse should document what postacute care is needed, the discharge instructions and education given to the patient, the names of the family members involved, and the level of understanding of the patient and the family.

Question

If a managed care payer refuses payment for treatment, are any of the providers liable if the denial is not appealed?

Answer

Managed care payers who deny payment for treatment consistently emphasize that they are denying payment only, and it is up to the healthcare professional to make treatment decisions. If a payer denies payment for treatment and the physician or the hospital feel that the payer is wrong in its denial, the physician and/or the hospital may have a duty to the patient to appeal the denial and provide additional facts and stronger arguments to justify the treatment.

In the seminal case regarding the liability of an MCO versus the treating physician, *Wickline v. State of California,* 192 Cal. App. 3d 1630, 239 Cal. Rptr. 810 (Cal. App. II Dist., 1986), a patient sued her managed care insurer after the payer's utilization review consultant, a board-certified general surgeon, authorized only a 4-day extension of the patient's hospitalization when the patient's attending surgeon had requested an 8-day extension. The patient had undergone coronary artery bypass surgery and had experienced complications. The hospital and attending physician did not appeal, and the patient was discharged at the end of 4 days. The patient continued to have complications that resulted in amputation of her right leg. The jury found the payer liable for negligently discontinuing the patient's hospitalization and awarded the patient $500,000. The appellate court reversed the decision, however. It found that the ultimate responsibility for making patient treatment and discharge decisions belongs to the attending physician, who therefore has a duty to protest or appeal a denial of necessary care.

A 1999 New York case further discussed the responsibility of a primary care physician to take all reasonable steps within his or her control to obtain patient care that is available under the patient's plan. In *Nealy v. U.S. Healthcare HMO,* 93 NY 2d 209 (1999), a 37-year-old man diagnosed with coronary arteriosclerosis and a coronary artery lesion was required by U.S. Healthcare to obtain a referral from a primary care physician before he could see a nonparticipating cardiologist. He allegedly was first denied an appointment with the primary care physician he chose because he did not yet have his health maintenance organization (HMO) identification number, and then was rejected because his form had the wrong primary care physician number. After examination, the primary care physician agreed to the patient's request to see the nonparticipating cardiologist who had performed the patient's angioplasty but did not submit the paperwork to obtain U.S. Healthcare's approval for 10 days. After U.S. Healthcare initially refused the referral because there was a participating cardiologist in the area, the patient finally obtained a referral to his cardiologist of choice. Unfortunately, he suffered a cardiac arrest and died the day before the cardiologist appointment. The New York Court of Appeals allowed the suit to proceed against both U.S. Healthcare and the primary care physician. The suit against the primary care physician phrased the allegations in fairly traditional malpractice/negligence terms: that the primary care physician violated the standard of care owed to the patient by improperly assessing the nature and extent of his condition and failing to take reasonable steps to provide for timely treatment by a specialist. The allegations against the primary care physician were separate from the allegations against U.S. Healthcare for the delay caused by its decision-making process with respect to coverage or benefits.

Nurses should remember that most payers will make decisions based on their concurrent review of the need for care, a process that is based largely on what is written in the patient's medical record. Complete and accurate documentation of the patient's condition, problems, and response to treatment is crucial and should be reflected in the notes of all members of the care team. Where differences of opinion between the managed care payer and the treating physician do arise, the patient must be kept informed about all of his or her options. The family should also be aware of all communications and the significance of such. The patient, physician, and hospital should ensure that an appeal is taken where appropriate. Even if the payer's final decision is contrary to the physician's treatment recommendations, the final choice about continuation of treatment always belongs to the patient. The record should reflect the discussion with the patient as to the risks and benefits of all options for care—remaining in the hospital, going home, or receiving other postacute care. Although the patient will likely consider which options will be paid for by the MCO and which options will be paid for by the patient, the final choice of the option belongs to the patient.

Question

Can a patient sue the MCO if it denies payment for care?

Answer

Many patients have attempted to sue their insurers for denying payment for care that was sought by the patient—care that in some situations was necessary to save the patient's life. Although some cases have found liability on the part of the managed care payer and in a few situations awarded huge damages against the payer that denied payment, most cases have precluded suit. Many of these cases were based upon the preemption clause under the federal Employment Retirement Income and Security Act (ERISA), 29 USC Sections 1001-1461 (1988). ERISA is a federal statute controlling employee benefit plans and mandates that any state law that attempts to regulate ERISA-governed plans is preempted due to federal control of the field.

If a managed care plan continues to deny payment for care after an appeal of the denial by the care providers, however, some courts have found that the MCO may have liability if the continued denial is unreasonable, despite ERISA. In *Wilson v. Blue Cross of Southern California*, 271 Cal. Rptr. 876 (Cal. App., 1990), the same court that decided *Wickline v. State of California* (see previous case) ruled that a payer may be liable for the death of a psychiatric patient who committed suicide 3 weeks after he was discharged from a hospitalization for depression, drug dependency, and anorexia after the payer refused to continue inpatient coverage. Despite the recommendation of the treating psychiatrist for 3 to 4 weeks of inpatient care, Blue Cross authorized only 10 days, based on its concurrent review guidelines. The appellate court sent this case to trial, finding "there is substantial evidence that [the utilization review] decision not to approve further hospitalization was a substantial factor in bringing about the decedent's demise" (*Wilson v. Blue Cross of Southern California*, 271 Cal. Rptr. 883 [Cal. App., 1990]). The court had determined that the patient's premature discharge from the hospital was directly related to the patient's suicide 3 weeks after discharge.

Some states have debated legislation specifically allowing lawsuits against MCOs for medical negligence claims. Texas was the first state to actually pass such a law, which became effective September 1, 1999 (Texas Health Maintenance Organization Act [Article 20A.12A,

Vernon's Texas Insurance Code and Article 3.70-31]). Although Texas ultimately allows such suits, it first provides that disputes be sent to an independent arbitration system. MCOs lobby vigorously against such laws, arguing that the ability to sue under the law will simply drive up costs.

Question

I have heard that federal law requires patients to get a list of home care providers and that a patient cannot be referred to the hospital's home health agency. Is this the same with managed care patients and how does it affect discharge planning for managed care patients?

Answer

The federal Balanced Budget Act of 1997 amended the Medicare Act to require expressly that as part of the discharge plan, a hospital must provide patients with a list of home health agencies that participate in the Medicare program, service the geographic area in which the patient resides, and request to be listed as available by the hospital. The purpose of this law was to prevent hospitals with home care agencies from channeling all patients to the hospital's agency. The hospital is also required to identify for patients any home health provider in the patient's discharge plan in which the hospital has a financial interest or that has a financial interest in the hospital. Medicare managed care plans may have contracts with some but not all home care providers and will authorize payment for home care only when the home care is provided by an agency with which it has a contract. The U.S. Health Care Financing Administration (HCFA) has suggested that hospitals not distribute their entire list of home health agencies to participants in Medicare managed care plans, since patients may believe that the listed providers all participate in their plan. Instead, hospitals may provide Medicare managed care patients with a list of home health agencies approved by their managed care plan. Therefore the patient may be able to choose between various agencies, but the agency chosen will have to be one with a relationship with the managed care payer, and the managed care payer will require that it receives sufficient information to authorize the care in advance.

Question

Can a patient be refused emergency care if the hospital believes that the patient's managed care plan will not pay for the care?

Answer

The federal Emergency Medical Treatment and Active Labor Act (EMTALA) states that any patient who requests emergency treatment from a hospital with an emergency room must receive at least a medical screening examination and treatment sufficient to stabilize any emergency medical condition. This law provides penalties both for hospitals and its staff (such as nurses) and for physicians who do not comply with its mandates. EMTALA was intended to prevent "dumping" of uninsured patients but applies to any patient who seeks treatment for an emergency from a hospital with an emergency department (ED) (Social Security Act, section 1867 [42 MSP 1395 dd]).

EMTALA may apply to patients whose health insurance is through a managed care arrangement if that patient comes to the emergency room of a hospital seeking screening or treatment. The EMTALA regulations and interpretive guidelines prohibit a hospital or its staff from taking any action that would discourage the patient from seeking emergency treatment, including calling the MCO for authorization until after the patient has been screened for an emergency medical condition and has had that condition stabilized.

Question

Can the hospital check the patient's insurance in the ED before providing care?

Answer

In November 1999, the U.S. Department of Health and Human Services, the Office of Inspector General (OIG), and the HCFA published a special news release that made it clear that hospitals must not delay screening or stabilizing patients while obtaining authorization from managed care plans. EMTALA, the antidumping statute, prohibits a hospital's inquiry about a patient's method of payment or insurance status, or use of such information, from delaying a screening examination or stabilizing medical treatment. The OIG stated that it is aware that some hospitals routinely seek prior authorization from a patient's primary care physician or from the managed care plan when a managed care patient requests emergency services, since the failure to obtain authorization may result in the plan refusing to pay for the emergency services. Although the OIG noted that hospitals are sometimes caught between the legal obligations imposed under EMTALA and the terms of the agreements with managed care plans, obligations under EMTALA are primary (OIG, 1999).

The OIG suggested the following practices to minimize the likelihood that a hospital will violate EMTALA:

- A hospital should not request and a health plan should not require prior authorization before the patient has received a medical screening examination to determine the presence or absence of an emergency medical condition, or before the patient's emergency medical condition is stabilized.
- A hospital should not ask a patient to complete a financial responsibility form or an advanced beneficiary notice or ask for a copayment before performing an appropriate medical screening examination. This request could deter the patient from remaining at the hospital.
- When a patient asks about financial liability for emergency services, staff must inform the patient that, notwithstanding the patient's ability to pay, the hospital is ready and willing to provide a medical screening examination and stabilizing treatment, if necessary.
- If a patient chooses to withdraw his or her request for examination or treatment, the hospital must: (1) offer the person further examination and treatment, (2) inform the patient of the risks and benefits of withdrawal before receiving treatment, and (3) attempt to secure the patient's written informed consent to refuse such examination and treatment.

Question

Can an MCO refuse to pay for emergency care?

Answer

There are two reasons that managed care plans most commonly give to deny payment for care provided in an emergency room. The first is that the managed care plan's requirements for preapproval or authorization before care were not met. Most hospitals and many physicians are able to negotiate contracts with managed care payers that exempt the provider from being required to obtain preauthorization from the MCO for treatment in cases of emergency. Some state laws specifically state that MCOs cannot require preauthorization from the MCO for treatment in emergency situations.

Unfortunately, a statement that a provider does not have to contact the managed care plan for authorization before emergency care is provided is not the same as a mandate that the MCO must pay for that care. The second reason that managed care plans commonly give to deny payment is that the patient's condition was not a true emergency, and therefore the care was not "emergency care." Many MCOs review ED diagnoses to assess whether the condition for which treatment was sought was an emergency or would have been amenable to treatment in a physician's office. If the condition was not a real emergency (e.g., otitis media in a child), the MCO may refuse to pay on the basis that the treatment provided was not treatment for an emergency. Some hospitals have negotiated and some states have mandated a minimum screening fee for cases treated in the ED that are found not to be emergencies, but the modest fee (e.g., $35.00) often does not come close to covering the costs of the hospital ED in providing care to a patient.

Question

If a patient is cared for in the ED and needs admission, can the hospital transfer the patient if the MCO will not authorize admission to *that* hospital?

Answer

EMTALA allows transfer before a patient's condition is medically stabilized only in the following two situations:
1. If a physician certifies that the anticipated benefits of transfer outweigh documentation of a patient's request for transfer to another facility.
2. If the patient opts for transfer to another provider, these guidelines should be carefully followed.

In addition, EMTALA requires that the following four conditions be met for a transfer:
1. The transferring hospital must provide treatment within its capacity to minimize the risks of transfer.
2. The transferring hospital must receive permission from the receiving hospital to transfer the patient. (A hospital with specialized capabilities may refuse only when it does not have capacity.)
3. The patient's medical record must be sent with the patient to the receiving hospital.

4. The transfer must be effected through use of qualified personnel and transportation equipment.

Question

What is the role of the case manager for a managed care patient?

Answer

Many hospitals hire case managers to manage a patient's case while in the hospital. The case manager is often responsible for tracking the patient's stay, expediting performance of tests, beginning discharge planning early during the patient's stay, transmitting information to the patient's managed care payer, and obtaining authorization and precertification for procedures and continued stay. In addition, the case manager may arrange for all services required for discharge or relocation of the patient, including equipment, home care, or transportation; coordinate efforts with the rest of the care team and the family; ensure that the home is safe; identify problems with discharge; obtain payer authorization for treatment; act as a liaison between the hospital and the insurance company; share information about the patient with the physician; work with the physician and care team to achieve the best outcome; and counsel the patient and family about resources necessary for postacute care.

Case management has become popular and perhaps even necessary due to the multiple interactions that occur between a provider, especially a hospital, and a patient's managed care payer. Many MCOS will authorize only a few days of care at a time, and the case manager is the person who is responsible for seeking additional authorization for payment.

In a lawsuit by a patient against a hospital, physician, or nurse alleging premature discharge, the case manager's notes will also be reviewed to assess whether the notes support the hospital's discharge of the patient. Similar to the nurses' notes, the case manager's notes should reflect the discharge planning process, the discussion with the patient and family as to the options with regard to discharge, that the patient and family were informed as to the risks and complications involved in each of the options, and that the ultimate choice as to discharge and postacute care was made by the patient.

Question

Are there any special discharge planning concerns for managed care patients?

Answer

As with any patient in today's healthcare environment, discharge planning for managed care patients should begin at the time of the patient's admission to a facility or before admission if possible. The staff nurse should be involved with the physician, case manager, and rest of the care team in assessing the patient's expected length of stay, the expected outcome, any special requirements at discharge, and what needs to be facilitated early on. For example, if the patient is expected to need rehabilitation after acute care (e.g., for a stroke), planning should begin at the time of admission, and the patient and family should be involved in discussions about appropriate rehabilitation facilities.

Lawsuits can be germinated by a failure to meet a patient's and/or family's expectations. The best way to avoid this is early and full communication with the patient and family to discuss realistic expectations. The patient and family should be informed of all aspects of the patient's care, with the ultimate decision about care in the patient's hands. The family should therefore be informed of what type of care the patient will require at home and whether this will require the family to purchase special supplies or equipment, and the family should be trained about care that they may need to provide at home. If a patient is going home with a colostomy and will rely upon a family member for assistance in changing the bag and cleaning the stoma, the family should be adequately trained in the hospital about that care. Patients also may not understand that their managed care plan will not cover certain items or postacute care and may become angry at hospital staff who do not put that care in place. The nurse, physician, and case manager in the hospital should be very clear with the patient about what items are and are not covered by their managed care plan and should inform the patient about the options for private payment if the patient is able.

Although family members or persons who may be injured due to a hospital's allegedly premature discharge may express a desire to sue the hospital, the hospital and its staff are generally not liable to anyone other than the patient. This is because, as stated previously, someone suing for negligence must demonstrate that the person sued owed a duty of care to the person injured. For example, *Purdy v. Public Administrator of County of Westchester,* 530 NYS 2d 573, 72 NY 2d 1 (CT App., 1988) involved a suit against a healthcare facility by a customer at a gas station who was struck and seriously injured by a car driven by a 73-year-old resident of a healthcare facility who suffered from a medical condition that left her susceptible to dizzy spells. The New York Court of Appeals found that neither the facility nor the patient's physician had a duty to prevent a resident from leaving or operating a vehicle off the premises.

In *Nunez v. New York Hospital,* New York Supreme Court IA Part 27, reported in *New York Law Journal* 7-30-90, a patient's daughter sued the hospital for reimbursement for expenses she incurred in caring for her mother discharged by the hospital to her home. The daughter claimed, among other things, that the home health aides provided either did not show up or left early, causing her to leave work, arrive late, or not go to work at all. The court dismissed the suit, finding that the hospital's only duty was to the patient and not to the daughter.

Question

What is the liability of nurses who provide telephone advice through managed care payers' "Call A Nurse" services?

Answer

As stated above, a patient suing a nurse for professional negligence must demonstrate first that the nurse had a duty of care towards the patient and secondly that the nurse breached his or her duty of care. Nurses who provide nursing advice to a person, whether in person or over the telephone, are presenting themselves as nurses and therefore have a duty of care to the caller. The questions that often arise are whether the nurse on the call line acted like a reasonably prudent nurse under the same or similar circumstances and whether the nurse's advice was a significant factor in causing the patient's injury or harm. Although it is always safer to assess someone in person before providing advice, managed care companies with "Call a Nurse" lines rely on clinical guidelines and the fact that most cases can be fit into the clinical guidelines. Nurses should be aware, however, that cases have been successfully brought against nurses who give telephone advice that turns out to have been incorrect.

Question

The nurse may receive multiple requests for information from persons claiming to be from the patient's managed care company. Can that information be released?

Answer

When someone obtains healthcare insurance, whether through an MCO or otherwise, he or she customarily is required to sign a form authorizing the insurance company to request and obtain all of the patient's medical information. The insurance company needs this information to determine if the services provided should be paid for. Nevertheless, a nurse should be reluctant to discuss a patient's medical information over the phone with someone with whom he or she is not familiar. The best approach is to ask the person to put the request in writing on company letterhead, with the name and title of the requester. A request for information can be faxed or hand-delivered if needed. The nurse can therefore ensure that the person requesting the information is who he or she claims to be and can consult with hospital administration if doubts still exist.

Question

Sometimes physicians or hospitals are given financial incentives by managed care plans to not provide care. Is there anything illegal about this?

Answer

In a recent case, *Pegram v. Herdrich*, 528 US 211, 147 L. Ed. 2d 164 1205 CK 2140 (2000), the United States Supreme Court upheld the legality of cost-containment incentives in healthcare under the federal ERISA law. This case was brought by a patient who claimed that the rupture of her appendix was caused by an unreasonable wait for an abdominal scan after examination by her physician, due to the physician's financial incentive to refer her only to a participating diagnostic center for the scan. After collecting a $35,000 malpractice judgment, the patient filed an ERISA suit, claiming that the doctor-owned managed care plan breached its fiduciary duty by creating economic incentives for physicians to deprive their patients of medically necessary care and retain the resulting profits for themselves. The Seventh Circuit Court of Appeals refused to dismiss the complaint, essentially blaming managed care for the accelerated decline of our healthcare system. The Supreme Court, however, found that the treatment and eligibility decisions the managed care plan made in treating (or failing to treat) her appendicitis were not fiduciary decisions under ERISA. Its opinion recognized that like other risk-bearing organizations, HMOs take steps to control costs, including issuing general guidelines for physicians and conducting utilization review. The Court stated that no managed care organization could survive without some incentive connecting physician reward with treatment rationing.

Question

It sometimes seems that MCOs have all the power when bargaining with providers. Can providers band together to negotiate against payers?

Answer

Providers must be careful in joining together to negotiate payment rates. Providers who collectively agree either to a certain price or to refuse anything less than a certain price can be accused of price-fixing under federal and state antitrust laws. Some hospitals and physicians have joined together to form *physician hospital organizations* (PHOs) for purposes of managed care contracting. These organizations must be careful only to relay the offer from the managed care plan to the individual physicians or groups, however, rather than negotiate rates on behalf of physicians who are not legally a single entity.

REFERENCE

Nunez v. New York Hospital, New York Law Journal, July 30, 1990.

Office of Inspector General: *Special advisory bulletin outlines hospitals' obligations to provide emergency services to managed care enrollees,* Washington, DC, 1999, Office of Public Affairs.

16

Ethics, Integrity, and Managed Care

Carol Taylor

KEY LESSONS IN THIS CHAPTER

- Managed care is sometimes blamed for the growing number of complaints about the current healthcare system.
- Nurses and other healthcare providers need a clear vision of moral healthcare, as well as a clear vision of their moral obligations as healthcare professionals.
- Managed care sacrifices patient and healthcare autonomy to maximize benefits to the group.
- Patients may be underserved in both traditional fee-for-service systems and contemporary managed care arrangements.
- Nurses must apply ethical decision making in their everyday practice.

How many of us entered nursing with the simple and sincere motivation "to help others." How many of us today leave work feeling good about our ability to make a critical difference in the lives of those entrusted to our care by helping them achieve valued health goals? If many of us are feeling increasingly frustrated by our growing inability to meet the reasonable expectations of today's patients and their families because of limited time and other resources, we must step back, reflect, and decide how we will respond. At stake is nothing less than the health and well-being of those we serve and our profession's moral integrity.

Ethical competence should be established as a core competence for all health professionals, on a par with intellectual, technological, and interpersonal competence. Ethical competence should serve as a criteria for admission to the health professions, hiring, advancement, and firing (Taylor, 1995). This author has also described some of the specific ethical challenges confronting nurse case managers in today's market-driven health environment (Taylor, 1997; Barnet and Taylor, 1999; Taylor and Barnet, 1999). This chapter explores the broad ethical challenges posed by managed care, traces their evolution in a brief discussion of how healthcare delivery has evolved in the United States, and concludes with some practical recommendations for reflection and action. Before reading further, you may want to take a few minutes to read the reflection questions in Box 16-1 and if possible, discuss your responses with colleagues.

THE BROAD ETHICAL CHALLENGES POSED BY MANAGED CARE

Managed care is neither morally good nor bad, and it is not a single entity. It can assume many forms as a result of its reason for being. At the very least, there is a critical difference between for-profit and not-for-profit versions of managed care. Those considering joining (or becoming employed by) a managed care organization should investigate the following (Zoloth-Dorfman and Rubin, 1995):

- Who is doing the managing?
- With what intention and goals?
- Under whose authority?
- And with what effect?

Recalling managed care's origins in *effectively* arranging healthcare for slaves, miners, and others who lacked access to physicians, some champion managed care as our best hope for securing basic healthcare services to underserved populations. Others insist upon demonizing managed care in general, believing it to be the source of everything that is

---

BOX 16-1
Moral Reflection Questions

- What is it *reasonable* to expect of a country's healthcare delivery system and of any organization that presents itself as a provider of healthcare services?
- Are there any nonnegotiables of moral healthcare that when threatened or absent demand redress?
- What is it *reasonable* for my patients, their families, and my colleagues *to expect of me* in the context of the professional responsibilities I have assumed? (Another way to frame this question is to ask, What promises have I made, explicitly or implicitly, by presenting myself to others in a professional capacity as a healer?)
- To what degree am I faithful in meeting these expectations on a regular basis?
- If I seem to be failing to meet these expectations on multiple fronts, what goods am I jeopardizing (e.g., the trust that makes healthcare work, safety, quality, collaborative practice), and what do I plan to do about this?
- What forces are constraining my ability to meet reasonable expectations (personal, professional, institutional, societal factors)?
- What needs to change, and how can I work with others to make this change happen?
- What are the consequences of my not working with others to secure needed change?
- Am I morally culpable if I allow an immoral system to continue?

currently wrong with healthcare. Although many surveys report high levels of patient satisfaction with MCOs, a number of political cartoons reveal the public's willingness to blame managed care for a growing number of complaints about the healthcare system.

TRENDS IN HEALTHCARE DELIVERY IN THE UNITED STATES

Table 16-1 illustrates trends in healthcare delivery in the United States by highlighting changes in the way healthcare is designed, delivered, financed, and evaluated. The continuum of changes is mapped along the following three time frames:

1. The rise of modern medicine: the period from after World War II to 1965, when the U.S. government began financing healthcare for older Americans and Americans with disabilities

TABLE 16-1
Trends in Healthcare Delivery: The American Experience

World War II-1965	1965-1983	1983-Present
Healthcare Human good→commodity???	Human good →right→commodity ???	Human good →right→commodity ???
Healthcare Delivery System Social service	→	Complex medical enterprise/ industry: development of for-profit healthcare
System of Care Individual practitioner	Modern hospital/healthcare systems	Integrated delivery networks
Technology Limited	→	Vastly increased
Economic Resources Adequate	→	Inadequate (perception of adequacy differs)
Financing Mechanism Fee-for-service (financial incentive to do *more* rather than less)	Rise of employer-based insurance model and government-financed medicine: Medicare/Medicaid	Managed competition (capitated payments, salary withholds, bonuses; financial incentives to do *less* rather than more)

Continued

TABLE 16-1
Trends in Healthcare Delivery: The American Experience—cont'd

World War II-1965	1965-1983	1983-Present
Access		
Out-of-pocket	Out-of-pocket	Out-of-pocket
Third-party payers	Third-party payers	Third-party payers
	Medicare/Medicaid	MCOs
Regulatory Mechanism		
License, voluntary accreditation	JCAHO, HCFA, NCQA	Complex matrix of accountability
Orientation		
Disease/illness care (rescue medicine; medicalization of childbirth, dying)	→Healthcare: holistic health/healing wholeness of being vs. wholeness of body	Healthy communities Integrative healthcare
Appropriateness (Sharpe, 1997)		
Clinical judgment	Desirability	Cost-worthiness→regulation (In one Canadian province: appropriateness = "Whatever the government will pay for")
Standards: clinical judgment		Standards: evidence-based practice and cost
Locus of Decision Making		
Physician	Healthcare professional and patient	Healthcare professional, patient, payers (increasing role for third parties)
Ethics		
Paternalism: good of individual patient (Hippocratic ethic)	Paternalism→age of patient autonomy; good of individual patient weighed against good of society Physician autonomy diminished→problems with futile care	Distributive ethic: move to displace focus from the good of individual patient to good of group; good of individual patient weighed against good of shareholders in publicly traded for-profit investment company
Ethic of HCP-patient relationship	Ethic of HCP-patient relationship and public health ethic	Ethic of HCP-patient relationship, public health ethic and business ethic; organizational ethics
Professionalism		
Strong sense of professionalism	→Eroding sense of professionalism	→Trade mentality

HCFA, Health Care Financing Administration; *HCP,* healthcare professional; *JCAHO,* Joint Commission on Accreditation of Healthcare Organizations; *MCO,* managed care organization; *NCQA,* National Committee for Quality Assurance.

2. The development of modern medicine: the period from 1965 to 1983, when cost containment efforts (initiation of diagnosis-related groups [DRGs]) and commercial interests began to play a leading role in shaping healthcare delivery
3. Postmodern medicine: the period from 1983 to the present, in which healthcare became increasingly commercialized and *commodified.*

Healthcare as a Concept

The United States has yet to decide if healthcare is one of the following: (1) a basic human good and therefore an *obligation of a moral society,* (2) a *right,* or (3) a *commodity* that can be sold in the marketplace. Throughout all three time spans described previously, there is evidence of these three conceptual ideas about healthcare. Although much of the popular rhetoric increasingly presents basic healthcare as a necessary condition for human development and growth in today's society, the United States has yet to implement health policies and legislation that guarantee healthcare as a right—especially for marginalized populations.

In the current healthcare system of managed competition and steadily (and now dramatically) increasing premiums, market forces play a major role in determining the distribution of healthcare. Increasingly the safety nets, which in the past ensured some level of care for the poor, are disappearing, and there are even greater disparities between care available to those with and those without adequate healthcare insurance. The numbers of uninsured Americans are increasing steadily.

Healthcare Delivery System

Since World War II, healthcare delivery has expanded from a social service mechanism delivered by individual practitioners to a complex medical enterprise or industry. The effects are far reaching. It makes a huge difference if nurses view themselves as deliverers of service versus owners of a proprietary skill that is a commodity sold in the marketplace to those who can afford to pay. Nursing as a service is committed to those in need to serve the goal of human health and well-being. Nursing as a market commodity is a means to secure wealth or other social goods, such as reputation, prestige, and power.

System of Care

In the period immediately after World War II, individual physicians were the major point of service for healthcare. Patients sought the services of their family doctors, who either treated the patient or referred the patient for care. During this time, physicians also played a leading role in the development of the modern hospital. As hospitals grew, they became the major vehicle for the disbursement of healthcare services. More and more physicians located their offices in suites in or near hospitals, and hospital administrators developed care networks, including clinics, inpatient services, and visiting nurse networks. As the focus of healthcare in the United States began to shift from a model of hospital-based acute illness care to community-based healthcare across the lifespan, the point of service evolved to integrated delivery networks. These networks coordinate healthcare services throughout the community and have resulted in a greatly diminished role for modern hospitals.

When physicians were the major point of service for all healthcare, family physicians often knew their patients well and even shared similar values. Healthcare was strongly community-based, and these communities tended to be religiously and culturally homogenous. Today typical communities in the United States are much more heterogenous, and integrated delivery networks virtually guarantee that patients will be cared for by physicians, nurses, and other healthcare professionals who are strangers. In this age of "stranger medicine," it becomes critically important for healthcare professionals to make serious efforts to understand and respect a patient's beliefs, values, and interests and to allow these to direct healthcare decision making. Similarly, if the patient's initial point of contact (and reviewer of the presenting complaint) is a nonclinician telephone receptionist, more opportunities exist for misdiagnosis and inappropriate referrals.

Technology

Few effective medical interventions were available to the public at the time of World War II. Within a comparatively short time, we have witnessed an exponential increase in effective pharmacological, surgical, and medical therapies, which are now supplemented by complementary therapeutic modalities such as acupuncture, meditation, and herbal therapies. New scientific knowledge and technologies are revolutionizing how we think about what it means to be born, live, and die. Human cloning, genetic screening, gene therapy, and research about aging continue to promise "better living." In the days of Hippocratic medicine when therapeutic alternatives were few, it was easy for healthcare professionals to make decisions for their patients and prescribe therapeutic regimens. Today more than one therapeutic option is usually available for any medical condition, and multiple factors influence what gets prescribed and funded.

Economic Resources

When effective medical interventions were few, economic resources were adequate. Today most people would argue that it is impossible to provide all the healthcare individuals desire without seriously compromising other human goods, such as housing, education, defense, art, and culture. Given that individuals place either greater or lesser importance on human health and well-being, it is important to engage patients in discussions about the economic consequences of healthcare decisions and to give them a leading role in weighing the respective merits of healthcare choices. For example, one patient with diagnosed high cholesterol levels may elect to pay for expensive anticholesterol medication himself if his health plan will not cover it, whereas another patient in the same plan hopes that dietary and lifestyle modification will secure similar benefits at a cheaper cost.

Financing Mechanism

During the rise and development of modern medicine in the United States, a *fee-for-service* financing mechanism was in place. Stated simply, physicians and healthcare institutions charged fees for the services they provided, and patients (or their healthcare insurers) paid these fees. Under this system, the financial incentives favored doing more rather than less, since providers were reimbursed for all services provided. A "self-interested" clinician or hospital was motivated to "overtreat" if the primary intent was to "make money."

As more and more Americans acquired health insurance through their employment or the government (Medicare or Medicaid, federal programs that respectively financed health-care benefits for older, disabled, or poor Americans), they failed to appreciate the rising cost of healthcare, since healthcare payments rarely came from their pockets. This attitude, coupled with the growing conviction that "if a little healthcare is good, more must be better," led to the dramatic escalation in healthcare costs that soon became unsustainable for the government or employers. At present, 13.5% of the U.S. gross national product (GNP) is allocated to healthcare costs.

In the 1980s, employers were tired of paying increasingly high healthcare premiums to insure their workers. The federal government began to demand an alternative to the costly fee-for-service financing mechanism. What resulted and is currently in place is *managed competition*. Under this system, the financial incentives are to do less rather than more, since the amount of money allocated to direct patient care is money not pocketed by the managed care organization or those providing care from the prefixed pool of money initially allocated for care.

Patients are potentially ill-served under both systems. Fee-for-service, with its incentives to do more rather than less, may lead some clinicians to overtreat for self-interested reasons, whereas the current managed competition system may apply incentives for clinicians to prescribe less care than may be medically optimal in order to realize a profit. For this reason, American patients have demanded full disclosure of their medical conditions and all their medical options along with the consequences of no treatment. Until the character of healthcare professionals and the infrastructure of the healthcare system make it reasonable for patients to presume that all healthcare professionals and organizations are motivated solely by a commitment to benefit the patient, educated and wise patients look to their own interests and are wary of those who would exploit their illness to their financial advantage. The obvious problem with this solution is that thousands of patients lack the knowledge and advocacy skills to adequately represent their interests.

Appropriateness

Perhaps nowhere do we see the changes in healthcare decision making so dramatically as in the different meanings attached to the term *medically appropriate*. Stated briefly, this term has evolved to include the following meanings: (1) appropriate because clinical judgment renders it so, (2) appropriate because of its desirability to the patient, and (3) more recently, appropriate because of its cost-worthiness (Sharpe, 1997). In one Canadian province, *appropriate* reportedly means "whatever the government is willing to pay for." In such a rapidly evolving system, knowledgeable patients are wise to ascertain the basis for clinical decisions and recommendations. In the past, patients followed medical orders simply because they were based on clinical judgment. With almost daily challenges in the media to what used to be considered excellent practice, today the public and healthcare payers are demanding evidence-based practice standards (demonstrate that what is proposed actually works), cost-worthiness, and desirability.

Locus of Decision Making

The locus of decision making for healthcare has evolved from "clinicians" to "clinicians and patients" to "clinicians, patients, payers and other involved parties." At each step of this transition, it is important to clarify the role played by each participant in the decision-making process and to understand how these changing roles facilitate the achievement of medicine and nursing's aims—promotion of the health and human well-being of the patients committed to our care.

Professional Ethics

As the culture of healthcare *decision making* has evolved, so has professional ethics. In the rise of modern medicine after World War II, paternalism was rampant. The Hippocratic ethic focused on the good of the individual patient as defined by the clinician. The clinician-patient relationship, a healing relationship, was central to this ethic. The primary principle of the Hippocratic ethic was beneficence, *"primum non nocere,"* or to act to benefit the patient or at the very least do no harm.

This ethic evolved into the ethic of autonomy, which still focused on the good of the individual patient, but now that good was defined by the patient. During the age of patient autonomy, clinician autonomy was compromised. Under conditions of increasing scarcity of health resources, this ethic changed into a focus on the good of the individual weighed against the good of society. How does what we are doing for this one patient affect our ability to meet the needs of *all* patients? Although the clinician-patient relationship ethic remained central, the ethic of public health played an increasingly important role.

Finally, today's emphasis on healthcare as a business requires adding business ethics to the equation. In a publicly traded for-profit investment company, the good of the individual patient is balanced against the good of investors. Medically beneficial care is sometimes denied to return a profit to investors. Many argue that this ethic is inappropriate for healthcare, but it is playing a major role today. A recent article in the *New England Journal of Medicine* suggested that it might be time for physicians to reject the Hippocratic ethic for a distributive ethic focused on the good of the group (Kassirer, 1998). This idea is at least partially responsible for the fact that many Americans no longer believe that healthcare professionals and institutions can be trusted to be committed to securing their interests. In this climate, increasing attention is paid to organizational ethics to foster institutional integrity.

FEE-FOR-SERVICE AND MANAGED CARE ARRANGEMENTS

Important ethical differences exist between traditional fee-for-service arrangements and managed care arrangements. These differences are highlighted by the comparison of their strengths and limitations in Table 16-2.

TABLE 16-2
A Comparison of Fee-for-Service and Managed Care Arrangements

Fee-for-Service	Managed Care
Strengths	
Primacy of healthcare professional-patient relationship	Cost containment measures are built into system design
Primacy of health and well-being of *individual* patient	Acknowledges that health/healthcare is but one of life's primary goods
Primacy attributed to both healthcare professional and patient autonomy	Potential to address needs of underserved groups
Limitations	
No mechanism to control costs; healthcare consumes ever-larger percentage of GNP, resulting in sacrifice of other human goods	Sacrifices patient and healthcare professional autonomy to maximize benefits to group
Financial incentives do more rather than less, resulting in some patients getting more treatment than desired	Financial incentives to do less rather than more, resulting in some patients getting less treatment than desired
Growing numbers of underserved individuals (percentage of uninsured or underinsured U.S. citizens)	For-profit managed care increases commodification/commercialization of healthcare, reduces healthcare to market commodity, and potentially objectifies people
	Growing numbers of underserved individuals (percentage of uninsured or underinsured U.S. citizens)

GNP, Gross national product.

THE MAJOR ETHICAL CHALLENGES RELATED TO MANAGED CARE

At the level of society, the primary ethical question is whether or not managed competition is an ethically defensible means to achieve the goal of a country discharging its obligation to provide basic healthcare services to its people. To the extent that managed competition reduces healthcare to a commodity to be bought and sold in the marketplace with resultant haves and have-nots, it is immoral. This judgment follows from the belief that although it is ethically defensible to allow financial status to dictate whether one walks, rides, drives, or is chauffeured to work, it is not ethically defensible to allow one's financial status to dictate whether or not one receives basic healthcare services. The ethical question for the public is whether managed care arrangements allow people to trust realistically that they will have access to healthcare that does not fall below acceptable standards of safety and quality. Ethical questions are also raised for the public as citizens and taxpayers whose votes elect representatives who set health policy and legislation.

    For nurses and other healthcare professionals, the chief ethical question is one of personal and professional integrity. What guarantee do nurses who work in managed care organizations, or in any sector of the healthcare system whose resources are restricted because of managed care contracts, have that they will not be forced to participate in sub-standard care? How can we practice with integrity, faithful to the primary ethical tenet, *the nurse's primary commitment is to the patient,* when we are denied access to the resources our patients and families need to achieve valued health outcomes? One way to describe this tension is *the problem of divided loyalties.* To whom are nurses primarily responsible? Patients? Well members of a managed care plan? Employers? Stockholders in a for-profit managed care organization? Themselves? Their families? Also, how do these priorities direct nurses' use of time, resources, and so forth?

Both individuals and institutions (health plans) suffer from the problem of divided loyalties. Box 16-2 offers a guide to values conflict resolution when multiple stakeholders are involved.

How nurses deal with this tension is crucial. Nurses feel that they need to abandon a commitment to making a difference in the lives of their patients in order to feel peaceful when they leave work each day. "So long as my criterion for being a good nurse is meeting the needs of my patients, I go home frustrated each day feeling guilty about my repeated inability to meet patient needs. I've now lowered my standard to giving an honest day's labor for a day's pay. I know I can do that." Although this maneuver may soothe our consciences, it does not bode well for the patients and families we treat.

One group of nurses in Massachusetts took dramatic action to enlist the public's support for their efforts to be able to practice with integrity when they united with physicians to protest the corporatization of the healthcare system. According to Judith Shindul-Rothschild, "Nurses and doctors know . . . that the unbridled greed of corporate health care is killing our patients, and squeezing every ounce of humanity out of our health care system. And we are not going to take it anymore. The revolution starts right here, right now, tonight" (*Am Nurse,* 1998, p 6). These nurses promulgated the following new set of principles for healthcare reform (Ad Hoc Committee for Healthcare, 1997):

- Medicine and nursing must not be diverted from their primary tasks: the relief of suffering, the prevention and treatment of illness, and the promotion of health. The efficient deployment of resources is critical but must not detract from these goals.
- The pursuit of corporate profit and personal fortune has no place in caregiving.
- Potent financial incentives that reward "overcare" or "undercare" weaken doctor-patient and nurse-patient bonds and should be prohibited. Similarly, business arrangements that allow corporations and employers to control the care of patients should be proscribed.
- A patient's right to a physician of choice must not be curtailed.
- Access to medical and nursing care must be the right of all.

The ethical question for managed care organizations and other institutions is also a question of integrity. How can they present themselves to the public as organizations committed to securing everyone's health interests when by design they lack the means to do so?

BOX 16-2
Methodology for Values/Conflict Resolution:
Georgetown University Center for Clinical Bioethics

Recognizing and Acknowledging the Conflict or Uncertainty
Although this step of the process seems self-evident, it is often the source of unresolved conflicts. Participants may deny the actual conflict or uncertainty and reject the idea that there are *legitimate* competing ethical principles and values. Resolutions begin by recognizing that others hold legitimate values and have ethical traditions that must be respected and taken into account. Once this step is made, the conflicts become evident and can be acknowledged publicly—regardless of the specific resolution each stakeholder initially finds preferable. Prerequisite: moral sensitivity and responsibility

Gathering Information
In this step of the process, participants attempt to learn all they can about the conflict itself. What is the source of the conflict and related uncertainties? What is at stake? What information is needed to facilitate resolution of the conflict? Who are the stakeholders, and what are their values and interests? During the data-gathering phase, it is essential to distinguish *factual judgments from individual or collective perceptions* that may or may not be true. Prerequisite: intellectual humility, openness, respect
- Identifying the Stakeholders
  Who are the stakeholders in the decision? That is, who will be affected by it, either through responsibility for making decisions or implementing the decision, or experiencing the outcomes of its implementation?
- Identifying the Stakeholders' Interest
  Each stakeholder should talk freely about his or her perspective on the issue in question. All stakeholders should be present at the table and should have a voice. Examples abound of discrepancies between perceived and actual values/interests of particular individuals and groups. The aim of this phase is to have people talk freely and fully, without contradiction or analysis, so that all the relevant perspectives and data get put on the table.

Articulating and Ranking Values
Begin by articulating and listing the cherished values of each stakeholder group. Rank these so that the most important values of each stakeholder are known to the group at large. Use some process to reach consensus about the core values, which then should direct the resolution of the problem at hand. Prerequisite: respect and trust

Achieving agreement on a decision will depend largely on the extent to which the participants in the discussion have gained an appreciation of and respect for the concerns and values of the varying perspectives they represent. Ideally, they come to respect and trust one another as honest, decent, well-motivated persons and not as members of hostile "interest groups."

Identifying the Issue
First, the group, after hearing the different perspectives, tries to define the disputed issue or issues as precisely as possible and identify the reasons for or root causes of the problem. The group should try to understand the problem as accurately as possible. Second, the group reflects on the various explanations for the problem that have been offered, tests them for their relative adequacy, and sees which best "fits" the data gathered in the first phase of the discussion. The aim of this phase is for all stakeholders to reach a common judgment on the best explanation of the issue, which will also involve the overcoming of partial ignorance or personal bias. Prerequisite: intellectual clarity

Modified from materials from the Woodstock Theological Center, Washington, DC, and Health Policy and Bioethics Consultation Group, Berkeley, California, 1998-1999.

Continued

BOX 16-2
Methodology for Values/Conflict Resolution:
Georgetown University Center for Clinical Bioethics—cont'd

Generating Possible Courses of Action

Crafting a response to the issue involves the identification of various plans of action, which are then critiqued in light of the most cherished values of the full group. Prerequisite: critical thinking and creativity

Making the Decision

Ideally a consensus is reached and a decision is made on the basis of a relatively adequate understanding of all dimensions of the problem and a generous concern for, not necessarily all, but the most cherished values of each of the stakeholder representatives. Prerequisite: responsibility and accountability

What should be done if a group of representatives cannot reach consensus and is deadlocked in opposing positions?

■ Redo the previous steps to make sure participants genuinely understand and empathize with the cherished values of each, so that they can prioritize the most compelling concerns to reach consensus.
■ Strive anew to creatively and imaginatively design a new course of action in which all the required values are promoted.
■ Ask the opposing parties if their disagreement is nonnegotiable (i.e., is a matter of serious violation of conscience) or whether they could move ahead with the majority's plan of action, even though it is not their preference.
■ Check the group's history to see if there is precedent for one or other of the opposed positions and how (and how satisfactorily) the issue was resolved at that time.
■ The group might be asked to agree on one of the opposed views on the condition that those who disagree would not be obliged to implement it themselves—if this is organizationally possible.
■ If time is not a major factor, the decision can be deferred to give opportunity for further thought and reflection.

Implementing and Evaluating the Decision

Once the decision is made about a possible course of action, it is important to determine how best to implement the decision given the interests and values at stake. Likewise, there should be some advance discussion about how to best evaluate the consequences of the selected course of action. The aim of this evaluation is to critique the adequacy of the process used to generate the resolution of this issue to facilitate further decision making. Prerequisite: responsibility and accountability

Modified from materials from the Woodstock Theological Center, Washington, DC, and Health Policy and Bioethics Consultation Group, Berkeley, California, 1998-1999.

ATTEMPTS TO IDENTIFY THE NONNEGOTIABLES OF MORAL HEALTHCARE

Nurses and other healthcare providers need a clear vision of moral healthcare, as well as a clear vision of their moral obligations as healthcare professionals. The Tavistock Group, a multidisciplinary and internal task force established with the express purpose of developing a shared code of ethics that would bring *all* stakeholders in healthcare into a more consistent moral framework more conductive to cooperative behavior and mutual respect, recently rejected the distributive ethic for healthcare professionals and called for a renewed commitment to the individual patient, within the context of efforts to secure the health and well-being of the community. The five themes of this document are as follows (Davidoff, 2000):

1. Healthcare is a human right.
2. The care of individuals is at the center of healthcare delivery but must be viewed and practiced within the overall context of continuing to work to generate the greatest possible health gains for groups and populations.
3. The responsibilities of the healthcare delivery system include the prevention of illness and the alleviation of disability.
4. Cooperation with each other and those served is imperative for those working within the healthcare delivery system.
5. All individuals and groups involved in healthcare, whether they provide access or services, have continuing responsibility to help improve its quality.

After publishing these themes and inviting feedback, the Tavistock Group presented the following version of the previous principles (Davidoff, 2000):

1. *Rights:* People have a right to health and healthcare.
2. *Balance:* Care of individual patients is central, but the health of populations is also our concern.
3. *Comprehensiveness:* In addition to treating illness, we have an obligation to ease suffering, minimize disability, prevent disease, and promote health.
4. *Cooperation:* Healthcare succeeds only if we cooperate with those we serve, each other, and those in other sectors.
5. *Improvement:* Improving healthcare is a serious and continuing responsibility.
6. *Safety:* Do no harm.
7. *Openness:* Being open, honest, and trustworthy is vital in healthcare.

The Tavistock Group offers these principles to guide the ethical judgments of everyone involved in the design, delivery, financing, and evaluation of healthcare about the roles they play. It is also helpful for us as nurses to ask if there are any universal moral obligations we all share by virtue of our professional commitments, which if violated demand action. The following list of moral obligations are *nonnegotiable* for nurses and all healthcare professionals:

- The healthcare professional's primary commitment is to the patient.
  - The healthcare practitioner practices with compassion and respect for the inherent worth, dignity, and uniqueness of every individual.

■ Healthcare practitioners can be trusted to act in ways that advance the best interests of the patients entrusted to their care.

 ■ The healthcare practitioner possesses the prerequisite competencies demanded by the professional role assumed and is willing to use these competencies and expertise to secure the interests of the patient.

 ■ The healthcare practitioner provides the information and support individuals need to make healthcare decisions to secure their interests.

 ■ The healthcare practitioner respects the privacy and confidentiality needs of patients.

 ■ The healthcare practitioner is a bridge to the resources individuals need to secure their health interests (advocacy).

■ The healthcare practitioner owes the same duties to self as to others, including the responsibility to preserve integrity, maintain competence, and continue personal and professional growth.

PRACTICAL RECOMMENDATIONS FOR REFLECTION AND ACTION

Consider the following recommendations as you evaluate your ability to practice with integrity in today's market-driven healthcare environment:

■ You are a powerful moral agent. Believe that you can make a difference. Understand that the difference you make will be enhanced if you work collaboratively with others.

■ Prepare yourself for your advocacy role by developing and monitoring your moral agency. Ethical competence can no more be safely presumed than intellectual, technical, or interpersonal competence. Box 16-3 highlights the essential elements of moral agency.

■ Practice the art of effectively confronting forces that jeopardize human health and well-being (safety and quality).

■ Value moral integrity, both your own and that of the health institutions for whom and with whom you work.

BOX 16-3
Moral Agency

1. *Moral sensibility:* ability to recognize the "moral moment" when a moral challenge presents itself
2. *Moral responsiveness:* ability and willingness to respond to the moral challenge
3. *Ethical reasoning and discernment:* knowledge of and ability to use sound theoretical and practical approaches to "thinking through" moral challenges; these approaches are used to *inform* and *justify* moral behavior
4. *Moral character:* cultivated dispositions that allow one to act as one believes one ought to act
5. *Moral values:* conscious and critical values that align with good moral character and moral integrity
6. *Transformative moral leadership:* commitment and proven ability to create a culture that facilitates the exercise of moral agency—a culture in which people do the right thing because it is the right thing to do
7. *Moral accountability:* ability and willingness to accept responsibility for one's moral behavior and to learn from the experience of exercising moral agency

In an era of cost-containment and compromised decision making and health outcomes, nurses must be aware of their ethical responsibilities to shape healthcare delivery. As patient advocates, nurses play a vital role in ensuring that all patients receive quality, compassionate healthcare. Society demands nothing less. Nor can we.

REFERENCES

Ad Hoc Committee for Healthcare: For our patients, not for profits: a call to action, *JAMA* 278(21):1733, 1997.

American Medical Association, Council on Ethical and Judicial Affairs: Ethics issues in managed care, *JAMA* 273(4):330-335, 1995 (Council report).

Barnet R, Taylor C: The ethics of case management: communication challenges. In Cohen E, DeBack V, editors: *Outcomes and collaboration in case management*, St Louis, 1999, Mosby.

Davidoff F: Changing the subject: ethical principles for everyone in healthcare, *Ann Intern Med* 133:386-389, 2000.

Kassirer JP: Managing care: should we adopt a new ethic? *New Engl J Med* 339(6):397-398, 1998.

Massachusetts nurses, doctors spark healthcare revolution, *Am Nurse* 30(1):6, 1998.

Sharpe VA: The politics, economics, and ethics of "appropriateness," *Kennedy Institute of Ethics Journal* 7(4): 337-343, 1997.

Taylor C: Rethinking nursing's basic competencies, *J Nurs Care Qual* 9(4):1-13, 1995.

Taylor C: Ethical issues in case management. In Cohen E, Cesta T, editors: *Nursing case management from concept to evaluation*, St Louis, 1997, Mosby.

Taylor C, Barnet R: The ethics of case management: the quality/cost conundrum. In Cohen E, DeBack V, editors: *Outcomes and collaboration in case management*, St Louis, 1999, Mosby.

Zoloth-Dorfman L, Rubin S: The patient as commodity: managed care and the question of ethics, *J Clin Ethics* 6(4):339-357, 1995.

17

Nursing Ethics in a Managed Care Environment

Ellen R. Mitchell

KEY LESSONS IN THIS CHAPTER

- Patient advocacy is an essential part of the role of the nurse case manager because it is the case manager's responsibility to ensure that the patient's needs are met.
- Although laws are written as rules and regulations, ethical values are subject to individual moral, philosophical, religious, and cultural definitions.
- Case managers, as nurses in general, maintain ethics as the foundation on which the profession stands.
- As patient advocates, case managers must identify the patient's priority needs and ensure that they are addressed, despite the possibility of no payment for these services.
- The ANA Code for Nurses (ANA, 1985) is the basis for the ethical practice of nursing and provides clearly for the role of all nurses, regardless of position, in the practice of their profession.

CHANGING TIMES

Significant changes in healthcare financing occurred in the last years of the twentieth century. A profusion of managed care organizations (MCOs) developed in response to increases in healthcare costs as a percentage of the gross national product (GNP) (U.S. Department of Health and Human Services, 1995). *Managed care* can be defined as any healthcare delivery system where an entity other than the healthcare giver or the patient determines the type of healthcare delivered. This entity intervenes to provide what it considers to be appropriate healthcare for the patient (Gerardi, 1997). Managed care systems frequently offer packages of healthcare benefits. They develop standards for the selection of providers and have formal programs for ongoing quality assurance and utilization review (UR). They frequently provide incentives for their members to use providers and procedures within the given plan (Guido, 2001). Purchasers of health plans, mainly businesses, have embraced the principles of managed care and are making arrangements with health maintenance organizations (HMOs) or other managed care companies to provide services for their employees.

Increased opportunities exist for nurses in the managed care arena. Virtually every major insurer in the United States offers some level of case management services. For the private payer, case management frequently focuses on patients with chronic illness or traumatic injury (Bower, 1992). These patients are considered to be high-cost cases. Case managers in these settings coordinate all necessary providers, services, and equipment to maximize patient care within financial limits. Patients can receive services through a single seamless system as they move through the care continuum (Guido, 2001). Although the focus of the payer is to contain costs, all case management programs have as their goal the provision of quality care and the attainment of positive outcomes.

Many experts agree, at least theoretically, that managed healthcare is an effective way to deliver care. In reality, however, managed care has become a method for financing the delivery of care and not for the delivery of care itself. Many steps taken by MCOs emphasize financial issues and fail to take into consideration the overall health concerns of the patient (Guido, 2001). These cost-cutting methods have raised several legal issues concerning managed care.

PATIENT RIGHTS

As more financial restrictions were placed on benefits, patients' rights and autonomy (Dzacky and Sheldon, 1999) have become topics of increasing concern. Patients frequently cannot choose their own provider but rather must select one from the healthcare plan, and preapproval must be obtained for many treatments.

Over the past several years, as a response to these and other issues, several initiatives have been taken in the legislative arena. In December 2000, the U.S. Department of Health and Human Services published rules adopting standards of the Privacy Rule in the Federal Register. The Privacy Rule is the second of a series of rules put forth in the Health Insurance Portability and Accountability Act of 1996 (HIPAA) (Federal Register, 2001). The standards establish requirements relating to the use and divulgence of protected health information and the protection of the rights of individuals with regard to their health information.

In March 1997, President Clinton appointed the Advisory Committee on Consumer Protection and Quality in the Health Care Industry. They were charged to recommend measures as necessary to promote and assure healthcare quality and value, and protect consumers and workers in the healthcare system (Advisory Committee on Consumer Protection and Quality in the Health Care Industry, 1997). Part of their responsibility was to draft a consumer bill of rights (Guido, 2001).

In 1999 the Health Care Financing Administration (HCFA) enacted new standards for the protection of patients' rights for all providers participating in Medicare and Medicaid funding systems. These standards included provisions for patients to be informed of their rights before the provision or discontinuation of care and to be part of the planning of care. Privacy, safety, and freedom from abuse or harassment were addressed, as were issues pertaining to confidentiality of records and freedom from restraints that are not clinically necessary (Federal Register, 1999).

Congress continues to draft legislation that more fully addresses patients' rights and other factors that influence the consumers' choice of healthcare plans and providers. As technological advances become more readily available and sophisticated, attention must be paid to the just and rational use of these interventions. The challenge will be how to effectively manage these resources and yet provide for improved access to care, cost containment, and quality delivery of care.

THE ROLE OF THE HOSPITAL-BASED NURSE CASE MANAGER

The continued growth and increasing complexity of managed care systems for healthcare financing and the delivery of care present many challenges for nurses in case management. The provision of services on a daily basis, in an ongoing effort to provide optimum care, can test the personal and professional integrity of nurse case managers (Taylor, 1997). The nurse case manager, in the performance of his or her job responsibilities, may be serving many masters. Every day, nurse case managers interact with families, patients, providers, payers, and hospital administrators. Accountability can change quickly in response to changing situations. Opportunities to achieve goals and ensure safe quality care to patients within the framework of ethical practice can be identified, however, and are discussed later in this chapter.

Nurse case managers are in the unique position of being able to influence patient care across a variety of settings. In this manner, they serve as tour guides and travel agents for the patient along the care continuum. This role is accomplished by interacting with multiple administrative agencies, including the payer, the institutions, and vendors of services in the outpatient arena in a variety of roles. Generally, nurse case managers are responsible for coordinating patient care from admission to beyond the point of discharge. They ensure the delivery of cost-effective, outcome-oriented, quality healthcare (Tahan, 1993).

Patient advocacy is an essential part of the role of the nurse case manager because it is the case manager's responsibility to ensure that the patients' needs are met. Nurse case managers, in their role as utilization review coordinators, frequently speak on behalf of the patient in the negotiation of services for that patient. As members of the multidisciplinary team, they act as a spokesperson for the patient to other providers within the system.

Nurse case managers may see themselves as primarily accountable to the facility for which they work and driven by the financial bottom line. They may be reluctant to advocate for the patient who needs additional time to achieve target outcomes after discharge (Taylor, 1997). If one accepts that the American Nurses Association (ANA) Code of Ethics for Nurses (ANA, 2001) is the underlying foundation for the ethical practice of all nurses, regardless of title, position, or role function, then one must accept that primary responsibility is for and accountability is to the patient. Any plan of care enacted by the nurse case manager on behalf of the patient must reflect that primacy.

THE DIFFERENCE BETWEEN ETHICS AND THE LAW

Laws are written as rules and regulations. They are intended as binding and formal mechanisms that guide society. The legal system is a general foundation that gives continuing guidance to healthcare professionals, regardless of their personal views and value systems. For example, the Nurse Practice Acts of individual jurisdictions are the defining legal code for nurses. They were originally developed to protect the public, define the practice of nursing, give guidance with scope of practice issues, and set standards for the practice of nursing (Guido, 2001).

Ethical values are subject to individual, moral, philosophical, religious, and cultural definitions. Both the provider and the recipient of care come to the system with their own systems of ethical values. Situations exist in which the value system of the provider can conflict with that of the individual. In these situations, one turns to the law as the arbitrator. The legal system provides guidance to healthcare providers regardless of that person's personal system of values and mores. For example, the law speaks clearly to the right of a competent person to refuse treatment, whether or not the provider agrees with this decision (Guido, 2001).

Groups also can have an ethical framework by which they abide. The ANA Code of Ethics for Nurses (ANA, 2001) is one example of a code governing the ethical behavior of a group.

Ethics Defined

The concept of ethics is concerned with motives and attitudes and the relationship of these attitudes to the good of the individual (Guido, 2001). Ethical principles are subject to personal, philosophical, religious, and moral interpretation by both the provider and the recipient of healthcare services (Guido, 2001). Ethical dilemmas can arise when an action or process conflicts with the individual's interpretation of ethical principles.

Nursing has long maintained that ethics are the foundation on which the profession stands. In 1950 the ANA adopted the Code of Ethics for Nurses (Box 17-1), and it has been revised periodically since that time. It presents to all nurses and to the public the expectations and requirements of the profession in ethical matters (ANA, 1985). The Code provides a framework for nurses to use in ethical analysis and decision making. A dynamic document, it addresses fundamental values of the profession, boundaries of duty, and aspects of duty beyond individual encounters (ANA, 2001). The requirements of the Code may often exceed those found in the law, and every nurse is expected to uphold and adhere to the precepts in the Code and ensure that colleagues do likewise (ANA, 1985).

> **BOX 17-1**
> **Code of Ethics for Nurses—Provisions: Approved June 30, 2001**
>
> 1. The nurse, in all professional relationships, practices with compassion and respect for the inherent dignity, worth, and uniqueness of every individual, unrestricted by considerations of social or economic status, personal attributes, or the nature of health problems.
> 2. The nurse's primary commitment is to the patient, whether an individual, family, group, or community.
> 3. The nurse promotes, advocates for, and strives to protect the health, safety, and rights of the patient.
> 4. The nurse is responsible and accountable for individual nursing practice and determines the appropriate delegation of tasks consistent with the nurse's obligation to provide optimum patient care.
> 5. The nurse owes the same duties to self as to others, including the responsibility to preserve integrity and safety, to maintain competence, and to continue personal and professional growth.
> 6. The nurse participates in establishing, maintaining, and improving healthcare environments and conditions of employment conducive to the provision of quality health care and consistent with the values of the profession through individual and collective action.
> 7. The nurse participates in the advancement of the profession through contributions to practice, education, administration, and knowledge development.
> 8. The nurse collaborates with other health professionals and the public in promoting community, national, and international efforts to meet health needs.
> 9. The profession of nursing, as represented by associations and their members, is responsible for articulating nursing values, for maintaining the integrity of the profession and its practice, and for shaping social policy.

From the American Nurses Association, *Code of ethics for nurses with interpretive statements,* Washington, DC, 2001, American Nurses Publishing, American Nurses Foundation/American Nurses Association.

Ethical Constructs

There are seven constructs that are routinely applied by nurse case managers. Some are used more often than others. All have their roots or can find their parallel in the ANA Code of Ethics for Nurses. Each is discussed separately.

Autonomy

Autonomy is the right of the individual to make his or her own choices. It involves the respect of the healthcare provider for the decisions of the recipient of care or his or her spokesperson, even if the provider does not agree with this decision (Guido, 2001). Under the law, informed consent is a principle that reflects the right of the patient to be autonomous.

In certain situations, such as those involving communicable diseases like tuberculosis, the right to autonomy is not an absolute and can be restricted for the public good.

The first precept of the ANA Code for Nurses addresses the provision of services with respect for human dignity (ANA, 1985). Recognition of the rights of the patient, especially self-determination, is inherent in this concept. Patients have the moral and legal right to determine what will and will not be done to them and for them (ANA, 2001).

Patient autonomy can be limited by limitations imposed by the patient's payer. Nurse case managers, in these instances, may find themselves negotiating with the payer for the needed treatment or procedure on behalf of the patient. The nurse case manager's responsibility to the organization for which he or she works may be hindered while these negotiations take place, since provision of appropriate care may occur in the absence of reimbursement (Dzacky and Sheldon, 1999).

It is within the scope of the nurse case manager's practice to support the patient and the family in the decision-making process, coordinate the provision of information to the patient and family, make referrals when necessary, and address problems in the decision-making process.

Beneficence/Nonmaleficence

Beneficence means that the actions one takes should promote good. Actions should serve to promote a person's best interests. Nurse case managers encounter this concept frequently in discussing the long-term outcomes of invasive or noninvasive procedures (Dzacky and Sheldon, 1999). The corollary to beneficence is nonmaleficence, which means that one should do no harm. In situations where the patient is unable to express his or her autonomy, the healthcare team, with the family, must decide what is best for the patient. This conflict occurs frequently in discussions of whether it is in the best interests of a patient to initiate a do-not-resuscitate (DNR) order. If the family does not consent to a DNR order, the healthcare providers may question whether doing everything possible for a patient is truly in the best interest of the patient (Dzacky and Sheldon, 1999). It is the role of the nurse case manager in these situations to gather the necessary experts and the family together to discuss all the potential outcomes of either decision. In this manner, it can be reasonably assured that the patient's family had the necessary information to make a decision in the best interests of the patient.

The ANA Code of Ethics for Nurses addresses the primacy of the patient. The nurse must recognize the place the patient holds in his or her family or community. In this regard, the nurse case manager must seek help to resolve the conflict. Nevertheless, the nurse's commitment is always to the patient (ANA, 2001).

Veracity

Veracity incorporates the concept that individuals should always tell the truth. In healthcare, this can involve the honest answering of a patient's questions, providing all options for care, and acknowledging when the information is not available or is not known. The ANA Code for Nurses addresses this in terms of the nurse's effort to protect the public from misinformation (ANA, 1985).

Financial constraints imposed by the healthcare system may pose challenges to the integrity of the nurse case manager. These challenges may include requests to deceive or the choice to withhold information from a patient or surrogate. In these situations, nurse case managers must remain true to both their personal and professional ethical codes. It is appropriate to seek compromise in these situations but only when compromise preserves the integrity of the provider, the nurse case manager, and the patient (ANA, 2001).

Fidelity

Fidelity is keeping one's promise or commitments, as well as not making promises one cannot keep. Situations frequently arise in discharge planning in which this becomes a challenge. There are times when the ideal plan may not be available because of either practical or financial constraints, and it would be neither prudent nor ethical for the case manager to promise services that could not be provided. Again, a compromise that preserves integrity should be sought. An example of this situation is presented at the end of this chapter.

Parentalism

Parentalism allows one to make decisions for another. It is also known as the *standard of best interest*. This principle is used when the patient is unable to participate in the decision-making process. If it is used as a convention to take the decision-making process away from the patient, its use should be avoided (Guido, 2001).

Justice

Justice holds that people should be treated fairly and equally. The ANA Code for Nurses (ANA, 1985) states that services should be provided to all; however, conflict may arise when there is competition for available goods and services. One example is when there are two patients awaiting transfer to the intensive care unit (ICU), and only one bed is available. The nurse case manager can work with the critical care team to determine if a more stable patient can be moved out of the ICU without compromising his or her recovery to accommodate the needs of both critically ill patients. In this manner, all the patients are served appropriately, positive outcomes are achieved, and the integrity of the healthcare team is preserved.

Respect for Others

The number-one precept of the ANA Code for Nurses is that the nurse "provide services (. . .) unrestricted by consideration of social or economic status, personal attributes, or the nature of health problems" and later states the nurse "collaborates with members of the health professions (. . .) to meet the health needs of the public" (ANA, 1985, p 1). Respect for others can be said to be the highest of the seven principles outlined here. It acknowledges the right of the individual to make decisions. It transcends cultural, social, and economic differences. It is the core principle of the 1990 Americans with Disabilities Act. Nurse case managers can daily reinforce this principle in their interactions with peers, other members of the healthcare team, patients, payers, and families (Guido, 2001).

PRACTICAL APPLICATION OF ETHICAL CONSTRUCTS

The following cases present situations in which the nurse case manager must make decisions based on standards of nursing practice, the efficacious utilization of resources, and the ANA Code of Ethics for Nurses (ANA, 2001). Each addresses specific foci of the role of the case manager. Advocacy and utilization issues will be examined from the viewpoint of both the payer and the provider. At the end of this section, the nurse case manager should be able to identify practical strategies for the ethical management of difficult situations.

Situation 1: Acute Pancreatitis

H.G. is a 53-year-old male admitted to the general medical unit of the hospital for the management of acute pancreatitis. The acute onset of his disease was precipitated by a rum binge, which he describes as having lasted for 2 days before admission. On admission, the nurse case manager performed an initial intake and assessment of H.G. to determine his needs.

Through the interview process, it is determined that H.G. is homeless and jobless. He sleeps in a mission, where he is able to have a hot meal, a shower, and a cot on which to sleep. He states he does not want to be referred to the municipal shelter system, as he feels he has had bad experiences there in the past. He panhandles whenever he needs cash. He states that he has active Medicaid benefits, and he produces a Medicaid card that identifies a managed care provider for those benefits. The nurse case manager confirms the payer source through the hospital finance office.

During the course of subsequent interviews, H.G. repeatedly states to the nurse case manager his feelings of hopelessness. He states that there is no point to his not drinking, since there is little he can do to change his current situation. A review of his history reveals that he has been admitted to one hospital or another five times in the past 6 months.

The nurse case manager makes a referral to the clinical social worker for assistance with H.G.'s need to access adequate housing and public assistance benefits. Additionally, the nurse case manager is able to convince H.G. to accept a referral on discharge to an outpatient day treatment program for the management of his alcohol dependency. Through daily contact with the payer's case manager, the nurse is able to negotiate the approval for his participation in this program. The patient remains involved with and in residence at the mission. A letter was provided on his behalf to further the initial efforts of the nurse case manager and the social worker and to help him remain on treatment. One month after his discharge from the hospital, a telephone call to the mission reveals that he is still on treatment and has so far successfully remained sober. He hopes to begin seeking employment soon and to get permanent housing (Mitchell, 2000).

Analysis

Nurse case managers are faced with significant challenges when trying to help people such as H.G. with their chronic addictive behaviors. One of the best tools nurse case managers have in the planning of care with complex needs such as chemical dependency and homelessness is the ability to listen (Mitchell, 2000). Respect for others, one of the seven ethical constructs previously discussed, transcends cultural, social, and economic planes. The fundamental principle that nurses practice with compassion and respect for human dignity, without regard to socioeconomic status, personal attributes, or the nature of the health problem, predicates this (ANA, 1985). Human beings respond to positive regard by sharing who they really are. They are not likely to share their feelings, thoughts, and behaviors when a nurse demonstrates stigmatizing behavior prevalent in society toward those who are homeless or chemically dependent (Mitchell and Lunney, 2000).

The role of the nurse case manager in this situation is to coordinate, integrate, and direct the delivery of patient care services (Cohen and Cesta, 1997). Emphasis is placed on early assessment, intervention, comprehensive care planning, and inclusive service referrals. Nurse case managers, in collaboration with other disciplines, develop plans of care to meet the unique needs of each person. The ability to be open-minded, flexible, and to challenge societal assumptions (Brookfield, 1991) are vital to the ability of the nurse case manager to provide for the plan of care for H.G and to effect a positive outcome.

Situation 2: Myocardial Infarction

C.S. is a 47-year-old male. He came to the emergency department (ED) accompanied by his family after he experienced chest pain that radiated to his face and arm for 2 days' duration. The chest pain was accompanied by shortness of breath and diaphoresis. His past medical history is noncontributory. His healthcare coverage, provided by the warehouse where he is employed, is a managed care product.

The electrocardiogram (ECG) reveals changes consistent with a myocardial infarction. Echocardiogram indicates mild to moderate left ventricular dysfunction, mitral and atrial valve regurgitation, and inferior akinesis. Cardiac enzymes are drawn. He is admitted to the critical care unit (CCU), diagnosed as having had an acute inferolateral posterior myocardial infarction. The plan of care includes stress testing and cardiac catheterization once he is stabilized.

While in the CCU, C.S. experienced continued chest pain and fever. He developed respiratory distress and was intubated. He was now diagnosed as having cardiogenic shock.

A long hospitalization followed, during which he required the placement of an intraaortic balloon pump, a tracheotomy for airway protection, and the placement of a percutaneous endogastric tube for nutritional maintenance and experienced several complications of ventilator dependency, including ventilator-associated pneumonia, acute renal failure, and congestive heart failure. Throughout the course of his stay, the nurse case manager remained in contact with the payer to ensure certification of the continued stay.

Six weeks after admission, C.S. is successfully weaned from mechanical ventilation and is on a regular diet. He is infection-free, and his cardiac condition is considered to be stable on medications. Grossly deconditioned as a result of his long hospitalization, C.S. is actively participating in multidisciplinary rehabilitation activities.

C.S. underwent cardiac catheterization, originally planned at the outset of his stay. He consented to the procedure, verbalizing understanding that the root cause of his cardiac event had never been identified because of the severe nature of his illness and the length of time needed for his stabilization. The catheterization revealed severe coronary artery disease, and the cardiothoracic surgeons recommended that he undergo a coronary artery bypass graft (CABG) surgery. In light of his long hospitalization and despite these findings, the recommendation is made by the medical and rehabilitation teams that the patient go to a subacute level nursing facility for rehabilitation before surgery, which will enable him to regain some of his premorbid conditioning and strength.

The hospital-based nurse case manager agrees with this plan as being in the best interests of the patient, and she discusses the plan with the patient and his family. They agree to and verbalize a willingness to participate in the plan of care.

The nurse case manager approaches the payer to request approval for the plan and to get a list of contracted providers. The payer makes the determination that rehabilitation would not be appropriate at this time and recommends that C.S. undergo cardiac surgery before his discharge from the institution, since it is likely he would require rehabilitation after CABG surgery anyway.

The nurse case manager, in the role of advocate for both the patient and the hospital, argues that C.S.'s already protracted hospitalization makes him a prime candidate for potential postoperative complications. In light of his frailty, the nurse case manager believes C.S.'s needs would be better served by participation in a mild cardiac rehabilitation program, which would help him improve his strength. The nurse case manager also requests approval for referral to a community-based dietitian to help C.S. improve his nutritional status to a level conducive to undergoing an extremely stressful surgical procedure. It is hoped that these interventions will serve to prevent another lengthy, costly stay and facilitate C.S.'s successful return to the community and ultimately to the workforce.

By using sound financial and clinical rationales, the nurse case manager is able to convince the payer of the merits of this plan. C.S. is approved for a 2-week course of conditioning rehabilitation in a skilled nursing facility. He is also granted referral to the community-based dietitian for counseling in preparation for his upcoming surgery.

Analysis

The case of C.S. clearly speaks to the role of the nurse case manager as advocate. The nurse's primary commitment is to the patient, and any plan of care developed must speak to the primacy of the patient. The situation described here, where the payer originally disagreed with the plan suggested by the multidisciplinary team, creates a conflict for the nurse case manager. Changes in healthcare financing and care delivery systems can create friction between economic interests and professional integrity. It would have been far simpler for the nurse case manager to acquiesce and allow the patient to undergo risky surgery at this time. An ethically competent case manager is able to act as a patient advocate (Taylor, 1997) and mediate conflict between the healthcare team and the financial provider of services in order to effect a positive outcome. In the case of C.S., the plan to go for rehabilitation and nutritional counseling before undergoing a rigorous operative procedure is developed in the best interests of the patient. This situation is an illustration of the ethical construct of beneficence, which states that actions taken should promote a person's best interests (Dzacky and Sheldon, 1999). It is a secondary benefit that this plan of care will likely serve to decrease the chance of a further protracted length of stay.

In this situation, two parties, both identified as case managers, coordinate care delivery for C.S. Employed by the payer, the financial case manager serves primarily in the role of utilization review coordinator. He or she communicates with the hospital-based nurse case manager to determine continued stay eligibility and discharge planning issues, including eligibility of services.

Financial case managers primarily, as in this situation, advocate for the MCO and may have a caseload of hundreds of patients. The hospital nurse case manager in this situation is unit-based and has a more hands-on approach to the delivery and coordination of care for his or her patient population (Cesta et al, 1998).

Situation 3: Cerebrovascular Accident

B.A. is an 85-year-old female. She is brought by ambulance to the ED after having been found on the floor of her fourth floor walk-up apartment by her daughter. She has left hemiplegia, is dysphagic and aphasic, and on diagnostic testing, which includes a computed tomography (CT) scan and a magnetic resonance imaging (MRI) scan of the brain, is found to have experienced a right-sided cerebrovascular accident (CVA), her second.

Once she is medically stabilized on an acute neurology unit, she is transferred to the acute rehabilitation floor. Her managed Medicare provider has approved a 10-day stay for B.A. to achieve her goals, with an agreement to review her progress at the end of the seventh day. The patient and the multidisciplinary rehabilitation team mutually agree to these goals.

Before admission, B.A. lived alone in her fourth-floor apartment. There is no elevator in the building. Her daughter visits her 3 times a week to do the grocery shopping and other chores. At other times, B.A. receives limited services from a home care provider as paid for out-of-pocket by the patient. The patient's daughter states that her assets are dwindling because of these expenses.

On the seventh day of the hospital stay, it is determined in team evaluation conference that B.A. is not going to be able to achieve her rehabilitation goals within the approved 10 days. It is recommended by her rehabilitation physiatrist that she be placed in a subacute rehabilitation setting—a skilled nursing facility where she would be able to take more time to achieve her goals.

The nurse case manager approaches the payer with this plan. In her role as utilization reviewer, she provides the clinical data of the first 7 days and the plan for the patient to continue rehabilitation activities in a subacute setting. The payer informs the nurse case manager that they will not approve the subacute level management, since they feel it is custodial care, but they will cover limited services in the patient's home. The nurse case manager reviews the patient's home status with the payer and states that a home care plan is neither practical, since it places the patient at risk of return to the hospital, nor safe, since she lives alone in a walk-up apartment.

Additionally, the next day, the nurse case manager is advised that the payer has carved out the entire stay on the acute rehabilitation unit, since the patient made insignificant progress.

The nurse case manager initiates an expedited appeal process. She involves the attending physician in the process, facilitating his contact with the payer's medical director. Concurrently, efforts are initiated for the patient to begin application to subacute settings.

After coordinating multiple contacts with the payer by the physician, it is determined that the patient will be authorized for a 30-day stay at a contracted subacute facility. The original denial of the 7-day acute stay was partially overturned, with 3 days paid at the acute rate and the remaining days to be paid at the skilled nursing rate.

On the tenth day of the acute rehabilitation stay, the patient was moved to a neighboring subacute facility to continue her rehabilitation activities.

Analysis

The nurse case manager in this situation must determine which of his or her roles takes precedence in this situation, which can lead to a feeling of role conflict. In the role of utilization coordinator, it may be argued that the nurse case manager must make every effort to work within the parameters of the options presented by the payer, especially in the face of an impending clinical denial. The home care plan option presented by the payer, however, is clearly suboptimal and unsafe for this elderly woman.

As an advocate for the needs of the patient, the nurse case manager must identify the patient's priority needs and ensure that they are addressed, despite the possibility of the institution not receiving payment for the patient's care. In this situation, the nurse case manager enlisted the support of the attending physiatrist, who was able to justify the stay of the patient and negotiate for approval of the subacute placement of the patient through telephone contact with the payer's medical director.

SUMMARY

In ethics, as in nursing case management, answers do not always come easily. The changes that are occurring in healthcare and healthcare financing present challenges to the nurse case manager that require critical thinking and a strong foundation in ethical principles. The ANA Code for Nurses is the basis for the ethical practice of nursing and provides clearly for the role of all nurses, regardless of position, in the practice of their profession. As Taylor aptly states, "ethical competence is not an option for nurse case managers. The health and well-being of all those we serve literally depend on their ethical competence" (Taylor, 1997, p 333).

REFERENCES

Advisory Committee on Consumer Protection and Quality in the Health Care Industry: *Consumer bill of rights and responsibilities: report to the President of the United States*, Washington, DC, 1997, US Government Printing Office.

American Nurses Association: *Code for nurses with interpretative statements*, Washington, DC, 1985, The Association.

American Nurses Association: The Center for Ethics & Human Rights: *Code of ethics for nurses*, Washington, DC, 2001, The Association.

Bower KA: *Case management by nurses*, ed 2, Washington, DC, 1992, American Nurses Publishing.

Brookfield SD: *Developing critical thinkers: challenging adults to explore alternative ways of thinking and acting*, San Francisco, 1991, Jossey-Bass.

Cesta TG, Tahan HA, Fink LF: *The case manager's survival guide: winning strategies for clinical practice*, St Louis, 1998, Mosby.

Cohen EL, Cesta TG: *Nursing case management from concept to evaluation*, ed 2, St Louis, 1997, Mosby.

Dzacky SC, Sheldon M: An acute-care model in the management of end of life issues, *Nurs Case Manag* 4:228-235, 1999.

Federal Register: *Patients' rights: major new conditions for participation in Medicare and Medicaid*, Pub No 36069-36089, Washington, DC, 1999, The Register.

Federal Register: *Final rule: correction of effective and compliance dates*, Pub No 12433-12434, Washington, DC, 2001, The Register.

Gerardi T: The managed care market: nurse case management as a strategy for success. In Cohen EL, Cesta TG, editors: *Nursing case management from concept to evaluation*, ed 2, St Louis, 1997, Mosby.

Guido GW: *Legal and ethical issues in nursing*, ed 3, Upper Saddle River, NJ, 2001, Prentice-Hall.

Mitchell ER, Lunney M: Analysis and commentary: you make the diagnosis: a case management plan for a chemically dependent homeless man, *Nurs Diagn* 11:80-83, 2000.

Mitchell ER: You make the diagnosis: a case management plan for a chemically dependent homeless man, case study, *Nurs Diagn* 11:46, 2000.

Tahan HT: The nurse case manager in acute care settings: job descriptions and functions, *J Nurs Admin* 25:58-63, 1993.

Taylor C: Ethical issues in case management. In Cohen EL, Cesta TG, editors: *Nursing case management from concept to evaluation*, ed 2, St Louis, 1997, Mosby.

United States Department of Health and Human Services: *The increase of healthcare expenses as a percentage of the gross national product*, Washington, DC, 1995, The Department.

V

Strategies for Success in a Managed Care Environment

A Systems Approach to Hospital-Based Nursing Case Management

Laurie J. Frahm and Linda Hertz

KEY LESSONS IN THIS CHAPTER

- Hospital-based case management addresses healthcare's need to provide outcome-oriented, cost-effective care.
- Nursing case management is based on a relationship of trust developed over time between the nurse case manager and the patient and the family or significant others.
- A systems approach hospital case management program can have a positive financial impact by managing frequent users of system resources.
- Patient education is key to effective outcomes for patients managed by case managers.
- Future case management systems will continue to manage patients across the entire continuum of care, taking a proactive approach to patient management.

Since the mid-1990s, many healthcare organizations have implemented hospital-based case management programs. Some moved in this direction in response to imperative changes in reimbursement related to increasing managed care penetration, whereas others shifted to case management in response to perceived or expected changes. The story of the shift and ultimate acceptance of case management of Immanuel–St. Joseph's Hospital Mayo Health System in Mankato, Minnesota followed a journey of discovery for this organization. As in many such journeys, vision led to change and a paradigm shift in terms of the way the organization did business.

BACKGROUND

To learn from our journey, it is necessary to go back to the early 1990s. Immanuel–St. Joseph's Hospital is a regional medical center in the rural midwestern United States. The hospital is a 272-bed, not-for-profit, secondary care facility within 80 miles of major tertiary care centers. Services provided include medical, general surgery, obstetrics (1200 births/year), psychiatry, and chemical dependency. Outpatient services include same-day surgery, physical therapy, a pain clinic, and a cancer treatment center. The emergency department (ED) is Level II with 24-hour coverage by physicians. Physicians admitting patients to this hospital are independent private practitioners.

The hospital has contracts with third-party payers, in which charges are heavily discounted. Processes, like those in most healthcare organizations of the 2000s, are disorganized or broken. Despite these processes, somehow charges are set and patients are billed. Insurance providers pay an agreed-on percentage of accepted, preauthorized charges. On a case-by-case basis, they may pay for additional days when clinically appropriate. Medicare and Medicaid pay the diagnosis-related group amount set for a rural setting. The only ones expected to pay the entire charge are patients who have no third-party payer, are not eligible for medical assistance (Medicaid), and receive no healthcare benefits from their employers.

The physicians are still being paid by fee-for-service. At this time, they do not have the financial incentive to hold back on resource utilization, since they bill and are reimbursed without any utilization or gatekeeping function to question their bills. They do carry some contracts that will only pay "the usual and customary" costs, which they may accept as full payment for some health insurance policies, or they may bill the patient for the remaining balance as required by other policies.

Nursing case management (NCM) was developed in this setting of fee-for service and minimal managed care penetration. Nursing administration was aware that there was a growing need for healthcare providers to be held accountable for their performance and for overall outcomes (McBeth and Weydt, 1996). The demand for accountability was sought by consumers, third-party payers, legislators, and healthcare providers. Outcome-oriented care and cost-effectiveness were no longer a goal but a mandate (Bower, 1992).

Capitation, a preestablished reimbursement amount per enrollee for a given time, was expected to be the reimbursement method of the future. Fee-for-service was slowly fading out, and managed care would soon be fully in place in the region. This change in reimbursement meant that the organization needed to begin to think about the integration of healthcare financing with the provision of that care (Barger, 1999). It had to begin to identify expected outcomes and then determine ways to measure against those prospective benchmarks. Costs had to be contained while favorable patient outcomes were maintained.

Strategies selected to manage cost and quality included preadmission certification, concurrent review, aligned financial incentives and penalties, and controlled access to providers. Emphasis was shifted to prevention, wellness, cost-avoidance, management of diagnostic groups, and development of best practices from aggregate data. As fees moved to capitated risk contracts, other key goals identified included providing the best care in the most appropriate, cost-effective setting. To meet this goal, the organization had to begin to think as a true healthcare system, with a focus on the continuum of care. For these reasons, it made sense for the hospital to use NCM for certain frequent users of expensive hospital resources.

From the onset, NCM saved the hospital money. Cost-saving was measured by taking a sample of chronically ill, case-managed patients and comparing hospital charges 6 months before and after case management was initiated. Although it would have been better to compare actual cost rather than charges, charge data was the only available financial, patient-specific data available at the time. Two years later, these same chronically ill patients were reevaluated. The hospital charges for 6 months before NCM, 6 months immediately after NCM, and the last 6 months were compared. The comparison revealed that hospital use had increased slightly from the initial 6 months with NCM, but hospital use and charges were still significantly lower than those charges before NCM. Thus overall charges (and assumed cost savings) were maintained over time. The financial operating cost of the NCM program was supported entirely by the hospital, even though those third-party payers without capitated contracts also benefited.

At the time of the introduction of the case management program, financial incentives were not aligned between the physician providers and the hospital. The hospital signed managed care contracts with increasingly lower rates of reimbursement, which resulted in being forced to continuously cut costs. Physicians continued to be paid for any services they provided, with no questions asked.

As patients became educated consumers, they began demanding more services. Insurance was paying the bill, so why be conservative? Managed care continued to penetrate the area.

CURRENT ENVIRONMENT

Managed care arrived in this setting but not in the way originally thought. Large employers signed contracts with preferred providers. To maximize the reduced reimbursements, employees were now required to seek services from these providers. Some were required to get a referral from a primary care provider to seek care from specialists, whereas others had coverage that allowed them to seek care from the provider of their choice. Despite all this, managed care has not lived up to expectations.

The majority of the citizens of this region are not in health maintenance organizations (HMOs). Their care is fee-for-service paid by other commercial insurance and, of course, Medicare and Medicaid. The state also provides more affordable health insurance for those whose income is more than that allowed for Medicaid. An individual premium is set, based on personal income, and the cost of this insurance is underwritten by a 1.5% state tax on the services of healthcare providers.

How is NCM operationalized in this environment? Is it still cost-effective?

THE MODEL

In this model, NCM is based in the hospital and is integrated with the community. The role is similar to that of an independent nurse case manager who works across the continuum, managing patients for long periods (Mullahy, 1998). Because of these long-standing relationships, the nurse case manager and the client develop a partnership. Immanuel–St. Joseph's Hospital discovered that trust developed within the context of the nurse-client relationship is crucial to the success of NCM. As the client's partner in many different healthcare arenas, the case manager has an impartial advocate role.

Areas of focus for the case management program include patients who have complex diagnoses in medical or surgical areas, diabetes, pediatrics, newborns, and behavioral health problems or chemical dependency. In chemical dependency, special emphasis is placed on services to pregnant women or women with young children, since they represent patient populations at great clinical risk. Case managers are baccalaureate-prepared registered nurses who are selected for their experience in working with these patient groups. The nurses who developed the program had master of nursing degrees.

The program is designed so that the nurse case manager manages the patient for the episode of illness over time and across healthcare settings. Nurse case managers identify patients through referrals from social workers, hospital staff, families, patients, physicians, chemical dependency counselors, home care agencies, parish nurses, long-term care facilities, government agencies, and others. High-risk patient selection criteria includes at least three ED visits or two inpatient stays or one inpatient and two ED visits within 6 months. Other criteria include one or more of the following:

- Chronic, destabilizing health condition
- Difficulty coping with health condition
- Impaired coping ability
- No caregiver support

Once a patient has been identified, the nurse case manager and client work together to identify goals. The nurse case manager coordinates communication with all healthcare providers. Coordination is a primary intervention that reduces fragmentation and duplication of services and decreases costs. Referrals are made to appropriate community services. NCM interventions are aimed at achieving the outcomes of management of disease, health maintenance or promotion, increased coping, and development of an appropriate support system.

Ideally the initial contact is made before leaving the hospital. This initial contact is followed by a home visit to observe the client in his or her own environment. Further contact may be at home, other community settings, the nurse's office, or by telephone, as the situation indicates. The nurse case manager often accompanies the client to visits with physicians. Many patients have several physicians, and interdisciplinary coordination of care and communication of care provided are critical to improving outcomes and managing costs. Sometimes this coordination may be as simple as requesting that a copy of the visit note be sent to all providers. Although conceptually simple, coordination of care may not have been done consistently before NCM.

NCM is based on a relationship of trust developed over time between the nurse case manager and the patient and family or significant others. It is performed across all settings, primarily in the community. The goal is to provide quality care in the setting appropriate to the patient's needs. Nurse case managers work with patients in any hospital unit or at home, a clinic, a group home, a long-term care center, and even the patient's work setting.

The benefit to the patient is obvious, as the case studies that follow demonstrate. There is an accessible care provider. Accessibility is maintained through the use of voice mail, pagers, and cellular phones. An example is the patient who places a call and speaks to the nurse case manager or leaves a message on voice mail. Leaving a message activates that nurse's pager, and the message is received. If a return call is needed, it is made at the convenience of the nurse, using a cellular phone if necessary.

Some patients are comfortable sending e-mail messages, which provide a sense of constant contact at any time. They know that the message will only be read during the day, but they feel that someone is always available when they want to talk. In a sense, they are "self-charting." This practice has been especially helpful for some mental health patients and patients who want the feeling of connection during the night or on weekends. Messaging by e-mail also allows "contact" when the nurse is on vacation. These contacts, of course, are not how help is sought in an urgent situation. All patients know how to access care in an emergency. NCM is not an emergency service, and patients are always instructed to go to the nearest ED should an emergency arise.

Most importantly, patients often do better in the hospital and have shorter lengths of stay. A shorter length of stay results in less use of acute care resources, which is critical in this time of dwindling hospital reimbursement, and less inpatient resources such as bedside nurses. These chronic patients who had been frequent users of the hospital are admitted less often, have a shorter length of stay when they are admitted, use fewer critical care beds, and make fewer ED visits. The benefit to the hospital is a reduction of financial loss if the patient has a heavily discounted reimbursement provider or capitated arrangement. Other benefits include greater access to services for those patients who truly need them. ED beds, inpatient beds, and staff are more available for patients with acute needs. Thus NCM remains cost-effective for the hospital where it is based. Because hospital resources are not misused, other providers and payers benefit financially as well.

Patients surveyed have expressed increased satisfaction with their healthcare. "I don't feel so alone with my illness." "I can always reach my nurse; getting in touch with my doctor is like calling the President." "I have a better understanding of my illness and what my medications are for."

Case Study: Medical Patient

I.R. is an 85-year-old, tall, lanky man hospitalized with a diagnosis of hypertension, anemia, nosebleeds, unsteady gait, and multiple lacerations on his arms and face from his cats. The primary care nurse was concerned because he was being dismissed from the hospital, and no one was accompanying him home other than the taxi driver. She believed he would be vulnerable at home and made a referral to NCM. The nurse case manager was able to make the initial contact while I.R. was still in the hospital. At that time, he said that he would be safe and did not anticipate any problems. He said he had a live-in woman friend who would be able to help him get situated at home. They had minimal support from their families, who rarely visited because of the number of cats in the small house. He changed his mind and agreed to let the nurse case manager visit him the next day at his home.

Six cats and a woman who was approximately 5 feet 4 inches tall and 270 pounds greeted the nurse case manager at the door. The woman had 4-plus ankle edema and an unsteady gait but a big smile as she extended her greeting. A.P. was excited to have a nurse coming to the home to check on I.R. and her. She voiced much concern regarding the cats and wanted to have just one, her original cat that was neutered. She indicated that I.R. was the cat lover, adding that they were like his children. I.R. added that he just could not get the females neutered; it was too expensive and would hurt them.

In the course of the NCM relationship over time, goals were mutually identified, and plans were implemented to achieve them. I.R.'s blood pressure was to be controlled and the number of nosebleeds decreased. He hoped to avoid any more hospitalizations. A nosebleed kit was developed that contained an antibacterial ointment, cotton for packing, and a nasal spray recommended by his physician. It seemed that whenever a cat had a litter, I.R.'s blood pressure increased, and his nose began to bleed. I.R. and A.P. started taking vitamin C and a multivitamin with iron. They used healthcare diaries in which they would record their questions, times and dates of nosebleeds, and anything they thought was pertinent to their health. They documented nurse case manager visits and her findings and shared these at their doctor visits. (The nurse case manager added A.P. to her caseload by association, which frequently happens.)

I.R. and A.P.'s cats were never allowed outside for fear they would get lost. There were no city laws regarding cats if they were in the home. The sheriff and the adult protective services would not get involved because I.R. and A.P. were legally competent. The humane society was not interested because the cats were being fed and cared for. The house, however, was becoming unsafe. The cats continued to multiply, and some were sick. They were running wild, and the odor was overwhelming. A.P. and I.R. frequently tripped over kittens. I.R. had numerous lacerations on his arms and face from holding them.

Sometimes in any setting the nurse case manager is called to do things that are not in the job description (i.e., "other duties as assigned"). I.R. finally agreed to have the nurse case manager remove some of the cats if a home could be found for them. A farm home was found. The nurse case manager was able to obtain four kennels from the humane society and rounded up and delivered most of I.R. and A.P.'s cats to the farm.

One of the keys to this case management system is the communication and the relationships that develop between the nurse case manager and the primary care physician or specialist. The nurse case manager becomes the eyes and ears of the physician, identifying client needs before they become a crisis situation. Assessments by the nurse might encourage a patient to make an appointment with his or her physician. Perhaps just a telephone call is required to get a medication adjustment. Patients are encouraged to make these calls. It does seem, however, that calls are returned more promptly if the nurse places the call.

Nurse case managers do not want to be in the position of taking medication orders (that is the role of a home care agency), so the patient or caregiver is the one to get the change over the telephone.

When the nurse case manager attends the physician visit with the patient, all persons present have a chance to speak and contribute to any changes needed in the treatment plan. Later, the nurse case manager can offer support for any changes that were made. In addition to attending physician visits, collaboration is enhanced through a computerized client record. Within the hospital and among those providers who are part of that system and have a need to know, patient records can be accessed. Accessing patient records is done only with prior written consent from patients, obtained during their first contact with the system.

All documentation by the nurse case manager is part of the computer record. The primary care physician, if part of the same system, can view the client's record in the hospital and at the clinic site. The nurse case manager can communicate with the primary care physician by e-mail or fax machine.

Case Study: Behavioral Health Patient

J.L. is a 58-year-old single woman with psychiatric diagnoses of schizoaffective disorder and body dysmorphic disorder. She has a long history of instability, with several hospital stays, and has lived in structured settings. Her psychiatrist requested NCM when she moved to this city about 5 years ago. The purpose was to provide support, coordinate services, and be a liaison with the psychiatrist. At that time, her mental health was maintained with several psychotropic medications and electroconvulsive therapy twice monthly. She had the support of a county social worker case manager who, among other things, manages her finances. She was able to rent her own apartment and has lived independently since then. She has responded well to the new atypical antipsychotics and no longer requires electroconvulsive therapy. For the past 3 years, she has been fairly stable, with no inpatient admissions. She is unable to work competitively but has done volunteer work in the community.

Several months ago, J.L. was diagnosed with breast cancer. She required a mastectomy followed by chemotherapy and a series of radiation treatments. The nurse case manager accompanied her to all of her various physician visits to share information, assist J.L. with decision making, and promote follow-up with the treatment plan. This participation also allowed the nurse case manager to reinforce the plans and instructions with J.L. and her out-of-town family members.

J.L. experienced a great deal of anxiety during this time and required increased contact with her healthcare team. She asked for and was given extra support. She worked hard to use all of her coping skills. With the coordination of care and sharing of reports among care providers, there was no fragmentation. The nurse case manager was also able to provide guidance to those caregivers who were unfamiliar with J.L.'s mental illness and behaviors under stress. J.L. also allowed women from her church to volunteer to drive her to her daily radiation treatments. That was progress for J.L., who tended to isolate herself and instead benefited from this support. It also demonstrates that the nurse case manager does not need to do everything.

During this stressful time, J.L. was not hospitalized except for her surgery and one overnight observation for her first chemotherapy dose. She remains in her apartment and is regaining confidence in her ability to maintain her status and is resuming her community volunteer activities. The nurse case manager increased visits to at least weekly during the cancer crisis and is now able to visit once or twice a month. J.L. will phone the nurse case manager for support as needed between visits.

Costly inpatient stays were avoided, and in that way the hospital benefited. J.L.'s care was provided in the most cost-effective outpatient settings, so her insurance company benefited. Some physician visits were also avoided because of the trust relationship between them and the nurse case manager, who provided reassurance that J.L. could get through this ordeal at home. J.L. has benefited because she had fewer copayments, avoided taxi expenses, and was able to remain at home. She verbalized satisfaction with her care and treatment and her joy at being able to stay home. Her out-of-town family felt relief that J.L. was given the support that she needed, since they were too far away to help.

OUTCOMES OF NURSING CASE MANAGEMENT

The hospital initiated NCM to reduce costs per case and other resources by managing frequent users of the system. Table 18-1 indicates resource utilization of 119 patients who were case managed. They represent all ages and diagnoses. ED visits and those charges, as well as inpatient admissions and average length of stay, were tracked. It was important to know if the positive outcomes could be maintained over time. Therefore data was collected before NCM, the 6 months immediately after NCM, and the last quarter of 2000.

As Table 18-1 shows, there was a decrease in the number of ED visits, as well as the average charges for each visit. The number of inpatient admissions was reduced, as well as the average length of stay. Table 18-1 also shows the average charge per case and the reduction in overall total charges for this group of patients. Total charges decreased markedly af-

TABLE 18-1
Nursing Case Management Outcomes

Use of Resources	6 Months Before NCM	6 Months After NCM	Last 6 months
ED visits	33	32	21
Average charge per ED visit	$137	$82	$59
Inpatient stays (days)	9.54	2.29	1.55
Length of stay (days)	10.13	7.00	6.13
Average charge per case	$8946	$2577	$1867
Total charges	$1,064,562	$306,620	$222,145

Outcomes data: n=119, period ending December 31, 2000.

ter a nurse case manager became involved with the clients. The savings to the institution were evident. The effectiveness of NCM was maintained over time with these patients. The patients continued to use healthcare resources in a more appropriate way, received the healthcare they needed, and had follow-up with their own nurses.

Clients with NCM have an increased knowledge of their disease and how to manage it. They communicate changes in their status with care providers in a timely manner, and become more proactive in their care. A patient with congestive heart failure will make adjustments that have been discussed when he or she has increased ankle edema or a weight gain within certain parameters, rather than wait for the situation to become a crisis requiring an ED visit or even admission to the hospital. Patients report concerns to their nurse case managers earlier and learn what to look for so they can become their own care experts.

NCM patients report feeling more in control of their healthcare decisions, have an increased sense of self-worth, and believe that people care about them. They are using a wider range of healthcare services, and they are accessing primary care earlier. When acute hospitalization is needed, their duration of stay is decreased and they use community home services more readily. NCM patients are more satisfied with their healthcare services as a whole.

All the nurse case managers in Immanuel–St. Joseph's Hospital system have seen patients manage a situation comfortably and confidently at home that previously would have resulted in an admission. That experience is a result of their own confidence and sense of control.

Initially the NCM program measured financial outcomes and assessed patient and caregiver satisfaction. Since the case managers were nurses and not accountants, it was important to them to measure functional outcomes. They questioned that although the program was "successful," were their patients really doing better or just staying away from the hospital for other reasons? When the program and results were shared with administration, they would ask, "What do you do with the patients?"

Different ways to measure interventions and outcomes were explored. The group of nurse case managers made the decision to use nursing diagnoses of the North American Nursing Diagnosis Association (NANDA). The group selected a list of standardized interventions appropriate to the scope of practice from the Nursing Interventions Classification (NIC) (Johnson and Maas, 1997). Outcomes were also chosen from Nursing Outcomes Classification (NOC) (McCloskey and Bulechek, 1996). The care plans are modified to fit each individual. Because the record is computerized and standardized language is used on the inpatient units, the care plan is modified when the patient is discharged and is continued by the nurse case manager in the outpatient setting. The care is truly seamless.

It will be easy to actually count which interventions are most frequently used and to determine which are most effective. This information is just beginning to be evaluated. By graphing the outcome ratings over time, the patient's journey toward his or her goal can be viewed in a new way. This information can be used individually or as aggregate data by medical diagnoses. This method of documenting and tracking outcomes has great potential for various ways in which to use the data gathered in future interactions with patients.

For example, a female patient with severe depression was involved in setting the outcomes she wished to reach and then in ranking her progress. The nurse case manager would also rank the progress, and the two would compare notes and discuss similarities but, more importantly, discrepancies. The patient could then address what interventions by the nurse case manager and actions on her own part could move her toward her goals. By looking at the graph, she had a visual picture of her status, and she actively found ways to increase her adherence to the treatment plan and achieve her goals.

BARRIERS TO SYSTEMWIDE NURSING CASE MANAGEMENT

One barrier to NCM has been the need to rely on individual staff members to recognize patients who would benefit from NCM. Leaving this case finding to individuals is not the most reliable method. The bedside nurses are overloaded and it is difficult to keep new staff informed of the service. Most patients were discharged without ever being assessed using the previously mentioned criteria for NCM. A computer report is being written to have the computer scan each admission for frequency of contact with the hospital system, ED, inpatient stay, or observation bed. By scanning this report daily, the nurse case manager can evaluate patients listed who meet frequency of use and review charts to determine which patients meet the other criteria, primarily lack of support. The result will be to have each patient held to the same standard of assessment for NCM services.

Presently the healthcare system in this setting remains diverse. This diversity multiplies the need for NCM. Each patient has an individual payment plan with its own rules and coverage. Many people are not aware of what type of coverage they have until they are in need of care. There is also a need for education of physicians and other healthcare providers regarding healthcare plans. Because nurse case managers are not aligned with any payer system, they can play the role of patient advocate. Their experience has been that by keeping the focus on the clients and their needs and helping them become the experts in their own care, the pieces fall into place, and all those involved with the clients benefit. Keeping the focus on the client is a strategy that works in any reimbursement system.

IMPROVEMENTS FOR THE FUTURE

The ideal setting for this type of NCM is the primary care clinic. By the time any patient has become a multiple user of care in the hospital, the patient is at the most costly position on the continuum of care. In the primary care clinic, all clients could be assessed using criteria that determines who would benefit from NCM. Nurse case managers positioned in the primary care clinic would be part of an integrated system of care. This system would work best if all providers, clinics, and hospitals had the same financial incentives, which would promote appropriate use of resources and result in less abuse of the system, with improved client outcomes and increased satisfaction for all. It would make financial sense for payers or employers to include the services of NCM because it has proven to be an effective and cost-saving intervention.

REFERENCES

Barger SD: Building healthier communities in a managed care environment: opportunities for advanced practice nurses. In Turner SO, editor: *Essential readings in nursing managed care,* Gaithersburg, Md, 1999, Aspen.

Bower KA: *Case management by nurses,* Washington, DC, 1992, American Nurses Publishing.

Johnson M, Maas M: *Nursing outcomes classification (NOC),* St Louis, 1997, Mosby.

McBeth AL, Weydt A: Innovative delivery systems: freedom, trust, caring. In Cohen EL, editor: *Nurse case management in the 21st century,* St Louis, 1996, Mosby.

McCloskey JC, Bulechek GM: *Nursing interventions classification (NIC),* ed 2, St Louis, 1996, Mosby.

Mullahy CM: *The case manager's handbook,* ed 2, Gaithersburg, Md, 1998, Aspen.

Community-Based Health Programs in a Managed Care Environment

Mary Krentzman

KEY LESSONS IN THIS CHAPTER

- American society faces an ever-growing population of chronically ill persons who struggle to deal with both medical illness and social issues.
- Community case management strives to guide patients toward the highest level of wellness, as defined by the patient and not the healthcare system.
- Risk identification is an important component of community case management and is a proactive way to avoid adverse health outcomes in high-risk populations.
- Organizations must develop their own high-risk triggers, which represent risk within their own population of patients.
- Community case management will become a major component of future healthcare delivery systems.

A new way of managing healthcare is emerging in the twenty-first century. The impact of managed care on our nation's health is mentioned in newspapers and on the television news almost daily. We are witnessing an old system of healthcare that is forced to reinvent itself and redesign its methodology. This redesign includes the development of a care continuum with integrated delivery systems that view acute care as a much smaller part of the healthcare process. Preventive health strategies and health promotion for populations at large are replacing the days of illness care. Primary care providers are important players, and risk-based strategies are used to construct accepted methods of payment for patient care (Turner, 1999).

The strategies of managed care are designed to control and reduce costs while maintaining quality of care (Barnum, 1999). Because economics drive many managed care decisions, patients, who require a particular amount of healthcare for a given illness episode, are receiving care delivery at different points in the care continuum. Many services that were formally administered in an acute setting now take place in the community. The coordination of patient care across a healthcare continuum, dreamed about and planned for by health professionals, is finally becoming a reality.

THE CHRONICALLY ILL

American society faces an ever-growing population of chronically ill persons who struggle to deal with both medical illness and social issues daily. The U.S. Census Bureau estimates that approximately 35 million Americans are presently 65 years of age or older (Bureau of the Census, 1998). A small percentage of these older individuals constitute the frail elderly, who find healthcare to be an intermittent struggle of acute events. Usually these acute events are without the necessary follow-up to promote stability and wellness. This type of fragmentation causes elderly individuals to be at high risk for using most of the monies available in healthcare today. The Health Care Financing Administration (HCFA) (1995) reports that approximately 10% of all Medicare recipients use 70% of all Medicare funds. These figures demonstrate a critical need to implement models of healthcare delivery that are efficient, accessible, and provide quality care for this high-risk population.

The presence of managed Medicare in the Northeast has generated a need for a strong case management approach with high-risk patients. The cost burden of caring for patients with chronic illness is continuously on the rise. Health maintenance organizations (HMOs) and providers involved in Medicare risk contracts are changing their priorities when dealing with chronically ill populations. A traditional model of curative medicine does not work with older individuals who have diseases that cannot be cured. The goals of chronic care management now are quality oriented and focus on symptom relief and prevention of functional decline (Fox and Fama, 1996). To meet these goals, social and community services that are normally not considered a part of a patient's medical care are essential for survival.

COMMUNITY CASE MANAGEMENT

Community case management is an innovative nursing strategy that seeks to improve the management of chronically ill individuals, using multiple health system resources. This case management approach is a *reactive* approach to managing the medical conditions of those who are high risk and a *proactive* approach to managing issues of health promotion. It concentrates on psychosocial, environmental, and economic domains. Today there exists a strong relationship between medical and social problems in the elderly (Powers, 1997). Often, how patients respond to health problems depends on material resources, physical surroundings, and social interaction with others. Case management provides the support needed to identify and deal with actual and potential problems while introducing preventive strategies for the future.

Community case management strives to guide patients toward the highest level of wellness as defined by the patient and not the healthcare system (Powers, 1997). Many elderly individuals interpret their health status or degree of wellness by their level of function and ability to self-manage. Corbin and Cherry (1997) report that individuals who obtain stability with their chronic disease processes are able to live independently and have improved quality of life. The community case management model promotes quality of life and self-management skills through assessment, early mediation, and problem identification. Program design supports the evaluation and coordination of the most appropriate level of care based on individual health problems and patient choice, with goals of providing quality, accountability, and cost-effectiveness.

Community Case Management as a Model of Care

The Hartford Physician Hospital Organization (HPHO) in Hartford, Connecticut has extended a social commitment to its surrounding communities by developing a community case management program to follow patients identified as high risk for adverse events. The program is a physician-based initiative, financially supported by the HPHO, to manage Medicare risk members whose primary care physicians (PCPs) are associated with Hartford Hospital. Program goals include reducing acute events (inpatient admissions, emergency department [ED] visits), increasing support systems to maintain patients in the community, and enhancing the patient/physician/nurse relationship.

The design phase of the program brought together a group of professionals that included physicians and nurses at executive, administrative, and provider levels. Specific strategies used in the design process engaged physician and health plan participation, noting that each brings different strengths to the table. Early program development began with the identification of physician *early adopters*, defined as physicians who have large risk member panels and are eager to support a plan that provides nursing case management services for their patients at risk. In addition, they need to have large numbers of patients in the community. These physicians realized that many elderly patients with chronic health problems fail not only because of disease exacerbation but also as a result of social and economic issues that are out of control. Registered nurses, in a case manager role, partner with PCPs and high-risk patients to provide support by closely monitoring chronic health conditions, teaching self-management techniques, and providing the necessary resources to support patients in the community.

An initial interview process began with individual medical directors, representing physician groups within the HPHO, who selected registered nurses for the case manager role. Three registered nurses were hired to be case managers, and each became part of a collaborative team, attending medical management meetings and managing high-risk patients for their individual physician group. Strong clinical skills, nursing expertise in the management of high-risk populations, and familiarity with program development are required for this case management position.

Defining the Case Manager in the Community

As the role of the case manager evolved, initial workflow processes were developed to interface with providers and payers to ensure communication and support inpatient care. Program visibility was accomplished as case managers met with physician groups, home health organizations, area skilled nursing facilities, residential care facilities, adult day care centers, and social service departments. Specific multidimensional interventions were developed to define case management responsibilities and allow case managers to function as resources in the community. These interventions include the following:

- Individual home assessments
- Patient and family education
- Coordination of healthcare providers
- Referral to community agencies and supports
- Patient advocacy and empowerment
- Health promotion and monitoring
- Individual and group monitoring sessions
- Liaison with payers
- Outcomes measurement

IDENTIFICATION PROCESS

Risk identification is a proactive way to avoid adverse health outcomes in high-risk populations. Boult et al (1998) stress the importance of recognizing that seniors who need concentrated interventions require the use of multiple sources of information to be correctly identified. As the cost of providing healthcare continues to escalate, managed care organizations (MCOs) are seeking new ways to provide quality of care by accurately identifying high-risk members and improving service delivery.

An HMO in Connecticut that had a history of collaboration with the HPHO became involved with the community case management program and offered a willingness to explore alternative strategies to manage high-risk members. This insurer, through contract agreements, already provided membership and claims data to the HPHO on a regular basis. The information included current member lists and total dollar amounts for inpatient stays, ED visits, and PCP/specialist expenses.

Additional important screening data supplied by the HMO included moderate and high-risk scores from returned health risk assessment (HRA) forms sent to all members joining the managed Medicare program. The HRA is a self-reported health status questionnaire that identifies individuals with health needs or medical conditions that cause them to be at risk of using health-related services. Information obtained from this form includes medical diagnosis and comorbidity, activities of daily living (ADLs), instrumental activities of daily living (IADLs), durable medical equipment, and social support. Using the patient data discussed, the case management team developed designated triggers within the database to potentially recognize patients at high risk (Box 19-1).

Reviewing the data, physicians and case managers added physician referral as another important trigger in patient identification. PCPs, using the information in Box 19-2, submitted names of patients who were not identified by the previously described process but who were perceived as failing in the community.

As patients are identified as needing case management services, comprehensive information is exchanged between the physician and case manager detailing important patient care issues. Patient charts are reviewed for a list of medications, information on previous

BOX 19-1
High-Risk Triggers

Top 5% medical expenditures quarterly and annually during the past year
High or moderate HRA scores submitted by the HMO
More than one inpatient admission within the past year
An inpatient admission with a length of stay over 10 days within the past year
More than one ED visit within the past year
85 years and older

BOX 19-2
Second-Level Triggers

Multiple diagnoses and comorbidities that require numerous specialists and services
Lack of or incomplete information on environmental and financial resources
Knowledge of family conflict or poor support systems
Difficulties with memory loss or cognition
Inability to care for self

hospitalizations or ED visits, results of diagnostic studies, and health screening activities. Case managers then contact patients to discuss any immediate health concerns, introduce the program, and schedule an assessment home visit.

Assessment and Problem Identification

Assessment home visits made by case managers are one of the most critical components of the evaluation process. Deficits are easier to identify when patients are observed in their own environment. Home visits procure information that include a patient's demographics, medical history, current health status, environmental needs, psychosocial and physiological health, health-related behaviors, healthcare supervision, and prescribed medical regimen (Box 19-3). Data obtained from the interview process disclose safety concerns, financial difficulties, and cognitive problems. Other significant information includes a patient's perceived needs and support systems, knowledge of disease management, and capability of performing ADLs. During this evaluation, case managers identify actual and potential problems and work collaboratively with patients to develop mutually agreed-upon goals and interventions.

Screening Patients

A complexity screen that defines self-rated health status, number of ED and inpatient admissions, safety concerns, disease processes, functional status, polypharmacy, social sup-

BOX 19-3
Community Case Management Assessment Guidelines

Demographic Data
Age
Ethnic group
Marital status
Family members/significant others
Educational status
Occupation/retired
Health insurance/payer
Physician/specialists
Recent hospitalizations/skilled nursing facility/ED

Medical History
Arthritis, cancer, cardiovascular disease
Diabetes, endocrine disease, epilepsy
Kidney disease, neurological disease
Osteoporosis, peripheral vascular disease
Psychiatric illness/alcoholism/drug dependency

Current Health Data
Annual physical examination
Influenza/pneumococcal/tetanus shots
Prostate specific antigen/mammogram/Pap smear/
   bone density
Colonoscopy/sigmoidoscopy
Vision/dental/hearing
Podiatry

Health-Related Behaviors
Nutrition
Sleep/rest pattern
Physical activity
Personal hygiene
Substance abuse

Environment
Socioeconomic status/finances
Residence/safety check
Neighborhood

Psychosocial
Current community resources
Religion/cultural beliefs
Human sexuality
Abuse/neglect

Physiological
Hearing/vision/speech
Dentition/mouth
Cognition (MMSE, SF-12)
Pain
Integument
Neuromusculoskeletal function
Endocrine function
Respiration
Circulation
Digestion/hydration
Bowel function
Genitourinary function

Health Supervision

Prescribed Medication Regimen

Other

ports, number of physicians or specialists, and age is completed on all patients identified for community case management services (Box 19-4). The screen produces an intensity of service score used to determine the frequency of communication and visits needed to monitor a patient safely in the community. Three levels of intensity of service are available after an initial patient assessment is completed. Case managers implement interventions of monitoring, teaching, coordination, and referral at predetermined time frames according to individual severity levels.

Patients with high intensity of service scores (31 or more) are in need of immediate interventions and are considered the most acute. These patients may have multiple

BOX 19-4
Community Case Management Complexity Screen

Self-Rated Health Status		Disease Category*	
Very good	0	Arthritis	1; 5
Good	1	Asthma/chronic obstructive	1; 5
Fair	3	pulmonary disease/pneumonia	
Poor	5	Cancer	1; 5
		Cardiovascular disease/CHF	1; 5
ED Visits in Last 6 Months		Dementia	1; 5
0 visits	0	Depression/anxiety	1; 5
1 visit	2	Endocrine disorder	1; 5
2 visits	4	Kidney failure (acute/chronic)	1; 5
3 or more visits	6	Neurological disorders	1; 5
		Peripheral vascular disease	1; 5
Hospital Admissions in Last 6 Months		Psychiatric illness/alcoholism	1; 5
0 admissions	0	Other	1; 5
1 admission	2		
2 admissions	4	**Functional Status**	
3 or more admissions	6	Independent	0
		1 ADL	3
Polypharmacy		2 ADLs	5
0 medications	0	3 or More ADLs	7
1-4 medications	1	3 or More IADLs	3
5-8 medications	3		
8 or more medications	5	**Number of Physicians**	
		1 physician	0
Social/Financial Supports		2 physicians	2
Adequate	0	3 or more physicians	4
Minimum	2		
Stressed	5	**Age**	
Lack of	10	65 years	3
		65-70 years	1
Safety		71-80 years	2
Urgent safety need (always level 3)	40	Over 80 years	3
		Recommended Level of Intensity	
		0-10	1
		11-30	2
		31+	3

*1 = stable; 5 = unstable.

chronic conditions, cognitive deficits, two or more ADL deficits, polypharmacy issues, financial difficulties, and poor social support. An initial assessment may reveal unstable health issues that require an immediate evaluation by the PCP and close monitoring with frequent home visits and telephone calls by the case manager. Coordinating care may include referrals to a visiting nurse association (VNA) and other community services as needed. Patients with moderate (11 to 30) and low (1 to 10) intensity of service scores may have chronic but stable medical problems, difficulty with one or two ADLs, mild cognitive impairment, problems with medication management, financial strain, and difficulties with social support. These patients are usually stable and require a plan of care that includes monitoring in the home or with group visits, occasional telephone contact, patient education, and support.

Communication

Communication between the physician, case manager, and other community providers is essential for patients at all severity levels to provide comprehensive patient care. Once the plan of care is put into effect and chronic conditions begin to stabilize, a fluctuation between levels of intensity may be seen as patients begin to think differently about their health problems and treatment options and change self-care behaviors.

During an initial assessment, case managers explore options with patients and their family members. Because most patients wish to stay in their homes, finances and home care needs are closely evaluated. The coordination of available resources is invaluable, with some patients being eligible for state and federal entitlement programs and others using private pay services. Elements of a plan of care ensure that agreed-upon services are put in place, with monitoring initiated and adjustments made as necessary. Patient monitoring involves, but is not restricted to, home visits, physician office visits, group sessions, and telephone calls to the patient and family. Through this process, patients have the opportunity to improve their health status and graduate to a self-management level where they are monitored by telephone calls and may eventually be discharged from the program.

GROUP PROGRAMMING

As a natural progression of the community case management program, a select number of high-risk patients are seen at group programs. This intervention allows case managers to maximize their efficiency by interacting with a number of patients in one location. Also, it is a cost-effective way to provide one-on-one monitoring of patients while allowing for discussion of individual patient issues. The group format permits case managers to safely increase their caseload of patients and provide an opportunity for new physicians to refer patients to the case management program. At the same time, it provides an opportunity for patients to meet other patients who may be facing similar problems and issues and to learn from them and share those experiences.

Multidisciplinary Team Collaboration

Knowing that functional independence requires both positive feelings of self-efficacy and the ability to perform ADLs, case managers collaborated with physical therapists and established a strength and balance exercise program to be used as the theme for group settings. The clinical implication for such a program was clear, since current literature links muscle weakness with recurrent falls and failure to thrive in the frail elderly (Christmas and

Anderson, 2000). The program allows patients to come together at Hartford Hospital satellite sites on a weekly basis for assessment, monitoring, social interaction, health promotional activities, and exercise. If patients do not drive, case managers arrange for transportation to group sessions through local Dial-a-Ride services or family members.

Patients are individually screened by a physical therapist before their participation in the exercise group. This evaluation includes measurements of balance, gait, upper and lower extremity strength, endurance, and body weight ratio. The Mini-Mental State Examination (MMSE) (Folstein, Folstein, and McHugh, 1975) and selected questions from the SF-12 Health Survey (Ware, Kosinksi, and Keller, 1996) are brief scales also used in the screening process. A certified athletic trainer, experienced in cardiac rehabilitation, leads strength-training exercises with goals of halting bone loss and improving balance, flexibility, and strength. Music is used during exercise to increase enjoyment, with class participants choosing a wide range of song selections.

Each class begins with an extended warm-up to promote flexibility and range of motion while preparing muscles for exercise. The warm-up is followed by a 30-minute exercise section that includes exercises that can be done in a chair or while standing, using a chair for balance. The exercises are continuously tailored to meet individual patient limitations or needs. The class ends with a short cool-down period that uses the same slow and controlled warm-up exercises done earlier. Patients are asked to repeat these exercises at home at least twice during the week and record the dates in an exercise log. The group environment encourages patients to increase their activity level and learn safe exercise practices by receiving instruction on the correct way to perform strengthening and balance exercises.

Case manager activities during group sessions involve physical and visual assessments that include blood pressure, pulse, weight monitoring, and lung auscultation. Vital signs are recorded before each exercise program, with some patients receiving evaluations of pulse and blood pressure during and after exercise. Case managers are present within the group setting to support patients with balance difficulty during standing exercises and to monitor any untoward effects of the exercises.

Exercising in a group may be key to achieving improved feelings of well-being with the elderly. The group medium allows an opportunity for patients to socialize with their peers in an atmosphere of support. This socialization also promotes an increase in physical activity, since many patients faithfully attend each exercise session.

Health Promotion

Health promotional education sessions are often held after exercise class. Examples of different subjects discussed include medication management, diet, and stress reduction techniques, using dieticians, pharmacists, and massage therapists as guest lecturers. During these discussions, coffee, juice, and a diabetic snack are served. When a speaker is not scheduled, individual patients discuss a variety of subjects, with case managers available to answer questions and offer support.

FINANCIAL OUTCOMES

Outcomes have become one of the most frequently used buzzwords of healthcare today. The new focus of outcomes monitoring is moving toward wellness, with patients joining the ranks of interested parties. The HPHO developed preevaluation and postevaluation processes to produce outcome data in an effort to demonstrate that the community case management initiative is linked to improved patient care. The database used for this assessment was the Hartford Hospital medical database, which gives inpatient and ED cost data that occurred at Hartford Hospital. As much as cost is related to survival in healthcare today, this process began with the monitoring of medical costs and service utilization (inpatient admissions, ED visits and length of stay [LOS]) on all case managed patients at 6 months and 1 year before program entry. Financial data is currently being collected on case managed patients after 6 months and 1-year participation in the case management program and will be compared to the preentry data. Unfortunately, unlike the measurable boundaries of acute episodes of care, a less predictable care continuum may require longer time periods to see an impact and demonstrate positive trends of decreasing cost.

CLINICAL OUTCOMES

Along with cost, the case management evaluation process has focused strongly on clinical outcomes. Using multidimensional measurements, assessment data is collected by case managers at time of initial patient assessment and after patients have received 12 months of the case management intervention. These measurements include assessment of physical and mental functioning using ADL measurement scales, MMSE scores, and selected questions from the SF-12.

For elderly individuals, the ability to perform ADLs is essential to maintain independent living (Krach et al, 1996). As part of the evaluation process, case managers use self-rated information obtained by patient interview to measure a patient's ability to perform ADLs. Mental functioning is evaluated using the 10-item MMSE, a cognitive screening tool that is easily administered and highly reliable, along with questions from the SF-12 that relate to feelings of depression. These evaluations of physical and mental functioning allow case managers to review changes in health status periodically and make important decisions affecting resource needs and allocation. Other qualitative measurements include collecting data on basic preventive healthcare practices such as flu vaccine, pneumonia vaccination, and advanced directives.

Patients participating in the group exercise program receive more involved musculoskeletal testing that includes repeated measures of strength, balance, physical performance, endurance, and the ability to complete ADLs (Table 19-1). The data measurements for all patients attending this program at baseline, after 6 months, and after 1 year of program participation are collected by a physical therapist. Patients who have regularly attended exercise sessions have demonstrated an increase in strength and balance since joining. These functional outcome measurements are directed toward recovering and maintaining a patient's self-care potential and independence in the community.

TABLE 19-1
Community Case Management: Exercise-Strengthening Outcome Measurement

Measurement	Initial ___/___/___	6 Months ___/___/___	12 Months ___/___/___
Blood pressure			
Heart rate			
Respiratory rate			
Height			
Weight			
BMI			
MMSE			
Depression rating			
ADL			
Single limb stance Open eyes (sec)			
Gait speed (time in sec to walk 7.62 miles or 25 ft on smooth surface)			
Upper extremity strength grip dynamometry lb: (L)			
Lower extremity strength (time in sec to complete 5 sit-stands)			
2-minute walk (number of ft)			
Number of sessions attended			

BMI, Body mass index.

SATISFACTION MEASUREMENTS

Because the case management intervention depends on a close level of collaboration between the case manager, the PCP, and the patient, measures of program satisfaction also are evaluated. Satisfaction surveys were sent to all patients who had completed at least 6 months in the case management program and had a score of 23 or higher on their MMSE on admission to the program. Questions included in the survey asked patients how they felt about their health before and after entering the program, as well as if they felt satisfied with the program. A space was also included on the survey for patients to include comments.

Patient Responses to the Survey

The patients' responses to the survey reflected that they rated their health as improved since entering case management and overall were satisfied with the program. Many patients welcomed the opportunity to comment on their care, and some of these comments included the following:

I salute my nurse. Every time she left my house I felt better able to cope with my life. I was greatly impressed with her professionalism—at the same time never once losing the human touch . . . [B]ecause of my nurse's help, I am able to see the light at the end of the tunnel. I live alone—I'm wishing she can continue to check on me—my blood pressure, etc. I am [in my 80s] and am very grateful, not only to my nurse, but also to your wonderful organization. God bless you one and all.

My nurse is a very helpful and understanding person. She sometimes makes the impossible possible. She is a wonderful person to have around.

Physician Responses to the Survey

Physicians also were asked to complete a survey that examined the case management intervention, as well as the individual case manager's clinical practice. They provided favorable comments that noted high levels of satisfaction, as a result of being involved in positive case management experiences. The following physician comments are in response to being asked to give an example of where the interventions by a case manager resulted in positive outcomes for the patient:

I have had multiple positive outcomes working with my case manager (e.g., improved compliance with medications and follow-up office visits, increased understanding of the disease process, financial assistance, and community involvement). I believe that we complement each other and improve the care given to the patients we share.

As a result of working with the case manager, a patient with asthma and multiple medical and psychiatric problems has had decreased frequency of ER and office visits in the past year, despite being unwilling to give up [multiple pets in her home].

When physicians were asked about the ways in which the program could be improved, one physician's response was: "Clone the nurse!"

COMMUNITY CASE MANAGEMENT IN ACTION

Many times the most accurate demonstration of what community case management provides is told in story form. As case managers work closely with patients, they are able to coordinate community services and at the same time provide a service themselves. The following case study describes an elderly couple living in the community who need much support and shows how case management services are able to meet these needs.

Case Study: Promoting Independent Living

J.B. is an 84-year-old man who lives in a private home with his 79-year-old wife, S.B. J.B. has a medical history of insulin-dependent diabetes mellitus (IDDM), congestive heart failure (CHF), glaucoma, rheumatoid arthritis (RA), and gout. He has had three ED visits for hypoglycemia within the past year and has missed his last two office appointments with his PCP. Along with his numerous medical problems, he is the primary caregiver for his wife, who has advancing Alzheimer's dementia. Recently the police have been involved in multiple domestic disputes in the home, since S.B. becomes easily agitated and tries to assault her husband. J.B.'s PCP placed a referral to the community case management program to evaluate the home situation, develop a plan of care, and provide services for this couple.

Initial evaluation reveals an elderly couple living alone, with very little outside support. They have no children, and most of their close neighbors and friends are no longer living. Their home is in disrepair, with a soiled living area, cluttered furniture, and piles of newspapers in every room. They have no assistant devices to aid with ADLs, and only one of the three bathrooms within the home is functional. The food supplies in the home are sparse, high in sugar content, and of little nutritional value. Double locks are present on all of the outside doors, and there are no smoke detectors within the home.

J.B. prides himself on being the head of the house and has never had to hire outside help. It is only within the past year that he has started to realize that he is not able to keep up with things and feels that he may be losing control. He worries about his wife's recent behavior patterns and finds it extremely difficult to afford their prescription medications and other necessities. Despite these difficulties, J.B. repeatedly expresses his wishes to remain in his home with his wife as long as possible.

Initially the case manager evaluated S.B., assuming that her erratic behavior was a major factor in the deterioration of J.B.'s health. S.B. was very pleasant but disoriented during most of the interview. When tested for cognition, her MMSE score was 16. She apparently has not been taking any medications for quite a while, and there were no prescription medication bottles found in the home.

Immediate interventions included the following:

- A call to the PCP confirmed a list of S.B.'s prescribed medications, and the pharmacy was notified to refill the prescriptions, which J.B. picked up that afternoon.
- The case manager filled a weekly medication organizer later that day, and J.B. was taught how to dispense daily medication to his wife.
- A system of support was set up whereby the case manager telephoned S.B. twice a day and spoke with her by telephone as she took her medication.

This telephone monitoring was necessary for a 2-week period while S.B. became familiar with her daily medication routine, was able to appreciate the effect of the prescribed drugs, and began to trust in J.B. dispensing her pills. During that period, J.B. noted calmer behavior patterns in his wife, which strengthened his confidence as caregiver and reinforced his relationship with the case manager.

The plan of care was initiated and included the following:

■ A social work referral was made to the town social service department to evaluate financial status and determine eligibility for homemaker, transportation, and Meals-on-Wheels community services.

■ Smoke detectors were obtained and installed by the local fire department, as well as a complete safety check of their home.

■ Appropriate durable medical equipment was obtained and installed in their home. J.B. privately paid for this equipment (e.g., grab bars, shower chair).

■ Applications were submitted to obtain prescription medications from patient assistant programs through pharmaceutical companies.

■ Medical alert bracelets were obtained for J.B. and S.B. that listed their medical diagnoses and allergies.

During the first month of monitoring, frequent home visits were made to help J.B. stabilize his diabetes and begin teaching the major treatment elements of diet, exercise, and medication. These home visits included the following:

■ *Insulin self-administration:* Self-administration and syringe filling skills were evaluated, noting that J.B. was incorrectly filling his insulin syringes because he could not see. A prefilled insulin pen was obtained, and with patient instruction, J.B. was able to dial in his daily dose accurately. Because J.B. had been an insulin-dependent diabetic for many years, his injection technique was excellent, and supplemental education was provided on suitable sites and rotation schedules.

■ *Self-glucose monitoring:* J.B. had been monitoring his blood glucose infrequently at home. His self-glucose monitor (SGM) was very old and had never been calibrated. Physician prescriptions were obtained for SGM strips and lancets, with a new meter provided by the HMO. J.B. was able to see well enough to read this meter, and after receiving a demonstration on meter use, he was able to successfully obtain and record his fasting blood sugars daily.

■ *Patient education on hypoglycemia and hyperglycemia:* J.B.'s knowledge base was assessed, and a plan to provide supplemental patient education was implemented. This patient instruction included the signs and symptoms of hypoglycemia and hyperglycemia, as well as prevention and treatment of both conditions. Most importantly, J.B. was able to verbalize the optimal range of his blood glucose levels. Since hypoglycemia is a life-threatening complication in the elderly, J.B. was instructed in immediate treatments for low blood sugar. A referral to the HMO diabetes disease management program was made to provide weekly telephonic monitoring and support by a nurse diabetic specialist.

■ *Dietary management:* A referral to a registered dietician was made to review nutritional management. Individual dietary issues related to J.B.'s IDDM and CHF were reviewed by the case manager and were incorporated into meal planning.

■ *Foot care:* A referral from J.B.'s PCP was obtained, and an appointment with a podiatrist was made. J.B. was made aware that diabetic foot examinations and nail cutting by a podiatrist was covered under his HMO plan every 3 months. Patient education was provided on how to perform a self-foot examination, with the case manager completing a nursing assessment of J.B.'s feet monthly.

■ *Daily weight monitoring:* A scale with large digital numbers was obtained from the HMO. J.B. was instructed to weigh himself daily and report any weight gain over 2 to 3 lb to the case manager. Signs and symptoms of CHF were reviewed with J.B., as well as the importance of sodium restriction.

■ *Exercise:* J.B. and S.B. joined an exercise-strengthening group and began to attend weekly group sessions. During these sessions, medications were poured in a weekly medication organizer for S.B., and J.B. was able to review his daily blood sugar levels and weight with the case manager. J.B. swears that his balance and strength have improved greatly over the past 6 months, and S.B. appears to enjoy the group atmosphere and is able to complete most of the exercises without difficulty.

■ *Psychosocial support:* J.B. has been referred to an Alzheimer's caregiver support group and attends monthly meetings. He also receives peer support through the weekly group exercise program and frequently talks about feeling more in control of his life.

■ *Health screening:* Appointments were made with the PCP for both J.B. and S.B. to have a yearly physical examination. They both have received recent eye examinations by an ophthalmologist. Mammogram and prostate screening has been completed, and they are current with flu shots and pneumonia vaccinations.

J.B. and S.B. are able to live independently in the community and have a genuine quality of life, with the support of community services and monitoring by their PCP and community case manager. To ensure a safe future for this couple, case management services probably will always be required to maintain stability of their chronic illnesses and manage any further problems that arise.

Case management at the community level is one answer to the new direction for healthcare. A future of accountability and shared goals can join to ensure clinical quality and satisfaction while managing costs for patients, providers, and payers. The opportunity to excel in patient-focused, cost-effective care is waiting as community case management emerges as a major component of future healthcare delivery.

REFERENCES

Barnum BS: *Teaching nursing in the era of managed care,* New York, 1999, Springer.

Boult C, Pualwan TF, Fox P, et al: Identification and assessment of high-risk seniors, *Am J Manag Care* 4(8): 1137-1145, 1998.

Bureau of the Census: Population estimates, U.S. Census Bureau, Population Division, 1998, Available online: http://www.census.gov/population/estimates/state/st98 elderly.txt.

Christmas C, Anderson RA: Exercise and older patients: guidelines for the clinician, *J Am Geriatr Soc* 48(3):318-324, 2000.

Corbin JM, Cherry JC: Caring for the aged in the community. In Swanson EA, Tripp-Reimer T, editors: *Advances in gerontological nursing: chronic illness and the older adult,* New York, 1997, Springer.

Folstein MF, Folstein SE, McHugh PR: Mini-mental-state: a practical method for grading the cognitive state of patients for the clinician, *J Psychiatr Res* 12:189-198, 1975.

Fox PD, Fama T: Managed care and chronic illness: an overview. In Fox PD, Fama T, editors: *Managed care and chronic illness: challenges and opportunities,* Gaithersburg, Md, 1996, Aspen.

Health Care Financing Administration: *Healthcare financing review: statistical supplement,* Baltimore, 1995, Department of Health and Human Services, The Administration, Office of Research and Demonstrations.

Krach P, DeVaney S, DeTurk C, et al: Functional status of the oldest-old in a home setting, *J Adv Nurs* 24, 456-464, 1996.

Powers BA: Social support, social networks, and the problem of loneliness in elder care. In Swanson EA, Tripp-Reimer T, editors: *Advances in gerontological nursing: chronic illness and the older adult,* New York, 1997, Springer.

Turner SO: *Essential readings in nursing managed care,* Gaithersburg, Md, 1999, Aspen.

Ware JE, Kosinski M, Keller SD: A 12-item short-form health survey: construction of scales and preliminary tests of reliability and validity, *Med Care* 34(3):220-223, 1996.

20

Quality Management in a Managed Care Environment

Eileen Barton

KEY LESSONS IN THIS CHAPTER

- Fundamental to understanding quality management in healthcare today is an ability to address underuse, overuse, misuse, and variation in the delivery of healthcare.
- A framework for assessing today's healthcare systems includes an evaluation of the structure, the process, and the outcomes of care delivery.
- Strong, organization-wide performance improvement systems should be linked to the core mission and values of the organization.
- The Joint Commission on Accreditation of Healthcare Organizations (JCAHO) promotes a quality improvement framework that includes the steps of design, measure, assess, and improve.
- The Health Plan Employer Data and Information Set (HEDIS) is a standardized set of performance measures that assesses the quality of healthcare and services provided by managed care plans.

Managed care organizations (MCOs) are responding to the growing consumer demand for improved accountability and quality in healthcare, knowing that failure to recognize the public's increasing demand for both accountability and quality will hamper their ability to survive in today's competitive marketplace. Professional nurses employed by MCOs and those working for contracting providers must be knowledgeable about accreditation and the federal and state regulations that control the quality management activities of MCOs. They must also be prepared to articulate professional standards of practice when called on to participate in quality management activities. Clearly defining professional practice roles and holding themselves accountable for their achievements will strengthen nurses' position as providers of care and will enable them to be more effective patient advocates in planning for improvement initiatives.

CURRENT STATE OF HEALTHCARE QUALITY

Two recent reports have focused on issues central to the quality of healthcare in the United States. The first report was published in 1998, in response to a growing public movement to hold MCOs and other insurers responsible for improved measurement of healthcare quality. The Department of Health and Human Services released a report, which was reviewed by the Agency for Health Care Policy and Research (AHCPR) (1998a), *The Challenge and Potential for Assuring Quality Health Care for the 21st Century.* This report emphasized the fact that the United States, although possessing many of the world's finest medical facilities and providing high levels of care to millions, has nonetheless failed to address many important quality issues, specifically the underuse, overuse, misuse, and variation in care delivery. Because these problems are so pervasive in the healthcare field, we must understand their impact if we are to improve the healthcare delivery system. A brief overview of the key points of the report follows:

- *Underuse:* When certain tests, procedures, or treatments are withheld for any reason, the patient can suffer unnecessary complications.
- A 1998 survey conducted for the National Committee for Quality Assurance (NCQA) on behalf of HMOs found that 30% of women aged 52 to 69 had failed to have a mammogram within the preceding 2 years (AHCPR, 1998a).
- A 1997 survey by this group reported that 30% of eligible females did not get Pap smears. Such screening, they project, saves lives and reduces healthcare costs due to early detection. Nurses, in their day-to-day practice, are key to improving compliance to health screening measures (AHCPR, 1998a).
- *Overuse:* Unjustified services add to costs and in some cases actually lead to medical complications.
- Two frequently cited examples of overuse are caesarean sections and hysterectomies.
- The overuse of antibiotics is a well-known factor in increased microbial resistance, leading to the need for developing newer and more costly drugs.
- *Misuse of Services:* Negligence was blamed for 27.6% of injuries and 51% of deaths. Nurses have a responsibility to identify potential risk factors and work toward their reduction by promoting improved policies, procedures, and practices that minimize risk (AHCPR, 1998a).
- A study of New York State hospitals found that 1 in 25 patients were injured by the care they received and that death resulted in 13% of these injured patients (AHCPR, 1998a).
- *Variation of Services:* Practices vary significantly from one geographic area of the country to another and cannot be accounted for by patient status, resources, or preference.
- Lengths of stay in hospitals in the Northeast are considerably higher than those in western states.
- Caesarean section rates vary based on locale.

The second study, published by the Institute of Medicine (2000), is a scathing report on the quality of healthcare in the United States that places the entire healthcare industry on the defensive. Focusing on safety issues, the study made the shocking estimate that up to 98,000 preventable deaths occur throughout the nation each year and that 3% to 4% of hospitalized patients suffer adverse events (Institute of Medicine, 2000). These estimates, based upon morbidity and mortality studies conducted in various parts of the country, have been challenged by some, but there has been no challenge to the basic message of the report that healthcare systems must be compelled to improve safety.

The report also focused on the cost of these preventable medical errors. Patients and purchasers pay for errors through increased insurance costs and copayments. Many of these increased costs are attributable to the costs associated with providing unnecessary care.

The annual healthcare cost is estimated to be at least $15 billion. The cost of lost consumer trust, diminished satisfaction, pain, discomfort, and other factors are not included in this estimate.

Both reports made recommendations that emphasized the need to address these problems on a nationwide basis by establishing standardized sets of core quality measures and developing a framework and capacity for universal reporting of the results of a broad range of quality initiatives. The challenge to do this is formidable and requires more than professional commitment alone. What is needed is centralized leadership, financial support, and backing from all provider systems, including the federal government.

EVOLUTION OF QUALITY MANAGEMENT

In the early twentieth century, some physicians began to look at issues related to variations in care. Although some progress was made in the intervening years, it was not until the late 1970s that the foundation for healthcare quality began to evolve. Looking back, it is hard to believe that these concepts were so late in development and so slow to gain universal acceptance. Nursing was first to recognize and support quality management activities. Physicians as a group resisted opening their own practices to such scrutiny. As a result of this resistance, most quality management activities are mandated by outside regulators and accrediting bodies. Instead of healthcare professionals developing their own strategically focused quality management programs, the quality agenda is being played out in the media and the legislative arena. The following sections identify the initiatives that have taken place to date.

1970 to 2000

It was not until the late 1970s that Avedis Donabedian, MD, an academic physician from the University of Michigan, synthesized existing research and formulated a theoretical framework for patient care evaluation. He is best known for his Structure, Process, and Outcome Model of Quality Evaluation published in 1980 (Kongstvedt, 1996). Elements of this framework remain key to current healthcare evaluation systems. A brief overview of these elements and how they relate to managed care follows.

Structure

The *structure* of a healthcare program is defined as the physical characteristics of the healthcare organization itself. Aspects to be included in evaluating structural components include the following (Kongstvedt, 1996):

1. Ownership/contracting
2. Physical plant, including the technologies available to provide care

3. Qualifications/credentialing of professionals rendering care
4. Licensing/accreditation
5. Compliance to applicable codes, including fire safety and environmental safety
6. Recording/reporting and maintenance of medical records

Process

Process measurement is generally understood as the steps by which care is actually delivered in a given setting. Process criteria include diagnostic screening, treatments, and other tests and therapies that are part of a treatment plan. In the past, processes of care were measured indirectly by reviewing medical records, minutes of meetings, and policy and procedures that related to key aspects of care delivery. Today MCOs have been effective in measuring compliance by a number of key process elements, as well as comparing their performance to other providers. Process elements measured include mammography and Pap smear screening, immunization rates, prenatal testing and screening, as well as other population-specific indicators. Clinical pathways, flow charts, and other similar tools are also being used to reduce unacceptable variations in the processes of care.

Outcomes

The final aspect, the *outcomes* of care, can simply be defined as the result of care. Some examples of outcomes of care include mortality and morbidity rates, infections, and readmission rates. Individual hospitals routinely collect this data and track and trend rates over time. Unfortunately, that same data cannot readily be compared to other similar institutions unless the rates are risk adjusted for age, morbidity, and other variables. Accrediting bodies and other key forces, including consumer organizations, are now advocating for the development of comparative databases on a national level. The Joint Commission on Accreditation of Healthcare Organizations (JCAHO) has recently mandated participation in these databases and is now developing its own program of "Core Measures" that will compare processes and outcomes among providers (JCAHO, 2001).

In addition to Donabedian's contributions, other building blocks have contributed to modern quality management and performance improvement. In the late 1970s, there was an acceleration of quality initiatives, believed by some to be due to the improvement in information systems. Some aspects of these earlier successes have been incorporated into today's quality management systems. Figure 20-1 tracks the evolution of these initiatives.

Implicit Case Review

Although originally within the realm of the physician, over time individual cases came to be reviewed by professionals representing their own disciplines. Physicians, nurses, dietitians, social workers, and others reviewed and determined whether care was appropriate. Today case review continues to be an important tool of quality management; however, professionally accepted standards and guidelines and other established, accepted principles are used in addition to individual clinical expertise.

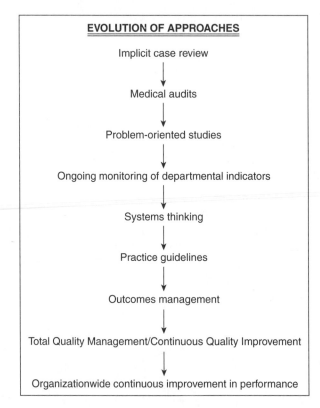

EVOLUTION OF APPROACHES

Implicit case review

↓

Medical audits

↓

Problem-oriented studies

↓

Ongoing monitoring of departmental indicators

↓

Systems thinking

↓

Practice guidelines

↓

Outcomes management

↓

Total Quality Management/Continuous Quality Improvement

↓

Organizationwide continuous improvement in performance

Figure 20-1 Evolution of approaches to quality management. (From Joint Commission on Accreditation of Healthcare Organizations: *Framework for improving performance: from principles to practice,* Oakbrook Terrace, Ill, 1994, Joint Commission Publications.)

Medical Audits and Problem-Oriented Studies

Medical audits and problem-oriented studies focused on the medical record, using indicators to determine compliance to specific criteria. If outcomes were achieved, the care was deemed to be appropriate. These audits did not take into account that other factors, not just direct hands-on care, affect patient care outcomes. As a result of these initiatives, measurement criteria now undergo vigorous testing and are more consistently applied.

Ongoing Monitoring of Departmental Indicators

Individual departments within a healthcare system evaluated their own performance. Departments were required to develop indicators to measure key aspects of services. Measurement results were tracked and trended to ensure compliance to a predetermined compliance rate. Departmental indicators continue to be included in quality management programs but are now considered a part of quality control, one arm of the quality management process.

Total Quality Management and Continuous Quality Improvement

Total quality management and continuous quality improvement (TQM/CQI) is the methodology driving quality management today. In its most basic form, TQM/CQI's foundation is based on the fact that healthcare organizations are made up of systems and that systems are only as good as their individual component parts. An organization that identifies key systems, monitors performance, and makes the necessary corrections to its systems and processes will deliver a stable and predictable product. Applied to managed care, TQM/CQI gives the organization focus and direction.

The "bad apple theory" (blaming a problem on an individual) is no longer acceptable. Today healthcare organizations examine the processes that support the practitioner to discover the root cause of the problem. (*Root cause* is the process of drilling down to the component parts that make up a given function or process. For example, a deficiency in the ordering, delivery, or education of the practitioner may actually be the root cause of an error.)

Using TQM/CQI, interdisciplinary teams comprised of direct care providers identify the root causes of a particular quality problem and develop effective plans for improvement. Systematic monitoring of key systems and processes is basic to the process. It allows for the implementation of timely corrective action plans. Successful implementation of this methodology depends on a strong commitment from top-level management to provide high-quality care. Central to the system is the focus on customer satisfaction, employee involvement, and continuous improvement. In organizations with well-designed TQM/CQI systems, top-level decisions are based on data driven by the process improvement system itself.

QUALITY MANAGEMENT IN MANAGED CARE

Overview

Nurses must be able to understand MCOs and how they approach their commitment to quality. In doing so, nurses can intelligently question managed care representatives, advise clients, and intervene appropriately if and when the best interest of the patient is in question. This background also serves as a foundation for nurses who seek employment in an MCO. Asking appropriate questions during an employment interview will give the prospective employee insight into how the organization views its commitment to quality. The following sections review the factors that drive the MCO to meet its commitment to quality and how quality management principles are incorporated into the managed care environment.

Commitment to Quality

MCOs can only survive in this competitive environment if high-quality care can be delivered to the largest number of recipients at the lowest possible cost. Therefore the MCO must organize itself to respond rapidly and effectively to both internal and external demands. Cost containment measures must be factored in without negatively affecting consumer expectations. The organization's survival depends on having sufficient information available to make the difficult choices between quality and cost.

A strong, organization-wide performance improvement system that is sensitive to consumer needs is a key factor in making these choices. To develop a strong program, top-level management must incorporate quality management principles into the core of the organization's mission and value system. Such a value system starts with top leadership and permeates all aspects of the organization, thereby providing a unified vision and focus for all divisions. Some MCOs are committed to quality, whereas others do only what is required to maintain accreditation.

A commitment to quality is easily recognized in daily interactions with an MCO. A concerned staff and a willingness to address perceived problems is the first sign that the organization is serious about its mission. Figure 20-2 shows the integration of the mission and value system into the organization's performance improvement process.

Framework for Performance Improvement in Managed Care

Two major frameworks are widely used in healthcare performance improvement. Both have been developed using established quality management principles, including the structure/process and outcome parameters previously described. The first framework is outlined in Kongstvedt's text, *Essentials of Managed Health Care* (1996), and delineates steps that emphasize the consumer and his or her basic expectations for care. The second framework, the

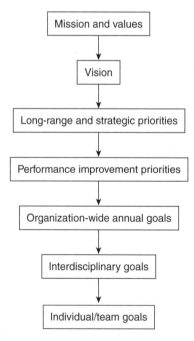

Figure 20-2 Integrated mission and vision. (From Kirk R: *Managing outcomes, process, and cost in a managed care environment,* Gaithersburg, Md, 1997, Aspen.)

JCAHO's *Framework for Improving Performance: From Principles to Practice* (1994), was initially developed for use in acute care facilities and is now used across the continuum of care.

Kongstvedt's framework (1996) emphasizes the following key steps:

1. *Understand consumer needs:* Consumers may be classified as external customers, internal customers, or suppliers. The internal consumers are the departments and services within the MCO, including the professional staff. Information relating to satisfaction surveys, complaints, focus groups, and other vehicles are used to pinpoint the expectations of the consumer group under study.

2. *Identify processes and outcomes that meet consumer needs:* The consumer expects the MCO to offer screening; preventive healthcare; management of chronic illness; and adequate, appropriate, and timely access to illness care. Systems and processes that meet these and other consumer expectations should be identified and targeted for evaluation.

3. *Assess performance compared with professional or best-of-class standards:* This step implies the assessment of those key managed care functions that are important to consumers. Results should be compared to benchmarks to determine whether care was appropriate and provided in a safe and cost-effective setting. (A *benchmark* is the optimum achievable level of performance for a given process or outcome.)

4. *Define indicators to measure performance:* Structure, process, and outcome indicators are developed to measure those targeted processes or outcomes of care selected for review and improvement. Case mix adjustment is applied when the results are to be used in comparative analysis between or among other providers. *Case mix* is defined as the specific attributes of a patient population (e.g., age, sex, severity of illness, comorbidities beyond the control of the health provider).

5. *Establish performance expectations:* An expected rate of compliance to each criteria should be carefully formulated, taking into consideration the organization's past performance, the relationship of the indicator to the desired outcome, and a review of the available literature.

6. *Monitor performance and compare with expectations:* Establish a system for monitoring key indicators. Determine compliance rates and compare to external databases.

7. *Provide feedback to providers and consumers:* Feedback mechanisms can include physician and other provider profiling and report cards that are made available to consumers, providers, and other key stakeholders.

8. *Implement improvements:* Implement practice guidelines, case management improvements, and other acceptable modalities that will improve compliance.

The second major contributor to the literature on performance improvement is the JCAHO (1994). The JCAHO has combined several widely accepted principles of performance improvement into a framework that can be applied across the continuum of healthcare. Its framework takes into consideration the external and internal environments and the cycle for improving organizational performance (Figure 20-3). Once again, the framework reinforces the importance of the organization's mission, vision, and strategic plan. The framework also emphasizes the role of information management and human resources as key to a successful performance improvement program. The cycle for performance improvement is the action

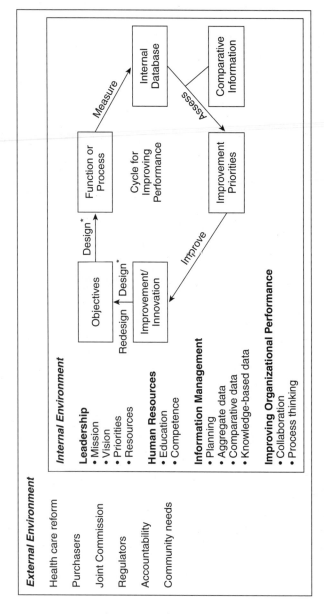

Figure 20-3   Framework for improving performance. (From Joint Commission on Accreditation of Healthcare Organizations, *Framework for improving performance: from principles to practice*, Oakbrook Terrace, Ill, 1994, Joint Commission Publications.)

*In the cycle of performance improvement, design means determining the objectives of a given organizational activity and designing and implementing functions and processes to meet these objectives. In establishing objectives, the cycle supports the use of the organization's mission, vision, and strategic plans.

arm of the framework and includes the following phases: design, measure, assess, and improve. This cycle can be entered into at any point and can be used for any function or process within the organization.

1. *Design:* In the cycle of performance improvement, design means determining the objectives of a given organizational activity and designing and implementing functions and processes to meet these objectives. In establishing objectives, the cycle supports the use of the organization's mission, vision, and strategic plans. In addition, customer need and current information about the process, including external databases, must be used in the design process. In this cycle, *design* refers to the design of a new process or the redesign of an existing process.

2. *Measure:* Measurement is the process by which data is collected for the purpose of assessing performance. Specific indicators are required for effective measurement and should be developed based on key functions within the process. Measurement is used to establish a level of performance, measure the effectiveness of performance improvement, or determine whether action is necessary.

3. *Assess:* Assessing data means translating data into information that can be used to make a judgment about performance. The results of the analysis may show that there are no problems in the process or that there are problems that require resolution. The assessment should also identify processes or functions that require improvement and the priorities among these opportunities.

4. *Improve:* The methods of performance improvement depend on the goals of the improvement process, how the process will flow, and how improvements can be measured. The plan-do-study-act (PDSA) tool can be used to implement any performance improvement process. Clinical process improvement tools commonly used in managed care include clinical pathways and disease management (DM) programs.

Useful Performance Improvement Tools

Dimensions of Performance and the PDSA tool are two commonly used performance improvement tools that can be used in any healthcare setting. Their use will reinforce the direction of most performance improvement projects.

Dimensions of Performance

In planning for any performance improvement activity, the following dimensions of performance can be used as a guide to analyze the process and formulate measurement indicators. The JCAHO incorporates Dimensions of Performance into its recommended *Framework for Improving Performance: From Principles to Practice* (1994).

Dimensions of Performance include the following (JCAHO, 1994):

- *Efficacy:* The use of the procedure or treatment in relation to the patient's overall condition. Would the procedure or process lead to the desired outcome?
- *Appropriateness:* The appropriateness of a specific test, service, or procedure. Is it necessary given the current standard of practice?
- *Availability:* Is the test available or has it been denied due to system problems or constraints on ordering?

- *Effectiveness:* Were procedures and tests performed appropriately, and were the desired outcomes achieved?
- *Timeliness:* Was the test provided in the appropriate time frame?
- *Safety:* The safety of the consumer/provider and others involved in the application of a procedure or treatment is taken into consideration.
- *Efficiency:* The efficiency with which the care or treatment is provided. Could it be accomplished with fewer resources or interventions?
- *Continuity of services:* The degree in which the care is coordinated among practitioners or levels of care.

Plan-Do-Study-Act

PDSA (Figure 20-4) is a process widely used in performance improvement. The process is associated with W. Edward Deming and is sometimes referred to as the *Shewhart Cycle* (Cesta, Tahan, and Fink, 1997). PDSA uses the scientific method as its foundation. The following is a brief overview of this commonly used tool:

- *Plan:* In the context of performance improvement, planning refers to the operational testing of a chosen improvement process. The plan answers the following questions. Who will be involved in the test? What will be involved? How will the test be implemented? What will be measured? What are the indicators of success?
- *Do:* Do means to implement the improvement process and collect measurement data.
- *Study:* During the study phase, the team analyzes the information collected to see if the plan is successful in reaching predetermined goals. A comparison between the results of the study and the established baseline is made to measure the degree of success.
- *Act:* A successful plan is incorporated into the standard operating process. The effectiveness of the action continues to be measured periodically to be certain that improvement is maintained.

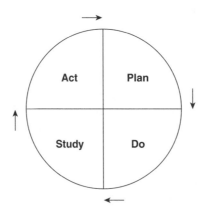

Figure 20-4 PDSA cycle. (From Joint Commission on Accreditation of Healthcare Organizations: *Using performance improvement tools in health care settings,* Oakbrook Terrace, Ill, 1996, p 5, Joint Commission.)

MANAGED CARE REGULATION AND ACCREDITATION

Although the first line of defense in maintaining and improving the quality of care in managed care is the individual licensed professional, there are many organizations, both public and private, that regulate or influence the way that care is delivered in the managed care environment. This section describes the contributions of the NCQA, the Health Care Financing Administration (HCFA), and other organizations that accredit and regulate care delivery.

National Committee for Quality Assurance

The NCQA was formed in 1979 by managed care trade associations, but it did not become an independent accrediting body until 1989. The NCQA has the following two main voluntary activities:

1. Accreditation of MCOs
2. Publication of measures of performance in the Health Plan Employer Data Information Set (HEDIS)

Since 1991, NCQA has expanded the range of organizations it accredits or certifies to include managed behavioral healthcare (MBHO), credentials verification organizations (CVOs), and physician organizations (POs). To date, the organization has accredited almost half of the HMOs in the nation, covering three quarters of all HMO enrollees. A growing number of major employers are now requiring NCQA accreditation for plans with which they do business. NCQA is currently the leading organization representing MCOs in the United States today (NCQA, 2000b).

Key National Committee for Quality Assurance Contributions: The Health Plan Employer Data and Information Set

Perhaps the most comprehensive contribution of NCQA is the development of HEDIS. HEDIS is a set of standardized performance measures that assess the quality of healthcare and services provided by managed care plans. The NCQA developed HEDIS in 1991 in conjunction with public and private purchasers, health plans, researchers, and consumer advocates. HEDIS, created in response to a growing need for consumers and purchasers to be able to rate plans in terms of quality, consumer satisfaction, costs, and utilization of services, has now been used by more than 90% of the nation's health plans (NCQA, 2000c).

In 1997 the HCFA also began using selected HEDIS measures for all Medicare managed care plans, certain risk and cost health plans, social health maintenance organizations (HMOs), and all Medicare Choice demonstrations. All Medicaid, commercial, and Medicare programs currently participate in at least 27 of the same measures across all categories of HEDIS measures. Except for HCFA-funded programs, all MCOs that participate in HEDIS measurements can determine if they want their organization's results made public.

HEDIS now contains over 50 measures, including measures relating to quality, healthcare management/utilization of services, and financial stability. Six of the more recent additions to the HEDIS measurement set focus on chronic diseases, including asthma medication use, chlamydia screening, cholesterol control, diabetes care, high blood pressure control, and management of menopause (HCFA, 2001a).

In addition to HEDIS, there are several other NCQA initiatives that focus on the quality of care, including the following:

- The association maintains a massive database of performance information. The database, Quality Compass, is based on HEDIS data sets. The 2000 edition of Quality Compass contains information on clinical performance, accreditation, and member satisfaction from 466 HMOs and point-of-service plan products covering 340 organizations. Another 101 managed care plans contributed their data for use in calculating averages and benchmarks. The report uses only standardized, independently audited information from the NCQA.
- In conjunction with Phizer, NCQA now publishes a new program, Quality Profiles, designed to provide the industry with information on successful performance improvement projects.
- NCQA has also formed a new Disease Management Advisory Council (DMAC). The purpose of this council is to provide expert advice on developing DM standards and relating them to MCO accreditation standards.
- Individual consumers can log on to NCQA's Website, www.NCQA.org, and request an online report card of selected MCOs. The data is compiled from accreditation surveys and Quality Compass projects.

NCQA publishes an annual report on the quality of healthcare. In the 2000 report (NCQA, 2000a), NCQA listed the accomplishments of the accreditation program and HEDIS initiatives. The report is based on Quality Compass data. Some of the accreditation program's accomplishments are as follows (NCQA, 2000a):

- Health plans that have publicly reported HEDIS data consistently for the past 2 or 3 years exceeded overall industry performance and have improved significantly over the period.
- Participation in Quality Compass grew substantially over the last year, and 85% of publicly reporting plans had their data audited.
- Health plans that are highly rated also have the most satisfied members.
- Health plans often make substantial improvements after the introduction of a new HEDIS measure, indicating that there is still substantial room for improvement in managed care.
- NCQA-accredited health plans significantly outperform unaccredited plans, and plans that publicly report their performance information significantly outperform plans that keep their data private.

Consumer Assessment of Health Plans

In 1998, NCQA and AHCPR joined forces to develop consumer satisfaction measurements that would be incorporated into the HEDIS Measurement Program (AHCPR, 1998b). AHCPR funded a 5-year project to develop tools to help purchasers identify the best healthcare plans and services. AHCPR took the results of that project and incorporated them into the HEDIS Measurement Set. The consumer satisfaction section in HEDIS retains the original project name—Consumer Assessment of Health Plans (CAHPS). The NCQA's publication, *The State of Managed Care Quality Report* (2000a), also provides a separate report on the results of consumer satisfaction ratings from 1998 and 1999. The report is summarized in Table 20-1. The results only include data from those MCOs that participated in NCQA accreditation and agreed to public reporting. Overall ratings are measured on a score of 1 to 10. Ratings of 8 through 10 are considered positive.

In April 2000, NCQA announced a refinement of its accreditation program to focus attention on patient safety. This new initiative appears to be in response to the Institute of Medicine report, *To Err is Human: Building a Safer Health System* (2000). Under NCQA's proposed standards for 2001, MCOs would be required to provide a comprehensive description of how they address patient safety issues, such as poorly coordinated care and adverse drug interactions.

Health Care Financing Administration

HCFA is the agency responsible for all federally funded healthcare programs, which means that the care rendered to Medicare and Medicaid beneficiaries under managed care contracts must be reviewed under established HCFA guidelines.

In 1992, HCFA and its peer review agencies embarked on a new quality of care initiative called the *Health Care Quality Improvement Program* (HCQIP) (HCFA, 2001b). This program was designed to analyze and improve national patterns of care. HCQIP now targets the following six areas:

1. Acute myocardial infarction
2. Breast cancer
3. Diabetes
4. Heart failure
5. Pneumonia
6. Stroke

TABLE 20-1
Consumer Assessment of Health Plans Member Survey Results: 1998-1999

Measure	1998	1999
Claims processing	76.9	77.9
Courteous office staff	91.1	91.2
Customer service	53.9	64.5
Getting care quickly	78.2	78.2
Getting needed care	73.22	74
How well doctors communicate	89.2	89.4
Overall rating of plan	57	56.7
Rating of all healthcare	70.3	70.2
Rating of personal physician	71.7	72.7
Rating of specialist	75.2	75

From the National Committee for Quality Assurance: *The state of managed care quality report,* 2000, Available online: http://www.ncqa.org/pages/communications/news/somcqrel.html.

The statewide professional review organizations (PROs) are contracted with HCFA. PROs disseminate indicator sets and educational material on a statewide level. Facilities then submit a performance improvement plan designed to improve compliance to these indicator sets. Periodically, PROs publish national and statewide results. Participating facilities also receive facility specific audit information for their own use in performance improvement initiatives. Medicare managed care programs are now part of this initiative. As part of the HCQIP initiative, each state PRO provides technical assistance and collaboration on quality improvement projects to every in-state Medicare + Choice Plan.

HCFA conducts oversight and evaluation audits of Medicare managed care HEDIS results and disseminates standardized HEDIS information to beneficiaries and purchasers.

QUALITY MANAGEMENT IN THE TWENTY-FIRST CENTURY

Fundamental improvements in our nation's healthcare delivery system are required if we are to deliver the care that consumers demand and deserve. To that end, the National Academy of Science was charged with the development of a 10-year plan that would provide direction and leadership in quality management. Its latest publication, *Crossing the Quality Chasm: A New Health Care System for the 21st Century* (National Academy of Science, 2001), outlines a strategy to improve care and prepare us for the inevitable expansion in the technology arena.

The first call from the Academy is to restructure the healthcare delivery system. The report indicates that "all health care constituencies, including policymakers, purchasers, regulators, health professionals, health care trustees and management, and consumers, commit to a national statement of purpose for the health care system as a whole" (National Academy of Science, 2001, p 5).

The Academy proposes the use of the key dimensions of performance to direct healthcare providers. It also promulgated rules to be followed in the redesign process. These rules support the patient's right to unfettered access to high quality care. Aspects of these rules are summarized as follows (National Academy of Science, 2001):

- Healthcare should be available 24 hours a day/7 days a week in response to patient needs. Other delivery modalities should be considered in addition to the office visit, such as the Internet and telephone.
- The system should reinforce the obligation to provide the patient with all of the necessary information to support informed decision making in both the *selection* and *provision* of healthcare.
- Care that is individualized and based upon the patient's values and preferences should be encouraged.
- Care delivery should be *safe* and *based on the best available scientific evidence.*
- The system should foster the integration of information across the continuum of care.

The Academy maintains that a major financial investment must be made to promote improved information systems that will support nationwide quality initiatives. To that end, it recommends that Congress establish a special fund to support quality initiatives that promote the aims of this report. The Academy also advocated that systems should be developed to promote evidence-based care practices, particularly in the realm of chronic disease. The dissemination of patient information through enhanced information systems is also a key priority (National Academy of Science, 2001).

The Academy goals outlined previously are comprehensive, far reaching, and a call to unify all aspects of healthcare delivery. With the publication of this report, and others still pending, consumers are more aware of the deficits of the nation's healthcare system. With this knowledge, they should be more inclined to support increased funding. This report's "call to action" may become the single most important quality improvement initiative to take place in modern day quality management. What is most significant is that all of us will play a role in the success of this major healthcare transformation.

REFERENCES

Agency for Health Care Policy and Research: *The challenge and potential for assuring quality in health care in the 21st century,* 1998a, Available online: http://www.ahcpr.gov/qual/21stcena.htm, accessed 2/3/01.

Agency for Health Care Policy and Research: *Consumer assessment of health plans, CAHPS: overview,* 1998b, Available online: http://www.ahcpr.gov/qual/cahps/dept1.htm.

Cesta TG, Tahan H, Fink L: *The case manager's survival guide,* St Louis, 1997, Mosby.

Health Care Financing Administration: *Quality of care in national projects Medicare HEDIS data,* 2001a, Available online: http//www.hcfa.gov/quality/3a1.htm.

Health Care Financing Administration, Quality of Care/Peer Review Organizations: *Medicare health care quality improvement program,* 2001b, Available online: http//www.hcfa.gov/quality/5b1.htm.

Institute of Medicine: *To err is human: building a safer health system,* 2000, National Academy Press, Available online: http://www.books.NAP.edu/books/039068371/html 132.html.

Joint Commission on Accreditation of Healthcare Organizations: *Framework for improving performance: from principles to practice,* Oakbrook Terrace, Ill, 1994, Joint Commission Publications.

Joint Commission on Accreditation of Healthcare Organizations: *Facts about core measures in ORYX,* 2001, Available online: http://www.jcaho.org/perfmeas/coremeas/cm-fmwrk.html.

Kirk R: *Managing outcomes, process, and cost in a managed care environment,* Gaithersburg, Md, 1997, Aspen.

Kongstvedt PR: *Essentials of managed health care,* ed 3, Gaithersburg, Md, 1996, Aspen.

National Academy of Science: *Crossing the quality chasm: a new health care system for the 21st century,* 2001, Available online: http://www.edu/books/0309072828/1.html.

National Committee for Quality Assurance: *The state of managed care quality report,* 2000a, Available online: http://www.ncqa.org/pages/communications/news/somcqrel.html.

National Committee for Quality Assurance: *An overview,* 2000b, Available online: http://www.ncqa.org/pages/about/overview3.htm.

National Committee for Quality Assurance: *Health plan report card,* 2000c, Available online: http://www.hprc.ncqa.org/methods.asp

21

Strategies for Accessing and Analyzing Meaningful Information

Lisa M. Zerull

KEY LESSONS IN THIS CHAPTER

- Case managers play an important role in coordinating care in a fiscally responsible manner.
- A simple way to begin data analysis is to use the performance improvement process.
- Data can be located in one of the following five broad categories: demographic, clinical, operational, outcomes, and comparative.
- Web-based technology is a foundational tool for outcomes management and tracking of best practices.
- Key outcome indicators should be identified based on annualized trends, as well as their impact on the patient population.

You now carry the title of Case Manager and have a job description to direct your activities and performance. You are expected to coordinate the clinical and financial aspects of care in a managed care environment. How is this carried out in your practice setting? Are you able to easily access data for analysis? Do you know what to do with the data once you receive it? Does technology support your efforts in analyzing data? What changes in patient care processes may result from data analysis? This chapter explores strategies for accessing and analyzing data using an acute care example.

In the last 15 years, the healthcare environment has undergone massive changes in structure, role, and process in response to dwindling financial resources. Two elements of care that have remained constant are the need to ensure quality-oriented and cost-effective care for patients. Add to this a continuing trend toward managed care, and you find healthcare organizations looking to case management to assist them in achieving desired clinical and financial outcomes. Case managers must not only be able to assess and collect data but also to manipulate data and report meaningful outcomes of care using the technological tools available in the twenty-first century.

Job descriptions for case managers may vary from setting to setting, but the overall expectation for the position remains the same. The case manager is responsible for the coordination of care while also keeping an eye on the bottom line. Although this may be the expectation, one must question how many case managers have *access* to both clinical and financial data. When asking for clinical and financial data, one should keep the following in mind. Does the case manager know what data to request? When the data is received, does the case manager know how to analyze the data? Finally, once the data has been translated into meaningful information, what changes can be made in care delivery to achieve more favorable outcomes of care? This chapter explores an organized approach to data analysis for a specific patient population within an acute care setting.

RATIONALE FOR ANALYSIS

The need for careful analysis of data related to care practices is critical to case managers who are responsible for the clinical and financial outcomes of care for patients. When beginning to look at a patient population, a primary question to ask is, "What is the goal—what do you hope to accomplish by analyzing data for this population?" Determine whether this goal is being driven by administrative or physician expectations and goals or whether there is opportunity to benchmark against best practice. Whatever the goal or expectation, take time to explore organizational expectations before designing the data analysis process.

Next, research the literature to find best practice patterns. Identify how expected outcomes are achieved. How does your patient population compare to the benchmark, or best practice? Ideally, you will want to look at the available patient data first, asking a variety of questions about care from a clinical and financial standpoint (data analysis), and then determine how best to impact patient care outcomes.

In Figure 21-1, a high-level flow diagram for analysis is presented to offer the case manager an overview of the data analysis process for a patient population. This diagram is applicable to any practice setting and population, particularly in a managed care environment. A discussion for each level is presented throughout this chapter.

GETTING STARTED

Most case managers do not feel confident with data analysis because this has not traditionally been a job requirement and may not have been part of their formal education. The idea of data analysis and research is unfamiliar, time consuming, and somewhat overwhelming. A suggested starting place for beginning to analyze data is to simply apply a performance improvement (PI) process, which can be used by any case manager, regardless of educational preparation.

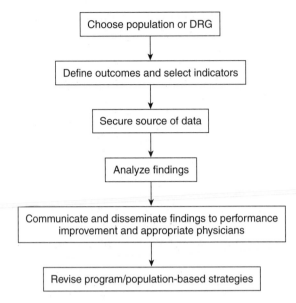

Figure 21-1 High-level flow diagram for analysis. (From the Department of Case Management, Valley Health System, Winchester, Virginia.)

1. Assess:
   - Determine the targeted service and/or patient population to analyze (e.g., diagnosis-related group [DRG]).
   - What data are available from the organization?
   - What data about this population are documented and entered into an automated system?
   - What data are essential to making care decisions and making changes in process of care delivery?
   - Who is responsible for entering data into available software systems?
   - What do you hope to accomplish by analyzing processes and outcomes of care for this population?
   - Who are the key players for this PI effort?
2. Plan:
   - What data sets will be requested?
   - Will both clinical and financial information be required?
   - Does the data reside in paper records or in automated applications?
   - Who manages specific sources of data (e.g., clinical staff, software programs)?
   - How will you obtain the necessary data/information?
   - Who will analyze the data?
   - What is the frequency for data analysis—monthly, quarterly, or annually?

- Will the case managers receive reports on paper or within a computer application?
- What education will be needed for individuals or a group of case managers to analyze data?
- What is the timeline for this effort?
- Will the task of data analysis impact case manager workload?
- Who will receive the outcomes reports with suggested changes in care patterns?

3. Implement:
   - The case managers receive data for analysis reporting outcomes of care or suggested changes to care delivery.

4. Evaluate:
   - Are the goals of care for a given patient population being achieved?
   - What are the opportunities for improvement?
   - What changes in the care process could move patients toward expected outcomes?

Another methodology for data analysis similar to the PI process is to ask some research questions, such as: What is happening here? What will happen if . . . ? How can I make something happen? (Diers, 1979; Polit and Hungler, 1995). These rather basic questions may simplify the data analysis process for the case manager who is apprehensive about analyzing data for a given patient population.

Both the PI process and suggested research questions provide a useful framework for data analysis. As data analysis strategies are designed, case manager educational preparation should be considered to ensure that all case managers understand and can apply the same process to their given patient populations. As part of a case manager orientation or annual competency, this author recommends offering education sessions targeting the data analysis process from a PI standpoint. Thus all the case managers have the same baseline of understanding for which to plan and carry out population specific data analysis.

DATA ELEMENTS/INDICATORS FOR ANALYSIS

The data found in healthcare information systems can be categorized based on use (Cole and Houston, 1999). The five basic data categories are presented as follows, with several examples for each category:

1. Demographic or descriptive data to define the population being analyzed (e.g., patient identification, diagnosis, gender, age, payer)
2. Clinical or physiological responses to treatment data (e.g., vital signs, weight, diagnostic results)
3. Operational/administrative data for strategic planning (e.g., salaries, expenses, scheduling)
4. Outcomes (e.g., decreased utilization of resources, decreased readmission rates, increased functional status)
5. Benchmarking or comparative data (e.g., case mix index, infection and mortality rates)

The selection of indicators should help the case manager and the overall organization meet the following (Spath, Smith, and Pelling, 1995):

- Organization's mission, vision, and values
- Requirements and data demands from payers
- Regulatory and accreditation requirements
- Organization's leaders' priorities for continuously improving quality

All healthcare organizations have defined specific indicators for measurement, both quantitative and qualitative, to meet their internal and external individual needs. The vision, mission, and strategic plans of the organization drive the internal selection of indicators to measure in order to meet population-specific or organizational goals. One example would be the number of open-heart surgeries for persons living outside the health system's service area to better determine marketing strategies and predict further growth to a surgical cardiac program. Regulatory agencies, such as the Joint Commission on Accreditation of Healthcare Organizations (JCAHO) and payers, such as Medicare, drive the external indicators to be tracked and measured requirements. An example is the data required by the Health Care Financing Administration (HCFA) to receive Medicare reimbursement for care (e.g., case mix index, mortality and morbidity). When possible reimbursement is in jeopardy, there is additional incentive for tracking and reporting specific outcomes of care.

In many settings, the director of case management may propose the indicators for measurement; however, the case manager for a given patient population should provide his or her expertise and input into the selection process for best results. Case managers are the most knowledgeable about their population and are key players in changing care processes that ultimately affect outcomes. Greater input on the front end of a data analysis project encourages ongoing committed participation and support.

The literature recommends that each data set or selected indicator should not be viewed in isolation, since one affects another (Spath, Smith, and Pelling, 1995; Cole and Houston, 1999; Woodcock, 2000). If data analysis is restricted to the use of descriptive data only, there is no link between interventions and outcomes (Cole and Houston, 1999). For example, if open heart surgery patients are sent home 3 days after surgery without any additional follow-up support, the costs for care may be minimal, leading one to believe that this care process is cost-effective. A retrospective comparative analysis of cost, support services after discharge (e.g., home health), and readmission rates, however, may identify that those patients who were discharged home with home health had the lowest readmission rates and the best outcomes overall.

Another common error with data analysis is for healthcare organizations to report outputs of care as outcomes of care. Outputs are the direct products of care (e.g., number of referrals, length of stay [LOS]), whereas outcomes are the end result (which may or may not be expected) of comparing multiple data sets. In some cases, outputs could also be outcomes of care. An example would be increased readmission rate for the same diagnosis within 10 days of discharge from the hospital. When compared to decreased LOS, the case manager might assume that the higher readmission rate was an outcome of decreased LOS or lack of follow-up care after discharge. The case manager would need to further analyze the discharge plans from the previous admissions to determine whether referrals to another level of care should have been made, thus possibly preventing the readmission.

A case manager can measure numerous indicators, and it is overwhelming and unrealistic to track and measure every aspect of care, as is often the case with novice case managers. Often the director of case management suggests the baseline indicators for measurement and then encourages input from a population specific team with representation from the case manager, physician, and other appropriate healthcare providers (e.g., social worker, physical therapist, dietitian, information support staff). When choosing indicators for measurement, it is imperative for the team to remain focused on the processes and outcomes of care that have the most impact on a given service or patient population.

ACCESSING INFORMATION

Once the determination has been made as to what data will be analyzed, the task of accessing and obtaining information begins.

Source of the Data

In any organization, there are multiple software applications kept in a variety of locations. Get to know key people in the Information Support (IS) department. Determine if there exists a listing of software programs in use within the organization, including a brief description of what data is entered into each program. Review the possible data sets, giving special attention to accessibility, relevancy, clarity, consistency, and validity (Lagoe, Kurtzig, and Hohner, 1999).

Box 21-1 provides possible questions to ask when reviewing data and determining indicators for measurement, targeting the areas of accessibility, relevancy, clarity, consistency, and validity of data.

Strategies for Accessing Data

Do your homework. First, during the assessment phase for data analysis, determine what data or information you are seeking. Ask for what purpose are you seeking this information, and how will the information be used? To whom will the information be reported?

Second, take a look at the culture in your organization. There is great benefit to organizing a formal group or committee for the purpose of multidisciplinary input, brainstorming, and delegating tasks. Consider including representatives from case management, utilization management, finance, information support, medical records, PI, and any other key players in the organization. If physician practice patterns are being reviewed, include at least one physician (or at least obtain physician input) on the planning team. Group participation facilitates implementation and buy-in of any new process, especially when changes in care provision may result. It is also imperative to enlist administrative support when seeking permission to access sensitive information, such as cost data and individual physician practice reports.

BOX 21-1
Source of Data Questions

Accessibility
- Do I have access to this data? If no, how might I obtain permission for access (e.g., provide written rationale, enlist administrative support)?
- What special considerations are there in obtaining this data (e.g., sensitivity, confidentiality)?
- Is the data available in hard copy, and/or can the data be exported into a computer file?
- In what language or platform does the data reside?

Relevancy
- What information would assist in making care decisions that impact quality and cost?
- What information is useful for or required by case managers, physicians, administrators, payers, and regulating organizations?

Clarity
- Is it possible to extract key data elements specific to the patient population?
- In what format can the data be organized?
- Do I have access to this data? If no, how might I obtain permission for access (e.g., formal request signed by an administrator)?

Consistency
- Who enters data into the software program?
- How often is data entered (frequency)?
- Are the data concurrent or retrospective?

Validity
- Is the information from a trusted source?
- How has the software program been reviewed for both reliability and validity?

Data Decisions

Determine if all patients for a given diagnosis or service are desired. Will you be looking at a population of patients, including all members of a defined group, or will you be looking at a sample of patients who are a subset of a given population? Research literature suggests a *minimum* sample size of 30 patients to prevent biased results; however, there may not have been that many patients in a specific population for the time frame under study, such as in a given month. With smaller sample sizes, be aware that one outlier patient could potentially skew the data, preventing the case manager from making any true assumptions about the given sample or population. For larger patient groups, a percent of the total may be appropriate. Consideration should be given to reporting not only totals and averages but also the mode (the most frequently reported value) and median (the middle value in a data set) to help control for outliers. For example, one outlier patient may have had a 20-day LOS due to physical complications, whereas all other patients in the sample had between 4- and 6-day LOS.

BOX 21-2
Data Sources

- Clinical documentation forms
- Medical records
- Automated documentation systems
- Finance/accounting department
- Support department reports (e.g., infection control, quality/risk management)
- Chart audit summaries
- Patient or staff surveys or questionnaires
- Targeted focus groups
- Telephone interviews
- Online patient feedback (patient uses the Internet to report key physiological assessment and functional status)
- Productivity reports of case managers (number of patient encounters, including individual, telephone, or group)

Data Organization

Data are entered into multiple software systems within an organization. Often the case managers are not aware of the data available to them. Do the case managers know what clinical or financial information they should request? Also, especially when cost information is included, do the case managers have access to the data? Too often administrators are hesitant to give case managers key data elements due to the sensitivity of the information. On the other hand, case managers may be given stacks of reports that can take many hours to collate and summarize. It is critical for the case manager and the director of case management to organize available data in order to have meaningful information for which to suggest changes in care delivery.

Data Collection Methodologies

Once you know what data is available, explore the possibility of capturing data sets from multiple software programs into one report so that data may be pulled together in a meaningful format. Box 21-2 provides a comprehensive list of possible data sources available in most organizations. The normal practice in most organizations is to receive multiple printed data reports from a variety of data sources with multiple pages and formats, including extraneous information on a monthly or quarterly basis. Often the reports were designed to meet past organizational demands, and the current recipients have not questioned the content, format, or frequency of reports. In addition, consideration needs to be given to new technologies and tools that would greatly improve the availability, efficiency, and organization of data.

THE WHO OF DATA ANALYSIS?

Data analysis and outcome studies used to be the responsibility of academicians and health services researchers outside of healthcare organizations. With the increasing emphasis on

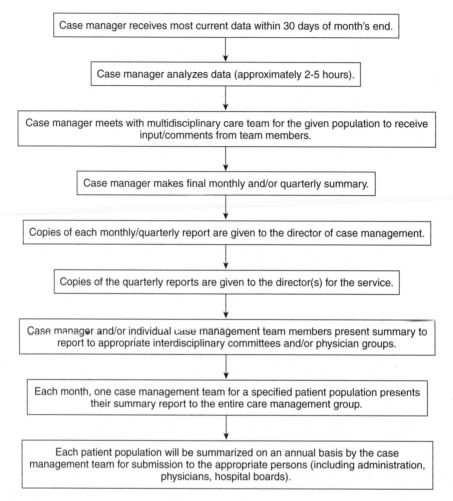

Figure 21-2   Outcomes analysis process. (From the Department of Case Management, Valley Health System, Winchester, Virginia.)

case management and the use of tools such as critical pathways, it makes more sense to have the case managers analyze data because they oversee both clinical and financial aspects of care and are extremely knowledgeable about the care delivery for their given population. It may be argued that the director of case management has the overall responsibility of and the time to carry out data analysis and PI. Although this may be true in some organizations, this author has found that given sufficient leadership and support from the organization and the director, case managers who are actively involved in data analysis for their given patient population can effect immediate and dramatic change in the care setting, thus impacting outcomes of both quality and cost. Caseload and workload responsibilities may need to be altered when the case manager is expected to take an active role in the data analysis process.

Figure 21-2 presents a flow diagram that gives an organized, step-by-step overview of the data analysis process. Although the process was created for an acute care environment, it can easily be edited to fit any case management setting.

OUTCOMES ANALYSIS FOR SPECIFIED PATIENT POPULATION(S)

Let us assume that the case manager now has access to and has received key clinical and financial information for a specific patient population. Is the information presented in a format that allows the case manager to analyze the data easily? The answer to this question is generally no. The ideal scenario would be for the case manager to use the latest technology to receive or import the data into a software spreadsheet for analysis. Consider the following two data options.

Tools for Data Analysis

Two tools for data analysis are presented. One uses the traditional hard copy printed report, whereas the other uses current automated technology.

Dashboards

A good starting point for case managers to receive data about their patient population is through a brief summary of patient information. Figure 21-3 shows an example of a "dashboard" for a diagnosis of Coronary Artery Bypass Grafting (CABG) Without Cardiac Catheterization (DRG 109). This dashboard summary is generated monthly, allowing the case manager(s) serving this population to compare at a glance, and in some detail, the types of patients served and the limited outcomes of care from a clinical and financial standpoint. A wealth of information can be perused by the case manager in this one-page summary.

Using this example of a one-page DRG dashboard, the case manager has a quick reference noting the following:

- Eighteen patients fell into the DRG 109 category—mostly men eligible for Medicare, and on average, the hospital lost $1095 per patient. The case manager does not know from this month's dashboard how this financial loss compares to previous time frames.
- The number of critical care days had decreased by 63%, yet the readmission rate had increased by 66%—a possible concern here was that those patients were sent home "quicker and sicker." When comparing this information with the disposition, the case manager noted that only one patient was discharged home with home health. A chart audit may be necessary to determine if any of the readmission patients might have been eligible for home care services, thus averting another hospitalization.
- A quick review of the physician profiles shows one physician's statistic (physician 278) with a profit of $5183 for one patient. From this data alone, the case manager cannot assume that this physician had the best care practices, since there is no consideration of patient severity for comparison.

St. Anywhere Hospital
CASE MANAGEMENT DASHBOARD
DRG 109: CABG Without Cardiac Catheterization
JANUARY 2001

AT A GLANCE

Number of Patients	18	
Number & % Medicare =	13	72%
Number & % Male =	12	67%

	LOS	Charge	Payment	Cost*	Profit
Average	7.4	27,376	17,047	18,142	(1,095)
Minimum	4.0	18,984	9,445	12,806	(3,361)
Maximum	14.0	47,976	43,562	27,792	15,770
Median	6.0	24,169	13,980	16,544	(1,933)

MISC INFORMATION

	Curr	Prior
Expected ALOS	7.4	7.5
Expected Mortality		2.2
Readmissions within 30 Days	3	2
Avg Days from Previous Disch	17	16
Complications (ICD9s 996-999)	4	1
CRITICAL CARE DAYS		
IC Days	17	26
CC Days	2	2
PC Days	0	2

MORE DETAIL

		AVERAGE PER PATIENT					
PHYSICIAN	# Pats	ALOS	Charge	Payment	Cost*	Profit	Age
310	6	8.2	29,812	18,192	19,395	(1,202)	67.8
272	4	7.0	22,080	15,257	15,174	83	69.5
273	4	8.5	31,842	18,932	21,034	(2,101)	74.5
305	3	6.0	25,635	13,865	17,066	(3,201)	75.3
278	1	5.0	21,304	19,344	14,161	5,183	41.0
	18	7.4	27,376	17,047	18,142	(1,095)	–

		AVERAGE PER PATIENT					
FINANCIAL CLASS	# Pats	ALOS	Charge	Payment	Cost*	Profit	Age
MEDICARE	13	7.3	26,328	14,015	17,692	(3,677)	72.8
BLUE CROSS	2	9.0	34,640	31,453	20,977	10,477	50.0
COMMERCIAL	2	7.5	28,805	26,155	19,202	6,953	71.0
SELF-PAY	1	6.0	23,614	9,445	16,209	(6,763)	61.0
	18	7.4	27,376	17,047	18,142	(1,095)	–

		AVERAGE PER PATIENT					
LENGTH OF STAY	# Pats	ALOS	Charge	Payment	Cost*	Profit	Age
4	2	4.0	22,457	16,192	15,440	751	66.5
5	6	5.0	21,435	14,683	14,438	245	66.8
6	3	6.0	24,301	12,392	16,392	(4,000)	69.0
8	1	8.0	30,964	14,094	20,407	(6,313)	79.0
9	1	9.0	25,620	14,208	17,254	(3,046)	85.0
10	1	10.0	40,515	14,322	25,600	(11,278)	72.0
11	1	11.0	36,963	33,563	24,402	9,161	75.0
13	2	13.0	41,880	29,114	26,028	3,086	66.0
14	1	14.0	28,520	14,779	20,158	(5,378)	66.0
	18	7.4	27,376	17,047	18,142	(1,095)	–

DISCHARGE STATUS

	# Pats	ALOS
Discharged Home	14	7.1
D/C to short-term general hospital	1	13.0
Discharged to skilled nursing	1	5.0
D/C to another type of institution	1	8.0
Discharged to home w/ home health	1	9.0

VISIT SOURCE

	# Pats	ALOS
Physician Referral	15	7.3
Transfer from hospital	3	8.3

DISTRIBUTION BY DIAGNOSIS

PRIMARY ICD9s	TYPE	ICD9	# Pats
CRNRY ATHRSCL NATVE VSSL	M	414.01	17
AMI INFEROLATERAL, INIT	M	410.21	1
AORTCOR BYPAS-4+ COR ART	S	36.14	11
AORTOCOR BYPAS-3 COR ART	S	36.13	5
AORTOCOR BYPAS-2 COR ART	S	36.12	1
1 INT MAM-COR ART BYPASS	S	36.15	1

SECONDARY ICD9S	TYPE	ICD9	# Pats
HYPERTENSION NOS	M	401.9	13
INTERMED CORONARY SYND	M	411.1	9
PURE HYPERCHOLESTEROLEM	M	272.0	8
ATRIAL FIBRILLATION	M	427.31	7
AC POSTHEMORRHAG ANEMIA	M	285.1	6
ANGINA PECTORIS NEC/NOS	M	413.9	5
HISTORY OF TOBACCO USE	M	V15.82	5
ATHSCL EXTRM NTV ART NOS	M	440.20	4
DMI WO CMP NT ST UNCNTRL	M	250.01	3
HYPERLIPIDEMIA NEC/NOS	M	272.4	3
EXTRACORPOREAL CIRCULAT	S	39.61	18
HYPOTHERMIA W/OPEN HEART	S	39.62	18
CARDIOPLEGIA	S	39.63	18
INTRAOP CARDIAC PACEMAK	S	39.64	18
1 INT MAM-COR ART BYPASS	S	36.15	17
CONT MECH VENT < 96 HRS	S	96.71	14
INCISION OF LUNG	S	33.1	1
REOPEN THORACOTOMY SITE	S	34.03	1
INSERT INTERCOSTAL CATH	S	34.04	1
INCISION OF MEDIASTINUM	S	34.1	1

COMPLICATIONS	TYPE	ICD9	# Pats
AC POSTHEMORRHAG ANEMIA	M	285.1	6
HRT DIS POSTCARDIAC SURG	M	429.4	2
POST TRAUM PULM INSUFFIC	M	518.5	1
COMP-OTH CARDIAC DEVICE	M	996.72	1
IATROGEN CV INFARC/HMRHG	M	997.02	1
SURG COMPLIC-RESPIR SYST	M	997.3	1
SURG COMP-DIGESTV SYSTEM	M	997.4	1
HEMORRHAGE COMPLIC PROC	M	998.11	1

CARE MANAGEMENT - DRG 109
# of Patients by LOS

*Cost is calculated retrospectively and is subject to change

NOT ACTUAL DATA

Figure 21-3 Case management dashboard for DRG 109, Coronary Artery Bypass Grafting Without Cardiac Catheterization. (From Case Management Performance Improvement Team, Valley Health System, Winchester, Virginia.)

- Expected LOS was on target at 7.4, with a median of 6.0 days, recognizing that 11 out of 18 patients had a LOS of <7.4 days.
- Physicians referred the majority of patients to cardiac service care, which does not seem to be a significant finding for a regional, tertiary care referral hospital.
- As expected from a clinical knowledge standpoint for this DRG, 17 patients had a primary ICD-9 code related to coronary atherosclerosis, thus resulting in a CABG procedure.
- The experienced case manager for this population has knowledge of the risk factors of heart disease as reflected in the secondary ICD-9 codes (e.g., hypertension, tobacco use, high cholesterol levels).
- The complication of posthemorrhagic anemia may warrant a closer review to determine if this complication could possibly be avoided by suggesting alternate treatment regimens.

In analyzing this month's data from the dashboard, caution needs to be taken when making assumptions from the data in isolation of other data impacting the outcomes of care (e.g., previous month, continued patterns of utilization). Several examples of this data were noted in this sample dashboard summary related to profit and readmit rate. The case manager would need to compare previous data with current data before drawing any conclusions. The comprehensive list of possible data analysis questions is presented in Box 21-3. These sample questions remind the case manager to look beyond the one-page summary to previous time frames for comparative data analysis.

Spreadsheet Technology

An alternative to a one-dimensional analysis of a patient population requires the use of a basic computer software application known as a *spreadsheet*. One example is the Microsoft Excel application, which has a PivotTable feature that summarizes selected data in a spreadsheet and then lists and displays the data in a table format (O'Keefe, 1998). Using the PivotTable function allows for an interactive comparison of multiple data elements for an individual patient or a population of patients. It allows the case manager to ask any of the questions presented in Box 21-3 and then easily manipulate the data with a limited number of keystrokes to answer the data analysis question. Some examples include the following (Mahn, 1999):

- Profile utilization, costs, and charges by physician or service
- Sort data by payer or financial class
- Obtain costs and/or charges by LOS
- Group by patient variables, including age, gender, and zip code

To use the PivotTable function, the case manager would request a "string delimited file" with one record per encounter, in which all data elements for each patient encounter are presented in a single row (Mahn, 1999). Case managers can drill down into data any way they want to look for patterns of utilization and cost. The primary advantage of using a PivotTable is that it reduces turnaround time waiting for reports from support departments while allowing the case manager to manipulate the data as desired (Mahn, 1999).

BOX 21-3
Suggested Questions for Analysis by Data Element

Point of Access
- From what point of access (e.g., emergency department [ED], urgent care, direct admit, transfer) did the majority of your patient population enter the health system?
- Was there a pattern/trend showing an increase in admissions through the ED? Through transfer? Through another source?
- Who are the physicians with the highest volume of admissions for the population? (Obtain list with all admitting physicians and percent of admission listed from high volume to low volume.)
- Is there a trend in referral base from another geographic location?

Patient Profile (List information by medical record number for identification.)
- What are the demographics for the "typical" patient in your patient population?
  - Age
  - Gender
  - Financial code/payer
  - Marital status
- What are the comorbidities in conjunction with the admitting diagnosis identified by ICD-9 codes? (e.g., what other underlying conditions exist as 2° or 3° diagnoses, diabetes, chronic obstructive pulmonary disease [COPD])
- What is the pattern for admission severity (i.e., how sick/acute were patients on admission)?
- Is this a readmission for the same or related diagnosis?
- Is there a clinical pathway for this patient population?

Readmission Rates
- How do the readmission rates compare to the last report for your patient population? Overall?
- Is this a readmission for the same or related diagnosis? (If readmission occurs <31 days from previous discharge)
- If readmission rate increased, did the LOS decrease?
- What were the reasons for readmission? Any patterns or trends?
- Were there critical care days involved with this readmission?
- What is the difference between hospital discharge date and readmission date? (On what posthospital day did the readmission occur?)
- Disposition with previous discharge (e.g., home, home health, skilled facility)?
- Was a follow-up telephone call or home visit made to the patient before readmission?

Critical Care Days
- Was there an increase or decrease in number of critical care days?
- Did one or more outlier patients accumulate the critical care days? (An outlier is any patient that exceeds average length of stay [ALOS] for a diagnosis by >5 days.)
- Were there critical care days involved in a readmission(s)?

Complications
- What are the predominant complications? Any patterns/trends?
- What is the actual versus expected mortality rate? Any significant increases or decreases?
- Is there a trend/pattern in nonresponder rate (e.g., did the patient deteriorate during his or her hospitalization)?
- Is there a trend/pattern in the number of ED visits within 30 days after discharge?

BOX 21-3

Suggested Questions for Analysis by Data Element—cont'd

Length of Stay
- How does the actual LOS compare to the expected LOS?
- What is the median LOS? (Report both mean and median to ensure that outliers do not skew the data.)
- How does the median relate to the actual LOS?
- How does the median compare to previous LOS for the patient population?
- Were there any outliers positively or negatively impacting LOS?
- Was there an increase or decrease in LOS?
- To what do you attribute the increase/decrease in LOS?

Disposition
- To what level of care (e.g., home, home health, hospice, skilled care) did the majority of your patient population transition to after hospitalization (i.e., disposition codes)?
- Was there a pattern/trend showing an increase or decrease in disposition to a specific level of care?
- What is the actual versus expected mortality rate? Any significant increases or decreases?
- Was a follow-up telephone call or visit made to the patient after hospitalization?

Financial
- What is the breakdown of payer type (i.e., volume and percentage)? Trends/patterns?
- What is the average cost? Trends/patterns?
- From which department(s) are the majority of your costs generated (e.g., radiology, laboratory, perioperative)?
- What is the average charge? Trends/patterns?
- What is the average reimbursement? Trends/patterns?
- What is the average variance from charge to reimbursement? Trends/patterns?
- What is the denial rate(s) by payer? Trends/patterns?

Practice Patterns
- What are benchmarks for this patient population?
- Who are the physicians with the highest volume of admissions for the population?
- How does each physician compare to the benchmark?
- How do physicians compare to their peers?
- Are there other services/individuals admitting to this diagnosis?
- Are there major practice differences (e.g., LOS, utilization)?
- Has there been a significant change in clinical practice for this patient population?

Operational Considerations Impacting Outcomes
- Were there significant staffing issues during this time frame (e.g., vacations, leave of absences) that might have impacted care provision/coordination?
- Were there environmental issues/challenges impacting care?
- Were any members of the care management team involved in tasks/projects other than those expected by role?

Performance Improvement
- What are the opportunities for improvement (either clinical or financial)?
- What are some suggested strategies the case manager and/or case management team can employ to improve outcomes?
- What improvements/outcomes have been achieved from the previous time frame/report?
- Are there additional or different indicators to be measured?

Tools for Care Management
- Is there a clinical pathway for this patient population? If no, would the development of a clinical pathway be beneficial for this population?
- Are there national practice guidelines for this patient population (e.g., hypertension or staging of congestive heart failure from sources such as the American Heart Association)?
- Were there significant variances identified for this time frame? If so, what are the variances? Any trends/patterns? How do they compare to previous time frames?

Both the one-page dashboard and PivotTable technology are useful tools that enable the case manager to analyze key data elements for a given patient population. Although the dashboard presents a quick summary reference for a patient population, the PivotTable provides the case manager with a more comprehensive tool to manipulate multiple data elements in an efficient manner.

OTHER CONSIDERATIONS FOR SUCCESS WITH DATA ANALYSIS

Successful care provision in a managed care environment depends on many factors. This chapter has addressed identifying data elements, obtaining access to data, and the data analysis process itself. Other considerations include the following:

- *Organizational structure:* Consider case management assignments and reporting relationships, as well as review caseload and workload expectations. Do the case managers report to a central case management department, or is there a benefit to having the case manager report to a service line or population specific director? This author's experience has found benefit to keeping a core case management department that provides direction and administrative oversight to the case manager role and data analysis process. Should the case manager be responsible for manipulating data for the purpose of population specific analysis, some adjustments may need to be made to ensure realistic workload and caseload expectations.

- *Education:* The associate-degree nurse and perhaps even the baccalaureate-degree nurse may not possess the knowledge base to perform data analysis. An education plan will need to be developed to ensure that all case managers have an equal understanding of their role and responsibility with the data analysis process.

- *Annual review of indicators:* At least once a year, the case manager (in conjunction with the director of case management) should review the clinical and financial indicators being measured for appropriateness and applicability. Again, review the literature for best care practices. How does your population compare to the benchmark? Where are your opportunities for improvement? Is this population still high volume, high risk, or high cost? Or should you consider another diagnosis or patient population to track and trend patterns of care?

- *Regulation of requirements and standards:* Careful consideration of regulations and care standards is necessary to ensure compliance and quality care. Include a review of these requirements in the education plan for case managers. Also, from a technology use standpoint, pay attention to the Health Insurance Portability and Accountability Act (HIPAA) mandated by Congress in 1996 to protect the security and privacy of medical information (HCFA, 1997). HIPAA greatly affects how patient information is generated, reported, and communicated.

- *Technology:* Consider whether the case managers have familiarity with available data and software systems, or will additional education be required so that everyone has equal understanding of the use of technology? Review computer hardware accessibility, availability, and portability. Will each case manager use a personal computer placed at a workstation, or is there benefit to using a laptop computer for greater portability? Consider computer software and connectivity. Ideally the computer should link to the mainframe system or network for access to the following:

- Patient care information (e.g., history and physical, laboratory and diagnostic test results, previous utilization information)
- Intranet and Internet, for ease of communication within and outside of the organization or care setting
- Word processing capability for the purpose of communication, reporting, and summarizing information. This capability requires the ability to access database and spreadsheet applications that allow the user to import or export information and manipulate data (e.g., PivotTable function).

The ideal technology for case managers would offer software (or the right to access software via the Internet) that automatically manipulates the data for a given population with predefined queries.

THE FUTURE

Internet or Web-based technology is being presented as the next generation in software development and will greatly change the way case managers access, analyze, and report information. Web-based software is a much less expensive option that allows the user to lease applications from the vendor on a monthly basis, instead of having to pay a large sum of money upfront to purchase server-based software. Other identified benefits of using the Internet include the following (Chidley, 2000):

1. Provides a mechanism for inexpensive communication, requiring only a computer and a browser
2. Crosses institutional borders, allowing interaction between multiple organizational and private computer applications
3. Removes the need for support from an internal IS department, since the software resides on the vendor's server
4. Requires minimal education for use by case managers, since most individuals have used the Web for other personal and professional purposes

When Web-based technology serves as the foundational tool for outcome management, best practices will be achieved in a timely manner, meeting the demands of patients, healthcare professionals, payers, and policy makers (Cole and Houston, 1999). Articles in the literature are beginning to add an extra letter to the title of case manager, such as *E-case manager*, with the expectation that case managers "act as health information navigators for their patients, especially those with complex or chronic illness" (Kibbe, 2000, p 32). The Internet provides another inexpensive and quick mechanism for accessing, analyzing, and communicating key patient care information.

SUMMARY

In this age of technology, it is surprising to find such a large percentage of healthcare organizations that continue to focus their PI efforts on LOS and charge information alone. Although it is important for these indicators to be tracked over time, there are multitudes of other indicators that greatly impact the outcomes of care for patients. Information technology will continue to evolve and be a key tool for case managers in the data analysis process. The ultimate scenario would be that as soon as data is entered into a system, either manually or through other technology (e.g., voice activation), an automatic feed would occur, allowing the case manager to access information in real time and online via the Internet. Software companies are taking Web-based technology one step further by actively designing wireless connectivity that allows information to be transmitted through radio waves versus being wired through traditional telephone lines (Kelly, 2000). Technology will continue to improve and evolve, just as we are continuing to improve and evolve in the field of case management.

It is phenomenal to be able to add data and in minutes have access to status reports and a digital dashboard personalized to meet personal requirements in the practice setting. Picture a scenario where no more reams of paper reports sit on a desk or in a file cabinet collecting dust. The case manager can easily manipulate data within a few minutes' time and has the ability to send reports via the Internet to physicians, other key healthcare professionals, and administrative staff. There is no need to depend on the IS department to process information requests, thus no waiting time to receive or report key information for decision making.

The case manager of the future will be an individual equipped with the knowledge of research and technology applications, the ability to navigate the Internet quickly, and the permission to have access to all applicable clinical and financial information for his or her assigned patient populations. Changes to care practices can be made quickly, resulting in exceptional clinical and financial outcomes of care.

REFERENCES

Chidley E: Case management goes on the Web, *For the Record* 12(23):26-27, 2000.

Cole L, Houston S: Integrating information technology with an outcomes management program. In Turner SO, editor: *Essential readings in nursing managed care,* Gaithersburg, Md, 1999, Aspen.

Diers D: *Research in nursing practice,* Philadelphia, 1979, Lippincott.

Health Care Financing Administration: Provisions of the Health Insurance Portability and Accountability Act of 1996 (HIPAA): commonly asked questions and answers, April 1997, Available online: http://www.hcfa.gov/regs/q&a-con.htm.

Kelly J: Going wireless, *Hosp Health Netw* 74(11):65-68, 2000.

Kibbe DC: How to search for and find useful healthcare information online, *Case Manager* 11(6):32-34, 2000.

Lagoe RJ, Kurtzig BS, Hohner VK: Healthcare data and their sources, *J Nurs Care Qual* Special Issue Nov:7-24, 1999.

Mahn VA: Administrators are from Mars . . . case managers are from Venus, Preconference workshop for the fourth annual Hospital Case Management conference, Atlanta, 1999.

O'Keefe TL: Microsoft Excel 97: illustrated advanced, Course technology, Cambridge, Mass, 1998.

Polit DF, Hungler BP: *Nursing research: principles and methods,* Philadelphia, 1995, Lippincott.

Spath PL, Smith ME, Pelling MH: *Outcomes management: using data for decision making,* Forest Grove, Ore, 1995, Brown-Spath & Associates.

Woodcock EW: Using the data you already have, *J Ambulatory Care Manage* 23(4):31-39, 2000.

22

Utilization Management

Susan M. Erickson

KEY LESSONS IN THIS CHAPTER

■ Utilization review refers to the techniques used to review appropriateness of healthcare utilization, whereas utilization management refers to programs used to improve the appropriateness of that utilization.

■ Traditional hospital reviews may be prospective, concurrent, or retrospective.

■ Some case management programs integrate utilization as a fundamental component of the role of the case manager, whereas others maintain utilization as a separate and discrete function.

■ Administrators should be aware that utilization review programs have a direct impact on the organization's bottom line.

■ Utilization review/management has been an effective strategy in the struggle to contain healthcare costs and ensure appropriate use of healthcare resources.

BASIC TERMINOLOGY

Utilization management (UM) and *utilization review* are terms that are used somewhat interchangeably to describe a range of activities and programs used by managed care organizations and acute care facilities to ensure appropriate use of healthcare services. Utilization review is sometimes defined as the *techniques* used to review the appropriateness of healthcare utilization, and UM is sometimes defined as the programs used to *improve* the appropriateness of that care utilization (Blackstien-Hirsch et al, 2001). Typical utilization review/management programs and activities include preadmission hospital review, continued stay review, outpatient procedure review, use of practice guidelines or clinical pathways, and case management.

The practice of utilization review first appeared in hospital settings in the mid-1980s in response to the implementation of diagnosis-related groups (DRGs) by Medicare. The advent of DRG-based payment compelled hospitals to begin internal review of the appropriateness of length of stay and level of care. Hospital-based utilization review efforts expanded in scope and amount as managed care became more prevalent in the 1990s. With utilization of hospital services accounting for 40% of total health plan expenses (Kongstvedt, 1998), managed care organizations increasingly required hospitals to follow specific review procedures. Today hospital utilization review programs are evolving toward a broader UM approach through close coordination with hospital-based case management and quality improvement efforts.

The term *utilization review* has also been used to describe the broad range of activities employed by healthcare plans to prevent inappropriate use of services by plan members. The American Accreditation Healthcare Commission/Utilization Review Accreditation Commission (URAC), which accredits utilization review organizations, defines utilization review as "(a) process performed by or on behalf of a third-party payer, that evaluates the medical necessity, appropriateness and efficiency of the use of health care services, procedures and facilities" (URAC, 2001). Escalating healthcare costs and wide variation in physician practice nationwide precipitated the development of UM within healthcare plans. Today over 90% of managed care organizations employ one or more of the UM activities listed earlier, and nearly 138 million Americans are in health plans subject to some level of utilization review (Wickizer, 1999).

From the mid-1980s to the start of the new millennium, utilization review/management has provided an effective means of controlling healthcare costs, and the work involved in these practices has evolved into a complex specialty.

HOSPITAL-BASED UTILIZATION REVIEW/MANAGEMENT

Traditional utilization review falls into one of the following three general categories: (1) prospective review (before the event or hospital admission), (2) concurrent review (during the event or hospitalization), and (3) retrospective review (after the event or hospitalization). In each instance, the hospital or healthcare facility determines the necessity and appropriateness of the medical service per internal standards and obtains approval (and ultimately payment) for the services from the payer source. Ideally this review is done using specific review criteria. Such criteria can be developed internally or obtained from published or commercially available sources (Doyle, 1990; InterQual, 1991; Utilization Management Associates, 1991).

Categories of Utilization Review
Prospective Review

Prospective review occurs through the preadmission or precertification process. Many payers require the admitting physician and the hospital to notify the plan before a member is admitted for inpatient care or specific outpatient procedures. Prospective review is often a condition for payment for diagnostic services, surgical procedures, or inpatient admission and is specified in the contract between the managed care organization and the hospital or provider.

Hospital review staff use established criteria to assess the appropriateness of the planned hospitalization or procedure and obtain approval (authorization) from the payer when such authorization is required. A careful system for tracking the status of precertifications in progress is established, including steps to follow when preauthorization is denied. Authorization for planned services is obtained before the admission or procedure for elective or prescheduled patients. This authorization is completed for all payers (primary and secondary) who require authorization, although priority authorization is focused on the primary payer.

The precertification process must be completed in a timely manner. When possible, preauthorization is completed at least 5 to 10 working days before the scheduled admission or procedure. This preauthorization lead-time allows adequate opportunity to obtain difficult authorizations or to reschedule cases if necessary. "Just-in-time" authorizations can necessitate last-minute cancellations or provision of service before authorization, outcomes that frustrate patients, providers, utilization review staff, and hospital administrators. Because last minute add-on cases are inevitable, routine preauthorization should be done through a timely, controlled process.

Concurrent Review

Concurrent review is the process by which the appropriateness of hospitalization for an admitted patient is evaluated. It includes initial review for patients admitted to urgent care or emergency departments within the last 24 hours or a continued stay review for patients previously authorized for admission. As for prospective review, the concurrent review staff use criteria to assess the appropriateness of the hospitalization or continued stay per internal standards and obtain authorization from the payer when indicated. Review staff may also review physician documentation concurrently to ensure that the information in the chart is complete and appropriate for the patient's condition and the services provided.

The detail of managing numerous reviews in progress can quickly become daunting. Each day, the authorization work in progress (WIP) will be authorized, denied, or will be pending (awaiting further information or response). The utilization review department must have clear procedures for follow-up on the common delays and types of denials as identified in Box 22-1. The tracking process should include a system, either manual or electronic,

---

BOX 22-1
Hospital Utilization Review

Common Reasons for Full or Partial Day Denials:
- Medical necessity
- Inappropriate provider
- Service not covered by plan
- No coverage
- Coordination of benefits issue
- Timely notification (technical)

Common Reasons for Delays in Authorization Process:
- No e-mail/call-back response
- Unable to reach payer
- Additional information required
- Never received request for benefits authorization

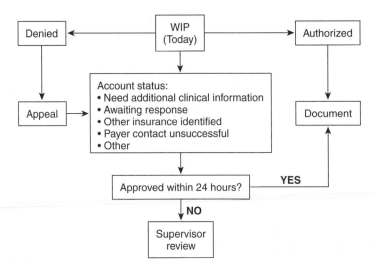

Figure 22-1   Concurrent hospital review work in progress (WIP). (Modified from Vanderbilt University Medical Center, Nashville, Tennessee, 1998.)

that transfers pending cases to specific "tickler" lists for follow-up. A rigorous system of checks must be put in place to ensure that all pending cases are tracked and resolved and that no cases "fall through the cracks."

Each day unresolved cases should be reviewed by the UM supervisor or another appropriate team member to identify a strategy for obtaining approval. The medical director should be consulted for cases in which medical issues require physician-to-physician discussion. A diagram detailing the flow of concurrent review WIP is outlined in Figure 22-1.

Retrospective Review

Retrospective review occurs in response to requests by payers or other entities for information after the hospitalization or procedure has been completed. It can include requests from Medicare or other payers for review of groups or categories of patients, or it can be an appeal of an individual account based on denial of payment. Retrospective review is also sometimes precipitated by internal concerns about types of patients, such as observation status patients, or denial of payment trends. Careful analysis of the number and type of denials by provider and payer can help identify problems with specific providers, payers, or internal processes. It is important to have a review team that includes staff from the front end (utilization review, admitting) and the back end (patient billing) look at retrospective trend data. A lack of understanding or communication about processes often results in denials. One large institution worked diligently to enhance its appeal process only to see an increase in the number of accounts written off for lack of medical necessity. Further analysis indicated that there was not a clear communication process for the appeal staff to alert the patient

---

BOX 22-2
Hospital Utilization Review: Caseload Priority

Concurrent Review (Highest Priority)
1. New admissions
2. Accounts not completed from the previous day
3. Newly discharged patients

Retrospective Reviews
1. High-dollar-value accounts
2. Mid-dollar-value accounts

---

billing staff to rebill once the appeal was approved. This lack of communication was easy to fix once the root cause was identified by the collaborative group (Mosier, 2000).

The overall goals for a hospital utilization review department are to obtain authorization before admission for all prescheduled patients, to obtain next-day authorization for all unscheduled admissions, and to obtain authorization for additional days of service before discharge. In addition, accounts that need appeals should be successfully completed within the required time frame, starting with the most expensive accounts. This prioritization of the hospital utilization review caseload is outlined in Box 22-2.

Enhancing Hospital Utilization Review Services: Diagnosis-Related Group Management

The increased penetration of managed care and the growing consumer awareness of healthcare over the past decade have increased the demand for hospitals and providers to demonstrate the delivery of high-quality, cost-effective healthcare. Profiling and report cards have become a way of life in the current healthcare environment, in which both consumers and payers are seeking value.

In the hospital setting, severity, cost, and case mix index (CMI) data for patients funded by Medicare and public healthcare programs are public domain, readily available for analysis and review. These data provide insight into how cost-effectively hospitals manage groups of patients of similar complexity or severity in terms of cost, morbidity, and mortality. Surprisingly, these data sometimes indicate that patients appear less severely ill, cost more to manage, and die more frequently than expected in their facility compared with patients at competing hospitals locally or nationwide. Typically this discrepancy is not about poor quality care but rather reflects that the reported CMI, severity, and cost-per-case do not describe the actual complexity of the patients.

When confronted with this dichotomy, physicians quickly indict "the coders." In fact, lower-than-expected CMI is usually caused by inadequate physician documentation in the medical record and lack of support for appropriate (higher-weighted) DRG assignments. This inadequate documentation is caused by physicians' failure to understand the need to fully document all comorbidities and complications and to use appropriate terminology. Coders cannot diagnose patients, and a medical record that lacks appropriate documentation cannot be altered after diagnosis. Thus patients who clearly were ill and received substantial care must be assigned, in the absence of appropriate documentation, a lower-weighted DRG code.

One example of this documentation coding gap is a cardiac patient who has the following signs and symptoms noted in the chart by the physician: "Patient in pulmonary edema, rales, S3 murmur, enlarged heart on chest x-ray, shortness of breath." Even if it is obvious (from nursing notes and so forth) that the patient has heart failure, the physician must write "congestive heart failure" to allow the coder to use that diagnosis in the DRG assignment.

Institutions that find their CMI to be lower than expected compared with benchmarks for similar hospitals nationwide can correct this problem through a proactive DRG management program. In this framework, the UM staff review charts concurrently and leave the physician a note (prompt) when key documentation is lacking. The physician can comply with the prompt, as in writing "congestive heart failure" in the previous example, or indicate that the prompt is not appropriate.

The desired result from this DRG management approach is not to game the system or upcode but rather to ensure that the documentation reflects the care provided and actual patient severity. Hospitals that have implemented this system often see an increase in CMI and severity commensurate with internal perception and national benchmarks. In addition, increased CMI results in additional revenue from DRG-based payers. In the final analysis, accurate CMI, severity, and cost data allow the hospital to be more fairly evaluated by managed care organizations and other payers in the quest for value partners.

Structure and Function Considerations

Hospital-based UM programs often evolve without careful planning. The work of UM is transparent to the organization and may not be well understood or valued. The primary goals, objectives, and functions of the UM department and review staff roles often become blurred and unfocused in light of responsibilities added on haphazardly through the years or after redesign efforts. The classic refrain of, "you're in the chart anyway" often begets additional quality, risk management, or other audit work for UM staff, as does burgeoning hospital interest in case management. In spite of numerous automated UM systems on the market, survey data indicate that about half of UM programs continue to function with cumbersome paper and pencil systems (Maryland Hospital Association Survey of Utilization Management Programs, 1999). Finally, program success (or failure) is often simplistically measured in terms of one or two broad measures, such as denial rates or variance days.

Given the impact that UM can have on overall hospital revenues, these structure and function issues should be given serious consideration to ensure an efficient and effective UM program. Careful analysis of key variables, such as goals, objectives, core work processes, roles, organizational structure, and measures of success, should be completed at least annually to ensure that the UM process is on target. Before any redesign of UM, such analysis should be done to evaluate current status, desired future, and the process for bridging the gap. A list of key structure and function questions for new or established programs is detailed in Box 22-3.

BOX 22-3

Structure and Function Considerations in Establishing or Upgrading an Acute Care Utilization Management Program

Purpose, Goals, and Objectives
- What are the goals and objectives for this program?
- Why is a UM program needed?
- What is the primary purpose of this program?

Function
- What is the scope of the work?
- How does UM relate to case management? To social work? To the quality program?
- Is the work (of these related departments) distributed and aligned to allow achievement of goals and objectives?
- Should the work (of these related departments) be bundled differently to balance workload, decrease duplication and fragmentation, create more holistic jobs, and optimize results?

Structure
- What organization structure positions UM for success?
- Should UM be linked with access functions (admitting), case management, quality, patient accounting, or other functions?

Roles
- Are job descriptions for utilization review staff clear? Are they distinct and collaborative from related job descriptions, such as case manager and quality review staff?
- Are criteria for performance evaluation clear, measurable, and achievable?
- Is there a medical director responsible for UM? How do staff interact with this person?

Staffing
- Is the staffing level appropriate (per national benchmarks) to achieve desired outcomes?
- If not, what work can be eliminated or deferred?
- Can nonreview staff complete clerical, time-consuming functions?
- During what hours will UM be staffed? Is weekend coverage needed?
- How is productivity measured and monitored?

Work Processes
- How are patient work lists generated?
- How is work assigned (by payer, specialty, floor, unit)?
- What checks are put into place to make sure all cases are tracked?
- What is the procedure to be followed for cases that cannot be authorized?
- What is the appeals process? How does UM communicate with accounting regarding billing/rebilling status?
- How do the front end (admitting/UM) and back end (patient billing) communicate the work in progress, potential write-off accounts, denial trends, and so on?
- Is an electronic tracking system needed?

Data
- What data are needed? By whom?
- How will data be collected, compiled, analyzed, and distributed?
- What forum will convene to review data? How often?
- Are appropriate stakeholders included in data review/analysis (e.g., admitting, patient accounting, UM, physicians, case management)?
- Is an electronic UM system needed?

In looking at successful UM programs, there are best practices that support positive outcomes. These best practices include the use of established review criteria, clearly defined roles, work processes and scope of work, adequate staffing, an involved medical director, an engaged oversight group, data available for analysis, and automated processes to support workflow. These best practices are summarized in Box 22-4.

Utilization Management and Case Management

Over the past decade, hospitals and healthcare systems have increasingly viewed case management as a strategy to ensure that cost and quality patient care outcomes are achieved. Surveys indicate that the majority of hospitals nationwide either already have or plan to implement case management programs (American Health Consultants, 1999).

This proliferation of case management programs has given way to a variety of models to match the unique needs and resources of the institutions involved. The relationship between UM and case management is often central to the structure of these models. Viewed simplistically, the work of UM and case management can be separate, collaborative, or integrated. The advantages and disadvantages of these approaches should be carefully considered.

In a model in which UM and case management programs are *separate,* they exist in the organization as unique departments. Often the departments report to different administrators, and there may be sharp boundaries and definitions for the work of each department. Because the work of UM and case management is highly interdependent, this is the least-desirable model. UM and case management, when functioning in "silos" (in isolation), however excellent their individual practices, miss an opportunity to productively work to ensure authorization and reimbursement for individual patients and to solve problems with trend data regarding avoidable days and denial patterns.

BOX 22-4
Utilization Management Programs: Best Practices

- Use of established criteria for review
- Clearly defined procedures for review, follow-up, and appeals processes
- An established system of checks to ensure that cases do not fall through the cracks
- Clear definition and reasonable boundaries for the scope of the work of UM, including collaboration with related departments (e.g., case management, admitting, quality, patient accounting)
- Clear definition of role and responsibility for the utilization managers
- Staffing levels consistent with national norms and appropriate for the defined scope/amount of work
- An involved medical director/physician advisor
- An oversight group with representation from key departments that is charged with review of program data and outcomes
- Clear, concise reports that track program performance and distribute it to key stakeholders
- Automated systems to support work flow

At the other extreme, a model exists in which the work of UM is *integrated* with the work of case management into a single role. In this model, utilization review staff plan discharges and monitor resource utilization in a utilization review/nurse case manager role. Another variation of this model is to require nurse case managers to take on traditional utilization review functions. This integrated model is often appealing superficially, since it allows an organization to "get started" with case management using existing utilization review and discharge planning staff. It appears to be cost-effective, since it seems to obviate the need for new full-time equivalents (FTEs).

In reality, this model often creates unrealistic roles. Utilization review is highly time dependent. Reviews must be done in a timely fashion to ensure proper approval. These timely, completed reviews are a measurable productivity target that review staff should be accountable for. The critical work of discharge planning may seem deferrable in the face of such a time-dependent, measurable target. (Re)review of charts, particularly for patients who do not have payers that require certification, such as Medicare, will likely not occur, as review staff struggle to meet competing and time-dependent priorities. If an institution wishes to extend the work of utilization review to a more revenue-generating DRG management model, the time needed to review the charts of DRG payers, prompt physicians, and ensure appropriate reimbursement is critical. Again, "working the charts" in this manner for DRG assurance may be highly compromised as certifications take priority and discharge planning becomes a potentially lower priority.

Perhaps most significantly, this utilization review/nurse case manager model dilutes the focus and power of case management. In a comprehensive analysis of case management services, the Nursing Executive Center of the Advisory Board Company noted that combining utilization review, case management, and social work (discharge planning) into one role is one of the major barriers to case management effectiveness (Healthcare Advisory Board, 2000). The motivation to achieve economies of scale by blending roles causes role confusion.

Nursing Executive Center research reveals that case managers in this arrangement spend a disproportionate amount of time performing routine tasks such as obtaining authorizations, determining what durable medical equipment company can be used or collecting data. As a result, case managers do not have time or focus for their more leveraged functions: stewarding patients through the case process, influencing and monitoring care giver practices, and coordinating with physicians and non-hospital entities (Healthcare Advisory Board, 2000, pp 1-15).

The middle ground and the most desirable model to align UM and case management is for these two processes to function in a highly collaborative, interdependent manner. In this framework, the core work of UM and case management is differentiated but highly connected and synergistic. Ideally, social work is incorporated into this collaboration to ensure that each discipline brings its expertise to assist the patient and to ensure that cost and quality outcomes are achieved. One version of this collaborative model is in place at Vanderbilt University Hospital. The focus of the three disciplines involved in case management, referred to as the *case management triad*, is described in Figure 22-2. In this model, the work of utilization review has evolved to a highly specialized UM/DRG specialist role. This UM department has achieved a denial rate below the national benchmark, has minimal funds written off for "no authorization" or "not medically necessary," and has seen an increase in CMI attributable to DRG management efforts (chart review and physician prompts). Furthermore, additional revenue resulting from the impact of accurate coding and an increased CMI on DRG payers is now captured and documented. These dollars were "left on the table" before the implementation of DRG management (Erickson, 1997, 1998).

Staffing Utilization Management

Having the right number of staff with the right complement of skills is key to the success of a UM program. In most acute care facilities, the work of traditional utilization review has increased in volume and complexity and has become more time dependent over the past decade with the increased penetration of managed care. The percentage of hospital admissions and outpatient procedures that require authorization has increased dramatically in most facilities. Concomitantly, there has been a proliferation of managed care plans, all

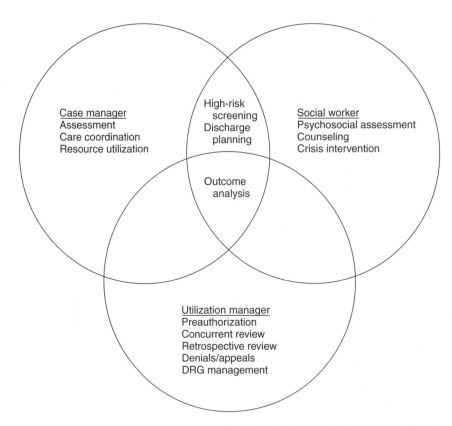

Figure 22-2   Case management triad. (From Vanderbilt University Medical Center, Office of Case Management, Nashville, Tennessee, 1993.)

with different review procedures and criteria. Utilization review staff must now become familiar with dozens of different payer requirements for review.

In many instances, the staffing of utilization review programs has been somewhat haphazard. Review staff often struggle with increasing workload volume and the myriad of health plan review requirements without additional training or resources. Often the role of traditional utilization review is redesigned to take on additional functions, such as quality review, discharge planning, and DRG management, with modest adjustments in staffing.

To ensure optimal UM outcomes and appropriate staffing levels, a careful analysis of program goals and objectives, workload, and number and skills of existing staff should be undertaken. Staffing and caseload volumes can be compared with national benchmarks (Box 22-5), which provide a generic comparison for evaluating staffing levels (Killey and Trutlein, 1992). Clearly the capacity for review staff to manage higher or lower caseload volumes relative to these benchmarks depends on the skill and experience of the staff, as well as the additional requirements of the role. If review staff are functioning as discharge planners, doing true DRG management, or completing numerous quality audits, the number of reviews they complete daily will be in the low-to-mid-range of the staffing benchmarks. A list of factors that affect review caseload capacity are detailed in Table 22-1. It is not unusual to hear reports of utilization review staff in utilization review/case manager roles who carry caseloads of 20 to 40 patients per day. If one considers the time requirement to complete just the review function, it becomes readily apparent that there is little time left for comprehensive discharge planning.

Administrators responsible for hospital utilization review programs should consider that UM, if done well, will directly affect the hospital's bottom line. There is a clear connection between authorization and reimbursement. High caseload volumes may be realistic for an experienced staff with traditional roles. If staff are not experienced, particularly if the review role has been expanded, high caseload volumes should be a warning that a component of the work may be suffering. To optimize results, there must be a match between workers and workload.

BOX 22-5
Utilization Management: Staffing Levels

Utilization Management Staff to Inpatient Bed Ratio
- Without discharge planning function (1:30)
- With discharge planning function (1:8 to 1:15)

Utilization Management Staff to Actual Inpatient Cases (InterQual, 1991)
- Without discharge planning function (1:40 to 1:50)

Utilization Management Staff to Health Plan Members (Kongstvedt, 1998)
- With hospital rounding (1:6000 to 1:8000)
- Overall range (0.01:1000 to 0.8:1000)

TABLE 22-1
Hospital Utilization Management: Staffing/Caseload Analysis

Factors Increasing Caseload Capacity	Factors Decreasing Caseload Capacity
Electronic review source	Manual chart review
Electronic data collection system	Paper tracking system
Review work done in one location	Travel to chart access
Rapid payer turnaround	Slower payer response
Scope of work limited to core review functions:	Review function plus additional functions:
Preauthorization	DRG management
Concurrent review	Discharge planning
Retrospective review	Quality review
Denial/appeals process	
Avoidable days tracking	
Data analysis	

A too-lean staff may compromise results and be false economy to the hospital in the long run. Finally, outcome measures that correlate with program and institution goals and objectives should be established and monitored to ensure that the program is achieving the desired results.

Evaluating Effectiveness

Hospital-based UM programs contribute to hospital financial security by ensuring that appropriate authorizations are obtained to facilitate billing and that bad debt is ameliorated through careful appeal of accounts denied for reimbursement. Working with case management, utilization review programs can further affect cost per case (and ultimately net revenue) through resource management. Utilization review programs that function in a DRG management framework ensure that physician documentation is complete and appropriate for the severity of the patient and the services provided. These efforts allow appropriate DRG assignment and often garner additional revenue. These areas of impact are significant for hospitals, yet UM programs may be underappreciated by hospital administrators. It is important for UM programs to define key measures of success and to measure and distribute these results within the institution. Existing outcome measures for UM programs may be inadequate to describe the contribution this program makes to the hospital's bottom line.

Traditionally, UM programs have monitored avoidable days and denial rates. It is important to track avoidable days as defined by both internal review and payer issued. When tracking denials, it is helpful to track the number of individual cases denied, the number of days denied, and the actual cost of payment denied. Similarly, for the appeal rate, it is helpful to track not only the number of cases appealed but also the number of days appealed and the actual number of dollars at risk before appeal. A system that can reconcile the actual rate of recovery from the appeal effort in terms of days, cases, and dollars helps determine the yield from the appeal process. Finally, it is critical to track the actual dollars that are ultimately

---

BOX 22-6

Utilization Management: Measures of Success

- Avoidable days—per hospital
- Avoidable days—payer issued
- Appeal rate (cases/dollars)
- Denial rate (cases/days/dollars)
- Write-off rate (cases/dollars)
- Authorization rate
  - Number/percent of patients requiring authorization
  - Percent of patients requiring authorization who were successfully authorized by discharge
- Sponsorship rate
  - Number/percent of patients without insurance at admission converted to sponsorship by discharge
- Case mix index*
  - Overall
  - Surgical
  - Medical
- Complications/comorbidity capture rate*
  - Overall
  - Surgical
  - Medical
- Paired DRG trends*

---

*For DRG management focus.

written off for reasons that fall within UM's domain, such as "not medically necessary" and "no authorization." All of these measures—avoidable days, denials, appeals, and write-offs—should be tracked by type and by physician. This information allows powerful trend analysis to determine what categories of problems are occurring and which physicians may require more coaching.

It is also useful to track the authorization rate. If UM is responsible for precertification, it is important to document the percent of patients who have a payer requiring authorization and how many cases and dollars this translates to annually. It is often surprising to see the increase in authorization work being done without additional staff as the percent of managed care payers in the hospital payer mix increase. In institutions where the UM department is responsible for sponsorship, identifying a payer for patients who are admitted to the hospital without any identified payer, tracking the number of patients without sponsorship and the number converted to sponsored before discharge should be tracked weekly.

If the UM department functions in a DRG management role, additional measures such as CMI and comorbidity and complication rates should also be monitored. These indicators should be tracked overall and broken down for medical and surgical cases. Finally, paired DRGs in which the option exists for higher- or lower-weighted DRG assignment should be monitored, and the proportion of higher- and lower-weighted DRGs should be compared with national benchmarks. These core indicators of success are detailed in Box 22-6.

PAYER-BASED UTILIZATION REVIEW/MANAGEMENT

Health plan UM has numerous components, including management of inpatient care, outpatient care, and specialty physician care; demand management; disease management; and case management. These programs form the basis for ensuring quality care and controlling costs within a health plan.

Demand Management

Demand management refers to the programs and services offered by health plans to reduce the requirement for health services by plan members. These programs can also serve as a marketing strategy for health plans by providing member-friendly services. Demand management programs include nurse advice lines, self-care programs, online medical information programs, and preventive services.

Nurse advice lines, also referred to as *triage nurse lines*, have been used by health maintenance organizations (HMOs) for many years. Nurse advice lines provide members with information about medical conditions and the need for medical care. Health plans may staff the lines with their own nurses or purchase the service from an existing company. Nurse advice lines are popular with specific segments of the healthcare market, such as seniors and pediatrics, and they can be effective in preventing unnecessary care in these healthcare populations.

Self-care programs allow plan members to access information from a variety of sources to become more informed about their medical condition and to make more appropriate decisions about when to seek care. Self-care strategies include health plan newsletters, self-care guides, and online services. Health plans often provide preventive or general medical education programs on plan Websites, with links to external sites on the Internet.

Health risk appraisals have long been used by health plans. Health risk appraisals query plan members about their health status. This information can then be used by the plan to assess risk. Plan members can be stratified accordingly so that high-risk members are referred for more intensive services, including case management.

Specialty Physician Management

In most health plans, the costs of nonprimary care professional services are higher than those of primary care services. These increased costs are typically driven by the fees associated with hospitalization but are also affected by the costs generated by consultants. In addition to the actual consultant fee, numerous tests and studies ordered by specialty physicians can increase costs. Health plans often establish systems to manage these specialty referrals and attendant costs. The most common methods are requiring authorization for the initial visit to a consultant and prohibiting secondary referrals. If the consultant believes that additional follow-up is warranted, this request must be communicated and coordinated through the primary care provider.

Facility Utilization Review

Prospective Review

The cornerstone of payer-based prospective review is precertification: requiring physicians and hospitals to notify the plan before admitting a patient for inpatient or outpatient services. Precertification is done for three reasons. First, it is done to notify the concurrent review system that a case is occurring so that follow-up review can be set in motion. Second, the case is reviewed to ensure that the most appropriate setting is being used. Finally, precertification allows data to be captured for financial accruals (Kongstvedt, 1998).

At the time of precertification, the plan will typically assign a length of stay guideline and verify eligibility of coverage. Verification of benefit at precertification is not binding, since ultimate eligibility for coverage is determined at the time the claim is processed. This gap between verification at time of certification and definitive verification at payment is a point of vulnerability for hospitals following review procedures in good faith. The hospital is sometimes left with unpaid accounts due to eligibility issues that the patient did not know about or disclose or that the plan did not identify on initial verification.

Two additional strategies that many health plans employ to manage utilization include requiring hospitals to send patients to specific (contracted) laboratories for preoperative testing and specifying which surgical procedures must be done on an outpatient basis. Health plans and hospitals both need to analyze the cost and benefits of inpatient versus outpatient surgery carefully. The cost savings expected from shifting cases from inpatient to outpatient settings are not always realized and the shift from inpatient to outpatient may not be satisfying to the patient. Finally, it is important for the precertification process to be linked to the health plan's case management effort. It makes no sense to precertify patients and recognize individuals at risk for a complicated course and not refer them for comprehensive case management services. Without a connection to case management, preadmission review merely generates a census list of inpatient admissions and misses an opportunity to intervene with at-risk patients in a timely manner. Preadmission review not connected to a UM or case management effort will not result in reductions in length of stay or facilitate alternative plans of care (Mullahy, 1998).

Concurrent Review

Concurrent review is used by the health plan to manage utilization during hospitalization. The most common techniques include length-of-stay assignment and tracking, rounding, and discharge planning by the plan UM nurses.

The UM nurse is a pivotal player in the success of a managed care program. The scope of responsibility of the UM nurse varies from plan to plan. In some plans, the UM nurse is primarily telephone-based and does information gathering and even "rounding" via the telephone. In other plans, UM nurses go on-site to evaluate hospitalized patients through chart review, physician discussion, and patient interview. In all instances, UM nurses should use established criteria to evaluate appropriateness of services. It is important that UM nurses know to use these criteria as guidelines only and adapt them appropriately in response to individual patient, provider, or facility issues. Patients and physicians can become irritated when guidelines are applied stringently without consideration of individual patient needs.

UM nurses need clear procedures for reviewing the daily log of hospitalized plan members with the medical director. Ideally this review can occur early in the day so that appropriate action can take place when indicated. Established plans with experienced UM nurses may opt for medical director review of only problem cases. This is usually the case in plans that cover a broad geographic area, in situations where the plan cannot justify additional personnel (e.g., start-up preferred provider organization), or if the hospital does not allow on-site review by plan nurses.

Ideally, plan UM nurses will make rounds on site in the hospital to obtain the most timely and accurate information, to most proactively engage in discharge planning and to detect hospital- or physician-specific practice variation that affects utilization. Because of the plethora of personnel involved with each hospitalized patient, it is essential that plan UM nurses coordinate efficiently with hospital-based UM, case management, and social work staff to optimize planning and minimize duplication of effort. Issues of patient confidentiality must also be addressed when plan UM nurses make rounds in the hospital setting.

Retrospective Review

From the health plan perspective, retrospective review occurs after the patient is discharged and involves either claims review or review of patterns and trends. For claims review, accounts are stratified by dollar amount, and valuable cases are reviewed. This review looks for congruence between services delivered and actual claims data. A plan reviewer may actually go on site to review medical records, or a request for record information may be made to the hospital.

Pattern or trend review involves compiling data on individual providers or hospitals to profile utilization, cost, and outcomes. The benefit of this analysis is the ability to provide feedback to providers regarding their patterns compared with those of their peers. Pattern and outcome analysis also provides the plan with data to use in decision making about the most appropriate setting for care for specific procedures (i.e., which hospital has the best outcome for the lowest charges and the shortest length of stay). This data can also be useful during hospital contracting in setting rates and expectations. The key to this analysis is to ensure the accuracy of the data so that providers will be compelled to change practice as appropriate.

Impact of Payer-Based Utilization Management

UM has been lauded as an effective means of cost control since its introduction to the managed care industry. Particularly in the early days of managed care, the easily corrected problems of redundant tests or questionable surgeries and procedures were avoided, and significant dollars to manage member health costs were saved. It may be that the easy opportunities for savings from second guessing claims have passed. Although hospital lengths of stay decreased significantly in the early 1990s, overall length of stay has been relatively stable during the past few years. Beginning in 1999, trends in utilization review have changed, and many payers now allow routine tests and procedures without review while retaining review requirements for a small number of procedures that are particularly costly or problematic (*Plunketts' Healthcare Industry Almanac*, 2001).

There has been ongoing debate as to whether UM has impacted patient access to care. One study of the UM data for 72,000 members covered by a large national insurance carrier between 1989 to 1993 addressed this question (Wickizer, 1999). This study noted that among general medicine adult patients, UM rarely denied admission outright. Less than 1% of cases reviewed had been denied admission. Patients having hysterectomies accounted for the largest number of admission denials. For these patients, there was a shift from the requested inpatient procedure to an outpatient procedure.

This study also noted that UM became more restrictive over time, particularly for patients with mental health conditions. In addition, among patients with cardiovascular disease, UM for patients who were admitted with a surgical diagnosis impacted length of stay and increased the relative risk for readmission. In these surgical cardiovascular patients, length of stay was decreased by 2 or more days in 9% of patients, and the relative risk of readmission was 2.7 times higher. For cardiovascular patients admitted under a medical diagnosis, UM had little or no effect on readmissions (Wickizer, 1999).

UM is at the heart of the managed care backlash and the issues related to patient rights. Over the past decade, many states have attempted to regulate UM through legislation. Maryland was the first state to adopt a stand-alone utilization review law in 1988. Today over 36 states have laws that govern aspects of utilization review. Typically this legislation addresses precertification and concurrent review and has a broad range of requirements relating to an appeal or ombudsman process (Gemignani, 1999).

SUMMARY

Utilization review/management has been an effective strategy in the struggle to contain healthcare costs and ensure appropriate use of healthcare resources. In theory, these review and management programs are valuable strategies to be employed by institutions and managed care payers to achieve these ends. The challenge is to keep these efforts aimed at maintaining patient care quality, as well as controlling costs. Utilization review staff provide an excellent supportive service to physicians and health plan members. Again, the challenge is to make sure that the review function is done in a collaborative manner, with the focus on optimizing patient outcomes.

UM will probably change significantly in the next decade as the healthcare industry continues to change. UM has evolved parallel to managed care in response to issues and needs and will continue to evolve in this manner as newer healthcare models emerge.

REFERENCES

American Health Consultants: Hospital case management and managed care growth link questioned, *Hosp Case Manage* 7(8):143-144, 1999.

Blackstien-Hirsch P, Cox JL, Ash Basinski, et al: The current status of hospital utilization review and management initiatives, 2001, Institute for Clinical Evaluative Sciences, Available online: http://www.ices.on.ca/doc/wp033.htm.

Doyle RI: *Healthcare management guidelines: inpatient and surgical care*, vol 1, Seattle, 1990, Milliman & Robertson.

Erickson S: Vanderbilt medical center redesigns case management, *Inside Case Management* 3(11):1-4, 1997.

Erickson S: The Vanderbilt outcomes management model, *Nursing Clinic of North America* 10(1):13-20, 1998.

Gemignani J: The utilization review controversy, *Bus Health* 17(7):39-40, 1999.

The Healthcare Advisory Board: *A necessary discipline: maximizing case management ROI*, Washington, DC, 2000, Nursing Executive Center.

InterQual: *The ISD: a review system with adult criteria*, Chicago, 1991, InterQual.

Killey SK, Trutlein JJ: A survey of human resources in managed care organizations, *Physician Exec* 18(6):49-51, 1992.

Kongstvedt PR: Managing basic medical-surgical utilization. In Kongstvedt PR, Plocher DW, editors: *Best practices in medical management*, Gaithersburg, Md, 1998, Aspen.

Maryland Hospital Association Survey of Utilization Management Programs: *Denials management conference syllabus*, Baltimore, 1999, The Association.

Mosier J: Vanderbilt University Medical Center: Personal communication, April 15, 2000.

Mullahy CM: Case management and managed care. In Kongstvedt PR, Plocher DW, editors: *Best practices in medical management*, Gaithersburg, Md, 1998, Aspen.

Plunketts' healthcare industry almanac: Major trends affecting the healthcare industry, Jan 2001, Available online: http://www.plunkettresearch.com/Plunkett/book_titles/HCIA/5-trends.htm.

Utilization Management Associates: *Managed care appropriateness protocol (MCAP)*, Wellesley, Mass, 1991, Utilization Management Associates.

Utilization Review Accreditation Commission: Utilization management, December 2001, Available online: http://www.urac.org/programs/health.utiliz.manage.htm.

Wickizer T: Effects of utilization review on healthcare quality and access, *Grant results report*, 1999, Robert Wood Johnson Foundation, Available online: http://www.rwjf.org/health/0199775.htm.

23

Outcomes Management in a Managed Care Environment

Lawrence F. Strassner

KEY LESSONS IN THIS CHAPTER

- Outcomes can be categorized in one of three ways: cost, clinical, and service.
- Performance measures are used to quantify how well activities within a process or the outputs of a process achieve a specific goal.
- Benchmark data can be based on either internal (organizational) indicators or external indicators.
- When possible, it is preferable to use cost data rather than charge data.
- It is generally better to start a process using general clinical outcome measures, followed by a more focused, detailed study.

As we begin a new millennium, healthcare will continue to feel the impact of the Balanced Budget Act of 1997, with a continued focus on decreasing healthcare costs while maintaining or improving quality of care. There continues to be a growing interest in outcomes, as well as a continuing increase in resources being expended to collect and interpret outcomes data. The need to measure and monitor outcomes will continue to grow in response to increased competition in healthcare. In addition, regulatory agency requirements for consistent reporting of process and outcomes data are growing.

Outcomes management is the use of outcomes data to protect and monitor the quality of healthcare services in an era of ongoing cost containment. Providers, hospitals, and payers share an interest in the science of outcomes management and use this data to document and defend the efficacy and quality of medical interventions. There are mixed reports about whether managed care and capitated reimbursement systems sacrifice quality while controlling costs. Nevertheless, outcomes management provides patients with the protection they need against too little care, or underutilization of healthcare resources.

OUTCOMES MANAGEMENT DEFINED

Outcomes management is a process that uses continuous quality improvement techniques to systematically assess and define the most effective care processes while considering the associated costs (Motheral, 1997; Pine, 1998). There are three different categories of outcomes: (1) economic/cost, (2) clinical, and (3) service. Service may also be referred to as *satisfaction with care.* Outcomes are multidimensional and can be immediate, intermediate, or long-term.

CASE MANAGEMENT AND OUTCOMES MANAGEMENT

Case management impacts all three types of outcome measures. As such, case management continues to gain considerable recognition as an effective strategy for providing high-quality, cost-effective healthcare. The effectiveness of case management in improving clinical costs and outcomes is evident in the following quote taken from an article in *Annals of Internal Medicine,* "People with diabetes are better able to maintain 'near normal' glucose levels, and thereby prevent or delay complications associated with the disease when their care involves a case manager" (Aubert et al, 1998, p 606). Case managers, regardless of where they are employed, are currently positioned and have the opportunity to apply outcomes management to their practice and play an even more important role in helping to change how care is delivered. Therefore this chapter describes the effectiveness of case managers in using the process of outcomes management in a managed care environment.

CASE MANAGERS IMPROVE COST, CLINICAL, AND SATISFACTION OUTCOMES

The professional case manager uses both clinical and financial outcomes to improve patient care. The case manager participates in cost reduction by preventing delays and expediting care processes. Strategies used to expedite care processes include preventing delays in consults or diagnostic tests, facilitating the transition from intravenous to oral antibiotics, and coordinating the discharge process, beginning at the point of admission. All of these interventions have a direct impact on the length of stay. The case manager helps decrease costly or inappropriate laboratory, radiology, pharmaceutical, and other medical interventions. One key mechanism used to monitor the appropriateness of resource utilization is through the use of standard orders sets, guidelines, protocols, and clinical pathways.

The avoidance of unauthorized treatments, tests, and admissions is also a function of case management and is often applied in health plans in which the case manager functions as a gatekeeper. In this context, the case manager may apply criteria for the authorization of admissions, treatments, and tests to effectively manage resource utilization and cost outcomes. Cost savings are also realized by negotiating with the payer to maximize an individual patient's benefits. Regardless of the strategies used, most case managers monitor and report the cost of care.

Case managers are an important member of the healthcare team in the improvement of clinical outcomes. Examples of how case managers contribute to the management and improvement of clinical outcomes include the following:

- Synthesizing the interdisciplinary team's assessment data and completing an integrated assessment of the patient and family's needs.
- Coordinating educational needs for patients and families before, during, and after an inpatient stay.
- Coordinating the multidisciplinary team, in collaboration with the physician, to promote the achievement of desired outcomes.
- Monitoring patient progress toward expected outcomes.
- Anticipating an actual or potential clinical problem and acting quickly to prevent or manage the evolving clinical picture.
- Monitoring, tracking, and analyzing aggregated clinical outcome data of specific patient populations. These data are then used to improve the process and outcomes of care.

SATISFACTION WITH CARE

Case managers have also demonstrated the positive impact they can have on patient, family, provider, and payer satisfaction with care and services. Patient and family satisfaction can be greatly enhanced as the case manager navigates the healthcare system for the patient, promoting easy access to the appropriate level of care. The case manager also assists patients in understanding treatment choices, alternatives, risks, and benefits. They directly solicit perceptions regarding satisfaction with care from the patient or family, as well as their satisfaction with care providers. They may be responsible for responding to patient complaints in a timely and appropriate manner. Provider and payer satisfaction are augmented as case managers improve communication and accessibility to the healthcare team and establish working relationships with referral sources. It is equally important for the case manager to monitor, collect, analyze, and integrate satisfaction measures with the cost and clinical outcome measures that demonstrate the value and effectiveness of case management.

PERFORMANCE MEASURES

Case managers clearly perform many role functions, which can result in effective reductions in the cost of care while enhancing quality clinical outcomes and improving patient, family, provider, and payer satisfaction. Case managers may also have the responsibility of measuring and monitoring this data. In this way, outcomes may serve as performance measures for case managers.

A performance measure is the quantification of how well activities within a process or the outputs of the process achieve a specific goal. The internal and external stakeholders who have a vested interest in the effectiveness of case management play a pivotal role in determining these specific goals. Examples of the prototypical internal stakeholders are the chief financial officer, chief medical and nursing officers, the director of case management, and the director of managed care. The external stakeholders include the payers and regulatory agencies, such as the National Committee for Quality Assurance (NCQA). When identifying performance measures related to specific goals, it is important to understand and identify the interrelatedness of structure, process, and outcomes. Critical to the success of any outcomes management effort is the measurement of the structures and processes of care and the ability to link these factors to the outcomes of care.

Criteria for Establishing Performance Measures

When establishing performance measures, the case manager must first understand the purpose, intended use, and relevancy of the performance measure to the organization. A fundamental step is to understand the value placed on economics or cost, quality, service, and satisfaction outcomes by key stakeholders in the organization. Is the intended use to improve services, manage the processes of care, avoid risk, or identify problems with current processes? Some measures and tools may already be defined for particular settings. Indicators of hospital quality defined by the Joint Commission on Accreditation of Healthcare Organizations (JCAHO) include the ORYX/Performance Measurement Requirements for Healthcare Organizations (JCAHO, 1997). Another example is the Health Plan Employer Data and Information Set (HEDIS) for health plan settings developed by the NCQA, which includes defined measures (HEDIS, 1998).

Establishing performance measures is also driven by market conditions. Some of the measurements depend on the setting in which care is being provided and the organization's level of risk for a particular patient population (Figure 23-1).

Case managers should have considerable knowledge of the current measures collected and reported in their organization. Identifying the impact of the implementation of the

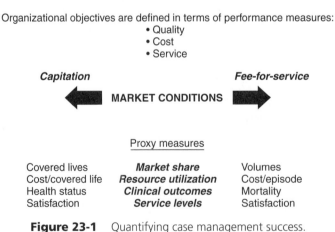

Organizational objectives are defined in terms of performance measures:
- Quality
- Cost
- Service

Capitation ←——— **MARKET CONDITIONS** ———→ *Fee-for-service*

Proxy measures

Covered lives	*Market share*	Volumes
Cost/covered life	*Resource utilization*	Cost/episode
Health status	*Clinical outcomes*	Mortality
Satisfaction	*Service levels*	Satisfaction

Figure 23-1   Quantifying case management success.

processes of case management on these measures may be a function of the case manager, and it will help the case manager begin to define where the measures will have the greatest effect.

Effective outcome measures should do the following:

- Have a clear and precise definition
- Be measurable
- Be under the provider's control
- Allow for confounding influences or patient factors

Risk Adjustment

The importance of using risk-adjusted data to compensate for severity of illness is critical. Risk adjustment refers to the statistical removal of any confounding factors affecting the outcomes data. Each patient's outcomes will depend on the following three factors: (1) patient-specific factors, (2) provider-specific factors (i.e., the quality of the care processes), and (3) random variation not attributable to any identifiable factor. Risk adjustment of the outcome measure or the removal of these confounding variables will allow for more accurate comparisons of the outcomes for similar populations of patients. In addition, this process will make the data more meaningful to physicians and other providers. For example, a physician reviewing a set of outcomes for a group of patients with congestive heart failure (CHF) can apply the data to all the patients if the data has been previously risk adjusted.

The performance measure must be actionable. It must have meaning and value to the providers by being translated into meaningful and useful information. There is no value in measuring things that have no real impact on the ability to manage the system or the provider's ability to practice effectively. The performance measure must also be reportable in a manner relevant to the stakeholder. This report may take a variety of formats based on the stakeholder, but the best report should fit on one to two sheets of paper, summarize the important data, identify outliers or deviations from the standard, and provide information on how the user may obtain more detail if desired (Kongstvedt, 1998a, 1998b).

Feedback to the stakeholders on a timely and routine basis by establishing routine reports requiring responsive action plans is key. The case manager should report the data at the departmental and organizational quality improvement committee and take responsibility for coordinating the action plans.

The performance measure must be obtainable with a minimal data collection burden. To ensure accuracy, the process of collecting, entering, and editing the measure must be well defined and consistently implemented.

The data should encompass an adequate time period. For example, if patient satisfaction is being measured, the data may need to be reported every quarter, since monthly reporting may result in too small a sample size. Other data, such as length of stay, may be appropriately reported on a monthly basis for the organization to stay on top of any potential problems as the data is tracked and trended. Data trends are more valuable than a single snapshot or single quarter's data, particularly when looking at practice patterns.

Quality indicator	Definitions	Threshold (calculated)	Source of threshold	Data source	Responsible party	Collection frequency (by day, week, month)	Reporting frequency (monthly, quarterly)
Functional status		80% physical 80% mental	Internal baseline	SF-12 tool	Case manager	Preadmission/ 1 month postprocedure	Quarterly
Transfusion required post-PTCA		Less than 2%	Internal baseline	Order entry/data repository	Utilization review	Monthly	Quarterly
Patient satisfaction		90%	Internal baseline	Patient satisfaction tool	Case managers	Upon discharge	Quarterly
Complication of procedure requiring subsequent surgical procedures		Less than 2%	Internal baseline	Medical record	Utilization review	Monthly	Quarterly
Wound infection		Less than 3%	Internal baseline	Infection control	Infection control nurse	Daily as indicated	Quarterly
Intrahospital mortality		Less than 3%	National benchmark	Medical record/ER record	Utilization review	Monthly	Quarterly

Figure 23-2   Outcome measurement template example for DRG 112: percutaneous transluminal coronary angioplasty (PTCA).

Benchmarking Versus Profiling

A final point to consider in establishing performance measures is the use of internal measurements and industry benchmark standards to set goals or targets. Internal measurements are one strategy used when the organization wants to compare its performance on a particular measure with its previous performance on that measure. For example, the organization may choose to monitor its own cost per case, comparing its cost from one period with another, with the goal of continuously reducing the cost per case without a particular final figure in mind. Industry benchmarking, on the other hand, refers to measuring against a selected and preestablished industry standard for a particular performance measure. Length of stay is typically measured in this way.

It is important to understand the difference between benchmarking and profiling as performance measures are identified and targets are set. Benchmarking demonstrates the "possible" and provides direction toward a particular goal. Benchmarking provides the case manager with information to engage physicians and other providers to build consensus around preferred interventions geared toward achieving the goal or benchmark. This process links the interventions to the expected outcomes.

Profiling tracks individual performance and measures the effects of interventions. It is used to build motivation for continuous improvement. For example, an organization may develop individual physician profiling reports, including the individual physician's performance in length of stay, cost per case, patient satisfaction, and quality outcome indicators.

Case managers may analyze and use both benchmark and performance data. Figure 23-2 provides an example of a tool that may be used by case managers when establishing outcome measurements.

CASE MANAGERS MANAGE COST OF CARE

Case managers facilitate efficient and effective care, where appropriate, to assist in decreasing the cost of care through the appropriate use of resources. Therefore case managers, like all members of the healthcare team, must be competent in the identification and monitoring of financial data measures. They must be able to identify areas for cost improvement, collaboratively engage physicians and other providers in discussions about the processes and cost of care, and use financial databases to demonstrate their effectiveness. The healthcare team may depend on the case manager to provide them with financial data that demonstrates where the cost savings opportunities are in their area of practice. The case manager may also be asked to provide hard data to support these opportunities. For example, a case manager might identify that the physicians admitting patients with community-acquired pneumonia use an expensive antibiotic. After reviewing the literature and discussing the issue with the clinical pharmacist, the case manager might report back to the team with other antibiotics, which are less expensive but produce the same outcomes as the more expensive antibiotic. Armed with this data, the team may decide to recommend the less expensive antibiotic as the recommend antibiotic of choice for patients admitted to their organization with pneumonia.

As a member of a performance improvement team, a case manager may use external benchmarking and internal data to identify cost savings opportunities for a particular diagnosis-related group (DRG) or group of DRGs. Most organizations have access to external regional or national cost data. Finance departments may obtain these data through linked databases or by hiring outside consultants who collect and report cost or charge data for the purposes of market analysis, strategic planning, identification of opportunities for improvement, and other uses. Before identifying cost outcomes, the case manager should review the cost or charge data currently available and share this data with the performance improvement team.

Figure 23-3 represents the use of internal "best" practices cost data and external benchmark cost data to identify potential cost savings opportunities for DRGs 358 and 359, hysterectomies. The cost savings analysis compares the current average cost per case for the organization with that of five Florida hospitals and both Medicare regional and national Medicare cost data for hysterectomies. Total potential savings are calculated using the difference between the

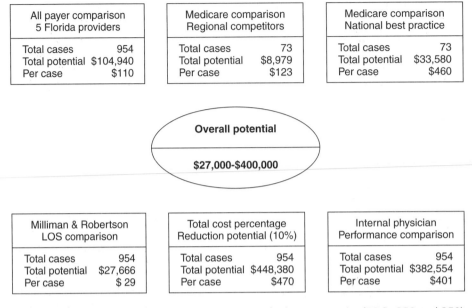

All payer comparison 5 Florida providers	
Total cases	954
Total potential	$104,940
Per case	$110

Medicare comparison Regional competitors	
Total cases	73
Total potential	$8,979
Per case	$123

Medicare comparison National best practice	
Total cases	73
Total potential	$33,580
Per case	$460

Overall potential

$27,000-$400,000

Milliman & Robertson LOS comparison	
Total cases	954
Total potential	$27,666
Per case	$ 29

Total cost percentage Reduction potential (10%)	
Total cases	954
Total potential	$448,380
Per case	$470

Internal physician Performance comparison	
Total cases	954
Total potential	$382,554
Per case	$401

Figure 23-3 Potential cost savings opportunities for hysterectomies (DRGs 358 and 359).

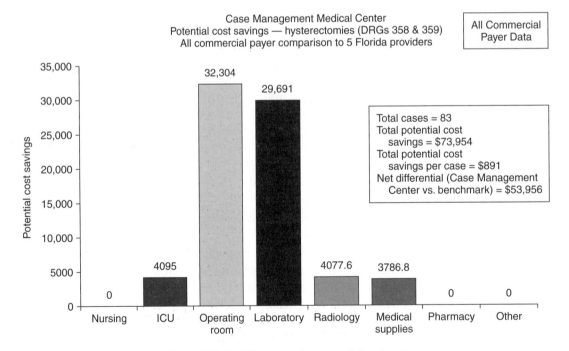

Figure 23-4 Where are the potential savings?

organization's average cost per case and the benchmark cost per case times the number of discharged cases. The per case savings is the difference between the organization's average cost per case and the particular benchmark.

The length of stay comparison approach focuses strictly on length of stay "well managed" or "moderately managed" Milliman & Robertson benchmark data (Doyle and Schibanoff, 2001). The savings are calculated using the difference in length of stay between the Milliman & Robertson benchmark data and the organization's average length of stay and assumes a reduction in nursing and ancillary costs for each day decreased, yielding a decrease in cost per case. The reduction potential approach assumes an overall decrease in cost per case by a predetermined percentage selected by the organization and will vary based on organizational goals, product lines, current performance, and reimbursement.

The internal physician approach uses the organization's own physician(s), with the lowest cost per case as the benchmark. The difference between the average cost per case of all other physicians performing hysterectomies and the internal lowest-cost physician is used to define benchmark cost per case and calculate total potential savings. Physicians often respond to this data more readily, since it already reflects a practice pattern within their own organization.

It is important and essential to provide a variety of methods to identify savings, since this approach points the physicians toward a target and helps engage them in dialogue about the opportunities for improving the cost of care. Physicians may prefer to have their data further stratified by severity of illness. By stratifying patients into severity levels, justification can be made for those cases for which the cost of care was higher. It would be expected that the cost per case would be higher for more severely ill patients who required a greater level of clinical intervention.

For example, by stratifying patients with CHF, the organization might identify that the most severely ill patients were using appropriate amounts of resources, whereas the less severely ill patients were overusing resources.

This exercise may identify that you have minimal or no cost savings opportunities in your less severely ill patients and that most of your cost savings opportunities may be found in your moderately ill patients. Most data that is purchased and many organizations that provide data to their clinicians adjust the data for severity. MedisGroups and 3M Health Information Systems are two vendors who provide software-based systems to categorize patients by severity of illness (Health Care Advisory Board, 1993). Many organizations have purchased systems to severity-adjust cost data used for physician profiling, case management, physician credentialing, quality improvement, and marketing.

Once the physicians acknowledge and understand the broad cost savings potential, they may then ask where or in what categories the cost savings opportunities are. To identify specific cost saving opportunities, the data must be analyzed at the next level of detail, which includes analyzing cost-by-cost "buckets," or categories. This is referred to as *drilling down*. In Figure 23-4, the greatest opportunity for cost savings for hysterectomies was found in the operating room and laboratory categories. The hospital was compared to the all-commercial payer, five Florida hospital benchmarks. As stated earlier, this points the clinicians in a direction but does not provide the precise practice patterns or define the structures within those Florida hospitals that are different. This step involves looking at the organization's internal laboratory and operating room cost and utilization data to determine where, if any, cost savings opportunities exist.

Physician Comparison Data

Although physicians may work within the same organization, they seldom realize the differences in practice patterns among themselves. To illustrate variation in practice and quickly identify areas for savings, the organization's internal cost and utilization data by cost bucket categories can be used (e.g., laboratory, radiology, pharmacy). At the utilization level, the physicians should be provided with the differences in utilization and cost by using the lowest cost internal physician practice as the benchmark. When you are able to say, "Dr. R's utilization per hysterectomy patient discharged includes one chest x-ray, two complete blood counts, and Ancef as the antibiotic of 'choice,' and your utilization is an average of 2.5 chest x-rays, three complete blood counts, and includes tobramyicin (higher cost) antibiotic as the antibiotic of 'choice,'" the physician may be more receptive to a discussion about how he or she might reduce his or her own resource utilization. To avoid the opportunity for the physician to comment that his or her patients are more ill than Dr. R's patients, only severity-adjusted data should be presented. There is no guarantee that you still will not be engaged in the severity or data integrity discussion, but you will have demonstrated your knowledge and attempt to address the issues of severity of illness.

Next, the case manager should work collaboratively with the physicians to identify and change practice patterns where appropriate and set cost per case targets. The case manager is often involved in orchestrating the changes in the care process. The case manager will also need the assistance of the finance department to factor the impact these practice changes will have on the cost per case. Once there is consensus on the cost targets and the changes in care processes (e.g., reducing resource utilization), a quarterly cost physician/case manager profile report, such as the one illustrated in Figure 23-5, may be used to monitor, track, and trend improvements. If needed, a more detailed "drill-down" utilization and cost report may also be used when assessing individual practice changes to agreed-upon defined goals or utilization targets. An example appears in Figure 23-6.

Another approach the case manager may use includes changes in practice formulated around a particular protocol. Using this approach, the case manager may have identified that there seems to be a high percentage of patients who develop atrial fibrillation after open-heart surgery. In reviewing the literature and discussing the issues with the clinical pharmacist, the case manager identifies that the prophylactic use of amiodarone could prevent the onset of atrial fibrillation postoperatively and therefore decreases the intensive care unit length of stay by 12 hours and the medical surgical inpatient stay by 18 hours.

Lessons Learned: Cost Outcomes Measurement

Case managers are not only accountable for identifying cost saving opportunities and managing care processes to produce the most cost-effective and efficient care, they are also responsible for monitoring, tracking, analyzing, and reporting the cost of care and cost savings. The following lessons have been identified as case managers take on this accountability.

DRG 481 or ICD-9 (41.01)

Bone Marrow Transplant, autologous (breast)

Quarter	Cases	LOS	Mode	Total	Routine	OR	Rad	Lab	Pharm	Supply	Therapy	Other	Contribution Margin
								Average Cost per Case					
Q1	10	10.52	10	$25,814	$8,710	$4,291	$2,022	$1,897	$995	$4,172	$1,356	$1,831	$1,780
Q2	4	12.43	9	$29,959	10,907	3,534	2,641	3,458	1,538	5,254	1,613	1,014	($500)
Q3	16	12.75	10	$30,901	11,679	3,696	2,094	4,047	1,531	4,992	1,528	1,334	$2,750
Q4	20	11.43	12	$26,819	9,705	3,420	2,548	3,002	1,095	4,917	1,266	866	($1,045)
Average		11.76	10	$28,373	$10,250	$3,735	$2,326	$3,101	$1,290	$4,969	$1,441	$1,261	$746
Benchmark targets		9.36		$25,851	$6,206	$4,189	$1,387	$1,076	$2,174	$7,949	$1,561	$1,305	$1,055

Bone Marrow Transplant, autologous (breast)

MD	Cases	LOS	Total	Routine	OR	Rad	Lab	Pharm	Supply	Therapy	Other	Contribution Margin
							Average Cost per Case					
3058	42	11.83	$25,792	$9,968	$3,422	$1,942	$2,671	$1,149	$4,075	$1,360	$1,205	$450
6357	40	10.5	$26,930	9,295	3,606	2,331	2,741	934	5,590	1,361	1,072	1,208
3884	31	11.55	$27,302	10,074	3,757	2,134	2,738	1,216	4,807	1,461	1,115	350
7219	9	12.22	$28,096	10,295	3,673	2,839	2,942	1,307	4,240	1,500	1,300	(1,308)
1330	48	11.94	$28,777	10,380	3,724	2,347	3,387	1,427	4,726	1,441	1,345	350
1568	33	12.06	$28,739	10,236	4,061	2,725	2,689	1,209	5,326	1,310	1,183	650
4051	25	12.72	$32,462	11,575	3,733	2,716	3,263	1,944	5,945	1,775	1,511	(724)

Figure 23-5   Physician/case manager profile (fictitious data).

Fiscal year 1998, Qtr 1   *Bone Marrow Transplant, autologous (breast)*   n: 25

Rev Proc	Item	Goal	Avg	Diff	Cost ea.	Cost for Population
4519912	Electrocardiogram (ECG)	1	1.15	0.15	$14.81	$55.54
4730108	Electrolyte panel, serum, emergency	0	1.35	1.35	20.22	$682.43
4730110	Chemistry, panel, serum	1	1.11	0.11	26.36	$72.49
4763020	HEME-8	6	2.59	(3.41)	27.69	($2,360.57)
4763022	HEME-8, emergency	0	1.44	1.44	15.00	$540.00
4763024	HEME-8 with electronic diff	0	1.02	1.02	18.98	$483.99
4763026	Prothrombin time	0	1.27	1.27	21.77	$691.20
4763332	Activated partial thromboplastin	6	4.00	(2.00)	11.73	($586.50)
4763342	Surveillance cultures	6	4.00	(2.00)	17.53	($876.50)
4765210	Fluconozal	14	8.00	(6.00)	25.00	($3,750.00)
4804510	Vancomycin	36	48.00	12.00	32.00	$9,600.00
4804599	SYPH sero: (RPR screen)	1	1.43	0.43	14.73	$158.35
4804599	Cytoxanserum level	5	4.00	(1.00)	18.22	($455.50)
4804598	NA/K emergency	10	12.00	2.00	12.99	$649.50
					Total:	$4,904.42

Figure 23-6   Resource utilization to targets.

Lesson 1

When looking at cost data, understand the difference between cost and charges. If your organization does not have a cost accounting system, you may want to focus on resource utilization (i.e., number and kinds of tests) and have your finance department identify the cost impact. Many organizations that do not have a true cost accounting system apply a formula ratio of cost to charges to estimate the cost of care.

Lesson 2

When examining cost data, focus the physician's attention on direct costs that have the most control and are most likely to have a direct impact. When starting your cost outcomes measurement process, exclude indirect costs, such as the cost associated with administrative overhead. Physicians will often get focused on indirect costs, particularly administrative overhead, and it may be difficult to engage them in a candid discussion about resource utilization and practice variations.

Lesson 3

Make sure that data is severity-adjusted and that you understand the methodology of this adjustment. You may want your finance department or statistician to assist you with the explanation.

Lesson 4

When presenting cost or resource utilization data to physicians, sort the data into meaningful diagnostic categories, such as by ICD-9 code or other meaningful diagnostic sorts. Often, sorting by DRG is too broad a diagnostic category to be meaningful. For example, DRG 209 includes total hip and total knee replacement surgeries. Although the care processes are similar, they are different enough to warrant an analysis of resource utilization and thus identification of cost-saving opportunities separately. Remember also that benchmarking data is not perfect and cannot give you the specificity that you need to understand the differences in practice patterns by each cost bucket in other organizations. Use the drill-down method of your own internal data to understand resource utilization by buckets that are unique to your organization. Be aware that some inaccuracy in the external benchmark cost bucket analysis (e.g., operating room, therapy) may exist as a result of how those organizations define and assign items to those various cost categories.

Lesson 5

The most important and final lesson learned is that this process must be driven and supported by physicians. They must actively participate in the process and believe in the integrity of the data. Without physician support, the case manager's ability to decrease cost savings will be severely impeded. The case manager will find this process laborious and frustrating and may see it only as a means or requirement to satisfy administration instead of a way to improve the cost-efficiency and quality of patient care.

CASE MANAGERS IMPROVE CLINICAL OUTCOMES

Clinical outcomes provide valuable guidance to patients, purchasers, and providers of healthcare. Outcomes management can improve the effectiveness and efficiency of clinical care and demonstrate value to the marketplace if designed and implemented successfully. To be successful in the management of clinical outcomes, case managers must link the processes of care to the outcomes and manage the processes of care to improve or maintain the desired outcome. Because healthcare involves a broad complex combination of processes that produce an array of interrelated outcomes, this task is not as direct or simple as measuring cost outcomes.

In healthcare, *clinical outcomes* are defined and measured in a variety of ways. Clinical status measures are usually defined as objective clinical measures. Some examples of clinical status measures include the following: (1) percentage of arterial blockage as measured by angiogram, (2) ejection fraction results, (3) blood pressure or pulse oximetery readings, (4) presence or absence of physiological signs and symptoms such as chest pain, (5) shortness of breath, and (6) complications after surgery or a diagnostic procedure, such as bleeding, renal failure, or stroke.

Functional status outcomes focus on the patient's ability to perform normal activities and social roles. They are measured using a combination of objective measures and patient self-report measures. Examples include limitations in usual role activities such as working, activities of daily living, or instrumental activities of daily living.

Quality of life outcomes include the patient's overall sense of well-being. Often these are measured as self-reported satisfaction, feelings, and perceptions related to the patient's condition. Examples may include level of pain, feelings of anxiety, levels of energy or fatigue, and risk of depression.

There are a variety of standardized outcome tools that are emerging to measure functional status and quality of life measures. One of the most widely used tools is the SF-36 Health Survey developed by Dr. Robert Ware in 1991 and available through the Health Institute at New England Medical Center (Ware, 1993). Another excellent reference for the case manager is a text by Lorig et al, *Outcome Measures for Health Education and Other Health Care Interventions* (1996).

Some measures that are collected and reported as clinical outcomes fall into a "gray area" that is mostly process-based. Examples of these type of process measures include the following: (1) access measures that provide data about how easy it is for a patient to gain access to medical services, (2) appropriateness measures that reflect whether a provider is providing care beyond what would be considered necessary, and (3) compliance measures that provide data on patient compliance to the treatment plan.

Although it is important to understand the various types of clinical measures, the success of the case manager lies in incorporating all categories of these outcomes measures into the outcomes management plan.

First Steps

The first step for the case manager, in collaboration with the healthcare team, is to define the patient population to be measured. For example, you may want to limit your outcome measurement to patients diagnosed with CHF, CHF patients classified as Class IV severity according to the New York Heart Classification, or those patients who have been hospitalized within the last year and have an ejection fraction of <25%. Because one purpose of your outcome data is to evaluate and improve clinical performance, you need to understand and define risk factors associated with the defined population. The case manager should work collaboratively with a statistician to appropriately aggregate the defined population from the database, which is essential to providing clinical outcome risk-adjusted data to the physicians and others in the organization.

It is generally better to start with broad general clinical outcome measures and as required, based on the data findings, complete a more focused detailed study. However, caution should be taken not to be so broad that the measure will lose value and meaning to the physicians and other providers. Start by brainstorming a list of potential outcome measures. You may want to start with the outcome and then work backward, identifying the milestones or clinical processes that are important to the achievement of that particular outcome. Some examples of broad general outcomes for the CHF population include the following: (1) patients who develop complications such as pulmonary edema or atrial fibrillation while hospitalized, (2) readmission within 30 days of hospitalization, (3) deterioration in self-reported physical functioning, and (4) use of calcium channel blockers by physicians. Consideration may also be given to using the Minnesota Living with Heart Failure Questionnaire as a measure of quality of life outcomes (University of Minnesota, 1994). Figure 23-7 provides an example of amputation as an outcome measure that incorporates the processes of care for a diabetic patient population.

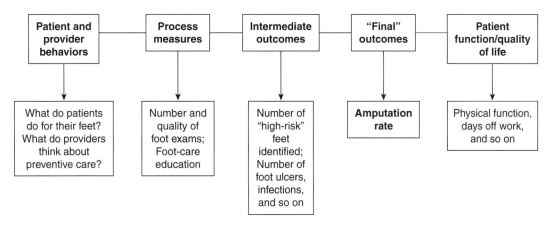

Figure 23-7 Linking process and outcomes.

Measuring Variations in Outcomes

To effectively impact clinical outcomes, case managers must be knowledgeable and competent in analysis of the variations in clinical processes and outcomes. There are two types of variations. *Common cause variation* often is described as statistically predictable variation that is uncontrollable and often caused by chance. *Special cause variation* is controllable and may be the result of system or human factors (Berwick, 1991). One of the roles of the case manager is to monitor, analyze, and reduce special cause variation through coordination of care and continuous quality improvement strategies.

There are three sources of special cause variation: operational, patient, and practitioner. Operational variation includes system issues within the organization or healthcare setting. Examples include documentation problems, nursing shortage, physical distance of the catheterization laboratory to the operating room, and unclear lines of communication.

Patient variations are patient-specific factors that could potentially impact the outcomes or processes of care. They are the risk factors identified during the process of selecting and defining your population for measurement. Some examples of patient variations include severity of illness, comorbidities, cognitive ability, and compliance to treatment plan. Practitioner variation is the result of judgment and technique of the practitioner. Some examples are omissions, errors, and delays.

Lessons Learned: Clinical Outcome Measurement
Lesson 1

Clinical outcome measures are often not available from a single data source or information system. Case managers will be involved in interfacing with a variety of data sources, such as quality management and utilization management systems, order entry systems, pharmacy or laboratory systems, and even manual methods of retrieving clinical outcome data.

Lesson 2

It is key that the selection of the clinical outcome measurements is the vital few versus the insignificant many. With a variety of methodologies to collect data also come a variety of data integrity risks. For each clinical outcome measure ensure the following: (1) clear concise definition of the measure, (2) define the methodology for calculating the results (e.g., for rate results, define the numerator and denominator), (3) the defined threshold and the source of that threshold, (4) the data source, (5) responsible party, (6) collection frequency, and (7) reporting frequency.

Lesson 3

Integrate the clinical outcome data associated with the case management program with the organization's continuous quality improvement program. These clinical outcome data may also be used to meet regulatory requirements, such as HEDIS or JCAHO. If this process is viewed as separate from quality improvement programs, it may not be given the level of support and resources required to successfully implement clinical outcomes measurement as part of the case management program.

Lesson 4

The use of a statistician in developing risk-adjusted models for each indicator and comparing risk-adjusted clinical outcomes is essential to change physician and other provider care processes.

Lesson 5

Clinical outcome measurements such as cost measurements must be driven and supported by physicians. They must actively participate in defining and analyzing the clinical outcomes data.

CASE MANAGERS IMPROVE SERVICE AND SATISFACTION OUTCOMES

Frequently, service and satisfaction outcomes are included within the clinical outcome measures of an organization. Regardless of where these measures are placed, it is important to understand the needs of and measure patient and family, provider, and payer satisfaction with care or services. Many organizations outsource their patient satisfaction survey. Generally the satisfaction data collected by this method may not have significant volume of the particular case management population or be timely and specific enough for clinicians to value. Organizations often do not use patient satisfaction information as regular feedback to administrative and clinical departments.

Patient, provider, and payer satisfaction are each affected through the processes of case management and as such should be measured and reported in the same fashion as cost and clinical outcome measures. Today payers and providers negotiate contracts that include satisfaction with care and services as part of the performance measures. Figure 23-8 provides an example of a report card that integrates quality outcomes and patient satisfaction.

Cardiovascular Surgeon/Case Manager Services Quality Scorecard

Outcome Measures	Criteria	Threshold	Results			
			Q1	Q2	Q3	Q4
Service quality						
	Improve 1½ standard deviation on 7 key questions					
	Improve 1 standard deviation on 7 key questions					
	Improve ½ standard deviation on 7 key questions					
	Meet minimum value of ___ on 7 key questions					
	Below minimum threshold value of ___					
Quality outcomes						
	Inpatient mortality after major cardiovascular surgery (DRG 104, 105, 106, 107, 108, 110, 111)	**Not to exceed:** 4.9%				
	OR complication: reop/bleeding CABG only Valve replacement only	**Not to exceed:** 0.43% 5.4%				
	OR complication: infection deep sternum CABG only Valve replacement only	**Not to exceed:** 0.9% 0.5%				
	OR complication: renal failure CABG only Valve replacement only	**Not to exceed:** 1.2% 1.6%				
	Percent of inpatients with lipid profile (ICD-9 diagnosis code of AMI/unstable angina)	50%				
	Percent of patients discharged on a β-blocker (ICD-9 diagnosis code of all AMI)	50%				

Figure 23-8   Satisfaction and quality report card.

There is no one standardized universally accepted patient satisfaction tool. Some organizations are adapting tools already in place in their organization to fit the particular patient population or focus of satisfaction. Others are using standardized or customized satisfaction survey tools from a variety of vendors, such as the Picker Institute's (2001) survey instrument. The Picker Institute's survey instrument focuses on questions related to access to care, respect for patient's values, communication between provider and patient, coordination and integration of care, and involvement of family and friends or significant others in the process of care.

Case managers interested in assessing patients' satisfaction with case management may consider questions including case manager competence, technical abilities, coordination of services, communication, accessibility, responsiveness, and knowledge of resources. There is a belief that what patients experience impact on the benefit of the medical or healthcare intervention. An example of the importance of patient experiences on outcomes is evident at a regional hospital in central Massachusetts that noted that reduced wait times for women with positive mammograms cut patient anxiety and improved cure rates (Larkin, 1998).

SUMMARY

Although case management has been in existence and practiced for quite some time, never before has there been such an impetus to demonstrate value through quantitative and qualitative measurement. The literature is beginning to consistently demonstrate that case managers reduce cost of care, enhance clinical outcomes, and improve patient, provider, and payer satisfaction with care and services. Case management is also contributing to the literature in evidence-based practice. As case managers continue to mature in their role of evaluating patient care and continue to develop sophistication in evaluation methodologies, they will strengthen their presence in healthcare for the next millennium. There is no doubt that case management will be an integral part of managed care strategies and, as a healthcare profession, will be a significant player in shaping future healthcare systems.

REFERENCES

Aubert R, Herman W, Water J, et al: Nurse case management to improve glycemic control in diabetic patients in a health maintenance organization: a randomized, controlled trial, *Ann Intern Med* 129(8):605-612, 1998.

Berwick D: Controlling variation in healthcare, *Med Care* 29(12):1212-1225, 1991.

Doyle RL, Schibanoff JM: *Healthcare management guidelines for inpatient and surgical care,* New York, 2001, Milliman & Robertson.

Health Plan Employer Data and Information Set: Annapolis Junction, Md, 1998, National Committee for Quality Assurance Publication Center, Available online: http://www.ncqa.org.

Health Care Advisory Board: *Outcomes strategy: measurement of hospital quality under reform,* vol 1, Washington, DC, 1993, The Advisory Board Company.

Joint Commission on Accreditation of Healthcare Organizations: *ORYX/performance measurement requirements for healthcare organizations,* January 1997, Available online: http://www.jcaho.org.

Kongstvedt PR: Using data in medical management. In Kongstvedt PR, Plocher DW, editors: *Best practices in medical management,* Gaithersburg, Md, 1998a, Aspen.

Kongstvedt PR, Plocher DW: Provider profiling. In Kongstvedt PR, Plocher DW, editors: *Best practices in medical management,* Gaithersburg, Md, 1998b, Aspen.

Larkin H: It serves you right: hassle-free healthcare builds loyalty, volume—and the bottom line, *Hosp Health Netw* 72(23-24):38-40, 1998.

Lorig S, Ritter G, Stewart A, et al: *Outcome measures for health education and other health care interventions,* Thousand Oaks, Calif, 1996, Sage.

Picker Institute: *Improving healthcare through the patient's eyes,* Boston, 2001, Picker Institute, Available online: http://www.harvard.edu/picker.org.

Pine M: Introduction to the measurement of clinical outcomes. In Kongstvedt PR, Plocher DW, editors: *Best practices in medical management,* Gaithersburg, Md, 1998, Aspen.

University of Minnesota: *Minnesota Living with Heart Failure Questionnaire,* Minneapolis, 1994.

Ware J: *SF-36 health survey: manual and interpretation guide,* Boston, 1993, Health Institute at the New England Medical Center, Available online: http://www.sf-36.com.

24

Disease Management in Managed Care

Donna Zazworsky

KEY LESSONS IN THIS CHAPTER

■ Although many definitions of disease management exist, in essence, disease management attempts to minimize costs and maximize resource utilization through a carefully scripted process-oriented approach.

■ The four essential elements of disease management are: (1) clinical management, (2) behavior modification, (3) information management, and (4) outcomes management.

■ A variety of risk assessment strategies exist that allow the practitioner to categorize the patient's level of risk based on the known risk elements related to their disease.

■ Evidence-based guidelines are a must in any disease management program.

■ Nurses must demonstrate their value in disease management programs and can do so through documentation of clinical, financial, and quality patient outcomes.

Disease management (DM) is not a new concept to healthcare. Providers have been delivering DM services for decades through targeted programs, such as diabetes self-care management clinics, cardiac rehabilitation services, and asthma programs.

Today, however, with the continued evolution of managed care, these episodically geared programs are not enough to meet the needs of a continuum-driven model. The focus must be systematic and integrated. Thus *disease management* becomes a new term with the intention to refocus providers toward the best practice framework with demonstrated structure, process, and outcomes for a defined population.

This chapter discusses theoretical models, identifies essential elements, and explores approaches of DM programs in managed care environments.

DEFINITIONS AND GOALS

DM has carried a variety of definitions. Plocher defines DM as:

a prospective disease-specific approach to delivering health care spanning all encounter sites and augmenting the physician's visits with interim management by non-physician practitioners specializing in the target disease. Disease management redirects intervention efforts for identified chronic disorders to the outpatient setting and compiles information from all sites of care for each patient with that disorder into a single longitudinal record (Plocher, 1996, p 318).

Zander ties DM to case management by stating:

DM is a method that attempts to conceptually and operationally organize care, essentially care of the chronically ill people, to achieve lower costs yet optimal clinical outcomes. DM is actually case management on the continuum level, with emphasis on prevention, and reduction of risk of exacerbation, hospitalization and further functional decline (Zander, 1997, p 86).

In essence, DM attempts to minimize costs and maximize resource utilization through a carefully scripted, process-oriented approach. Ultimately, DM aims to accomplish the following goals (Lamb, Mahn, and Dahl, 1996):
- Early identification of individuals likely to use extensive high-cost services
- Timely coordination and initiation of alternatives and the less expensive services, including primary care and community-based programs.
- Improvement or slowed decline in functional independence and quality of life
- Reduction in avoidable complications
- Reduction in avoidable hospitalizations and emergency department (ED) visits

THEORETICAL MODELS

Although the term *disease management* implies a reactive approach to health and wellness, an in-depth discussion on current models infers a proactive methodology when applied to a managed care population.

Population-Based Health Management Model

Peterson and Kane (1998) discuss a population-based health management model developed by the Hastings Healthcare Group that encompasses the following components:
- Acute care
- DM
- Risk minimization

In this model, the importance of linking health status, risk, and severity data with clinical and economic outcomes to determine predictors of health, disability, illness, disease complications, and probability of eventual outcome are critical for successful population management (Todd and Nash, 1998). Using this premise, the model encourages providers to embrace tools to target high-risk groups within each component and direct care accordingly.

For example, this model illustrates that when individuals within the population are in an acute care episode, the focus must be on disease-specific complication management such as an individual with Class 3 or 4 congestive heart failure (CHF) (as defined by the New York American Heart Association [NYHA] Guidelines). In this case, providers follow specific medical protocols to reduce the severity of acute symptoms (AHCPR, 1994).

When these individuals are stabilized, the focus then shifts to DM strategies that reduce the person's level of risk and the possibility of future acute episodes. Such strategies may include cardiac rehabilitation, nutrition counseling, and telephonic case management. Telephonic case management uses telephone or online interactions with patients to conduct brief assessments, monitor patient progress toward expected outcomes, and direct the patient as necessary.

Ultimately, risk minimization is the goal of any population-based strategy. The most common modalities for accomplishing this goal are through disease prevention and health promotion applications. Many managed care organizations (MCOs) support these applications through health screenings and patient education vehicles such as public seminars and calendars.

Figure 24-1 illustrates the dynamic interactions between the interdisciplinary team and DM interventions.

Chronic Illness Model

Lamb and Zazworsky (2000) approach a population health management strategy through an integrated chronic illness model. In this model, a continuum approach that integrates providers, services, and community with DM methodologies is used. Conceptually similar to the Hastings Population-Based Health Management Model, this model demonstrates the need to do the following:

- Focus on risk assessment and risk stratification
- Use appropriate medical and self-care treatment according to risk
- Monitor/track changes in risk status and outcomes

Lamb and Zazworsky (2000) operationalized this model by developing the FAST Approach to DM, discussed later in this chapter.

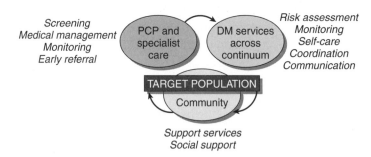

Figure 24-1 Integrated chronic illness care. (From Lamb GS, Zazworsky D: *Advance for Providers of Post-Acute Care* 3(11):28-29, 2000.)

ELEMENTS OF DISEASE MANAGEMENT

Eichert and Patterson (1998) describe the following four essential elements necessary for a systematic and integrated DM program:

- Clinical management
- Behavior modification
- Information management
- Outcomes management

Clinical Management

Within a clinical management system, certain tools are essential to implement a DM program. As illustrated in the previous models, the management of health depends on the health status, risk level, and severity of illness. Therefore the following three issues need to be addressed in this element:

- Risk assessment
- Evidence-based guidelines
- Documentation

To Risk Assess or Not to Risk Assess: That is the Question

DM programs usually (but not always) are directed at subgroups within a defined population. How does the MCO identify which subgroups need to be targeted? The answer depends on what the organizational goals and needs are. In other words, are the MCO's goals to:

- Meet regulatory requirements set forth by the Health Plan Employer Data and Information Set (HEDIS), the National Committee for Quality Assurance (NCQA), or Medicare?
- Reduce costs/losses?
- Improve clinical outcomes for better contracting potential?

Goals can be addressed through a number of different DM venues that may or may not require a risk assessment strategy. It is important, however, to obtain key stakeholder input and agreement on the structure, process, and outcomes of each DM program. These key stakeholders can be the chief financial officer, marketing and contracts, the medical director, and key MCO users/buyers.

Risk Assessment

Risk assessment becomes an essential tool when an organization must target resources more cost-effectively. In other words, the goal is resource allocation—making sure that patients are matched with the right service, at the right time, with the right provider, for the right cost.

For example, under Health Care Financing Administration (HCFA) guidelines, an MCO is mandated to provide DM programs in order to be a Medicare-risk provider. Specific diseases, such as CHF, a high-cost subgroup most commonly targeted within a Medicare risk population, is commonly targeted because of the high hospital readmission rates associated with the disease. The cost-benefit ratio of implementing a DM program for CHF has been successfully demonstrated many times (Venner and Seelbinder, 1996; Harrison, Toman, and Logan, 1998). A cost-benefit analysis may require a return on investment within the first year of implementation.

With appropriate and targeted risk assessment and stratification methods, high-risk patients with CHF are placed into a telemanagement/case management program. Such programs have been proven to reduce hospital readmissions (Venner and Seelbinder, 1996).

In another scenario, an MCO may be focused on commercial or Medicaid groups and is usually accountable for HEDIS and NCQA data. In this case, expected outcomes may include measuring and reporting outcomes related to clinical performance and member satisfaction. For example, if diabetic patients are targeted, identifying diabetes risk may not be the goal. Instead, diabetes compliance to annual retinopathy exams may be the preferred DM expected outcome. Programs to increase member compliance are usually implemented at the MCO plan level and directed toward all members with diabetes.

The Health Plan of the Upper Ohio Valley (UOV), a not-for-profit regional health maintenance organization (HMO), implemented a program early in 1998 that provided a simple coupon for an annual dilated retinal eye examination with an in-plan ophthalmologist. With this coupon, members were able to schedule an appointment with an eye specialist without a referral from the primary care physician. The coupon also waived any existing copayment usually required with this outpatient visit. In 1997 the percent of commercial members having a dilated eye exam performed was already high at 75.5%. This HEDIS measure increased to 80.5% for the same commercial population in 1998, the first year of the coupon program. The 1999 examination rate was 80.9%. The performance rate in the commercial population increased 5.4 percentage points from the 1997 baseline. The same HEDIS measure in the plan's Medicare population identified a baseline eye examination rate of 86.02% in 1997, 91.5% in 1998, and 88.12% in 1999. The performance rate in the Medicare population increased 2.10 percentage points from the 1997 baseline. The coupon program for eye examinations in the plan's diabetic population was the first integrated effort between the member, the primary care physician, and the ophthalmologist to screen for and monitor diabetes-related eye disease. The Health Plan UOV believes this effort may have also positively affected the rates of Hb A_{1c} and low-density lipoprotein cholesterol (LDLC) testing (Parsons, 2000).

Risk for What?—Selecting a Risk Assessment Tool

After determining that a specific DM program should include a risk assessment strategy, an appropriate risk tool and methodology must be selected. The organization must ask what type of risk it is assessing, or "Risk for What?" Answering this question is the backbone of the DM process. Therefore once key stakeholders have determined what the program goals are, the question of "Risk for What" should have also been answered. For example, if the program is to reduce the incidence of anemia in renal failure patients, risk assessment should focus on the risk for anemia.

Risk assessment tools are primarily divided into three types of risk:

- General
- Disease-specific
- Combined

General risk can be viewed as addressing the population or subpopulation (disease-specific) as a whole. For example, an MCO might review its Medicare group and ask the question, "Who is at greatest risk for hospitalizations or mortality?" Disease-specific risk addresses elements specific to the chronic illness in question. Finally, an organization might decide to use a combination of both.

Generic Tools

There are a number of risk assessment tools readily available to organizations, including the following:

- *PRA Plus:* The Probability for ReAdmissions Plus (Boult, Pacala, and Boult, 1995) is a predictive tool developed to identify seniors who are at risk for hospitalizations and uses elements that are based on the individual's perception of his or her health and how he or she is managing. This tool can be helpful for a general senior population or used in combination with other disease-specific tools to provide a more in-depth perspective of a particular subgroup such as patients with CHF.

- *SF-36:* The SF-36 Health Survey (Ware et al, 1993) is a generic measure that assesses health concepts that represent basic human values that are relevant to everyone's functional status and well-being. These generic health measures include health-related quality of life outcomes and are not age-, disease-, or treatment-specific. The instrument includes the following eight health concepts: (1) physical functioning, (2) role limitations due to physical health problems, (3) bodily pain, (4) general health, (5) vitality (energy/fatigue), (6) social functioning, (7) role limitations due to emotional problems, and (8) mental health (psychological distress and psychological well-being).

- *SF-12:* The SF-12 Health Survey (Ware et al, 1993) is a shortened version of the SF-36 and contains 12 instead of 36 health-related quality of life questions. It is applied to a population rather than to a subset.

- *Community Assessment Risk Screen (CARS):* Developed by the Coordinated Care Services of Carle Clinic Association, a statewide preferred provider organization in Urbana, Illinois and the Alzheimer's Institute of the University of Wisconsin–Madison Medical School in Madison, Wisconsin, the CARS tool identifies community dwelling elderly patients at increased risk for hospitalizations and ED encounters (Shelton, Sager, and Schraeder, 2000). This simple tool assesses health conditions, prescription medications, hospitalization, and ED/urgent care utilization.

Disease-Specific Tools

Disease-specific risk assessment tools look at the elements that place an individual at a greater level of disease severity. The following are two examples of disease-specific classifications:

1. *NYHA Classification* (Goldman et al, 1981)
   - Class I: Patients with cardiac disease but without resulting limitations of physical activity. Ordinary physical activity does not cause undue fatigue, palpitation, dyspnea, or anginal pain.
   - Class II: Patients with cardiac disease resulting in slight limitation of physical activity. Patients are comfortable at rest. Ordinary physical activity results in fatigue, palpitation, dyspnea, or anginal pain.
   - Class III: Patients with cardiac disease resulting in marked limitation of physical activity. Patients are comfortable at rest. Less than ordinary physical activity causes fatigue, dyspnea, or anginal pain.
   - Class IV: Patients with cardiac disease resulting in inability to carry out any physical activity without discomfort. Symptoms of cardiac insufficiency or of the anginal syndrome may be present even at rest. If any physical activity is undertaken, discomfort is increased.

2. *Chronic Obstructive Pulmonary Disease Grading* (Wedsicha et al, 1998)
   - Grade 1 or 2: Are you short of breath with strenuous exercise or when hurrying?
   - Grade 3: Walk slower than people of the same age on the same level or stop for breath while walking at own pace on the level.
   - Grade 4: Stop for breath after 100 yards or after a few minutes on the level.
   - Grade 5: Too breathless to leave the house.

Finally, combination risk assessments bring together known risk elements related to the disease. For example, diabetes risk is a combination of physiological (e.g., Hb A_{1c}, cardiovascular, renal, eye) and psychological (e.g., depression).

Another example is the Minimal Record of Disability Tool (National Multiple Sclerosis Society, 1985) used for people with multiple sclerosis. This standardized tool incorporates a neurological examination and questionnaires that trained interviewers ask face-to-face, recording results as direct answers or observations. Scores provide an overall status of the individual's level of disability with multiple sclerosis.

It is important to note that validity and reliability issues require consideration when choosing a risk assessment tool. The validity and reliability of the instrument should be well researched and confirmed before putting it into use. If the organization decides to design or combine tools, key stakeholders must be included in the process to ensure acceptance of the eventual outcomes.

Risk Methodology

Chart audits, interviews, and surveys (mail, telephone, face-to-face) are common examples of obtaining risk assessment information. In some cases, a combination of chart audits and interviews may be chosen. Each methodology brings its own benefits and barriers that need to be considered before finalizing a risk assessment tool and process.

Chart Audits. Chart audits can be complex and time consuming. Depending on the information to be collected, the following questions should be posed:

1. Does the information need to be collected by a trained health professional, such as an RN, physical therapist, or physician?
2. Is there a catalogue of terms that needs to be defined and approved before the audit? Who needs to approve it?
3. Who will pay for the audit? Is there outside funding sources/grants to assist with the funding?
4. Is the data going to be entered into a database? Who will perform data entry?

A pilot audit will prove beneficial to set targets for individual audits and track audit performance.

Interviews and Surveys. Interviews and surveys are another method for completing a risk assessment. Choosing which interview/survey method best fits the DM program, however, requires careful consideration. Surveys and interviews can be done by telephone, face-to-face, or by mail. The likelihood of compliance with any of these methods needs to be carefully weighed and considered.

If the MCO wants to take a broad population-based focus of its Medicare-risk enrollees, then mailing the SF-12 or the CARS annually to these members will be appropriate. The downfall issues are that return rates vary and do not reflect a random selection—which may not be representative of the population. The plan may use aggregate information to develop further programs and mail patient data directly to the providers. What the provider does with this information is unknown.

Some MCOs will use this information to target case management efforts, but again, it only addresses the group who completed the surveys.

Health Risk Appraisals. Health risk appraisals (HRAs) can be used with many different populations (Box 24-1). These appraisals are health promotion oriented and focus on potential risk for health problems such as diabetes, heart disease, cancer, and depression. They are popular with employer groups and many times are coupled with health screening, which may include blood pressure, heart rate, fitness testing, blood glucose, and lipid panel.

Key benefits of an HRA are that the individual report is proactive and can motivate individuals to change risky behaviors. Aggregate reports can guide employers to provide health education and self-care programs for the employees.

The pitfalls relate to employee participation, or lack of participation, and questionnaire subjectivity. In other words, are participants answering questions honestly?

Telephone Interviews. Telephone interviews require a special skill. Not only does the interviewer need to get the person to agree to answer the questions, but the questions must be asked consistently in the same way to reduce bias. Finally, the interviewer must be skilled to keep the conversation focused and avoid side conversations.

Telephone interviews work well with senior populations but not with the working population. Another thing to keep in mind is the technology of Caller ID, telephone blocks, and answering machines. All are vehicles to maintain privacy.

BOX 24-1
Health Promotion Case Study

A local school district approaches your healthcare organization to discuss the opportunity to provide an employee wellness program. As the manager of community services, you are contacted to meet with the school superintendent, the school nurse manager, the business manager, and the health plan representative.

At the initial meeting, the general discussion focuses on the desire to maintain the current health insurance plan, which is a self-funded program using a preferred provider organization (PPO) network. One component of the plan provides a $200 wellness benefit to cover an annual wellness physical examination, respective laboratory work, and a mammogram.

The school district is concerned because its monthly insurance premiums continue to increase annually due to outliers (employees or family members with high medical costs), yet the use of the wellness benefit is low. Therefore the school district is interested in establishing a proactive approach to control annual premium increases.

The school district and the healthcare organization begin to develop an agreement to manage the employee health through a comprehensive wellness program. The employee wellness program was voluntary and consisted of the following components:

- A comprehensive health risk appraisal (HRA) and group interpretation
- High-risk telephone follow-up
- Discounted annual physicals, laboratory, and screening mammograms
- Health education

The program was approved by the school board and implemented in all schools over a 3-month period. In Year 1, over 73% of the employees participated in the HRA program, with all high-risk individuals being notified either by telephone or letter. All participants were satisfied with the HRA program. The school board approved the program, which consisted of health education classes and the HRA, for Year 2.

The school district implemented the health education component in Year 2, with 80% of the schools participating in the group education classes. The HRA was administered again in Year 2 with approximately 20% participation—a dramatic decrease. Most people felt that one year was too soon to answer the HRA again.

Utilization of the physical examination benefit was still low and difficult to track. The school district continued to experience another annual premium increase. The discussion is now shifting to case management of the high-risk individuals and implementation of an employee assistance program.

Cost: $1500/year for HRA program, includes telephone follow-up
$100/health education class
Revenue: new referrals into medical group and diabetes program

---

The following are some helpful hints for conducting telephone surveys:

- Provide a script (Box 24-2).
- Train the interviewer and monitor initial and random calls thereafter.
- Establish a time frame for calls and have the callers keep a log to determine outliers.
- Track the rate of refusals.

Claims Data. Claims data is an easy method to get at targeted groups. Diagnosis-related groups (DRGs) and ICD-9 codes or other parameters, depending on the organization's database systems, can obtain this information. Some of the pitfalls, however, can be complex and time-consuming. Turnaround time for obtaining the data, cleaning the data of disenrollments or deaths, and integrating systems to reflect costs are common frustrations for DM programs.

BOX 24-2
Telephone Survey Script Example: Congestive Heart Failure Script

Introduction
Good morning (afternoon). My name is _____. I am a nurse from _____.
   I'm calling people who used one of our services in the past year. I would like to find out how you're doing and to offer you some new programs that you might find helpful. There is no cost to you.
   Would you have a few minutes to talk to me? This will all be confidential.

If No:
Would you be willing to arrange a time that I could call you back?

If Yes: Proceed
I'd like to ask you some questions about your health.

Proceed with Risk Assessment
Thank you for answering these questions. I will call you back _____ to let you know which service will best meet your needs.

Calculate Risk Score
Call Back: Follow decision tree for low, moderate, and high risk.
   Based on your answers, I recommend that you:

If Low:
Attend a class on congestive heart failure. I can schedule you on (date)_____.

If Moderate:
See a nurse at one of the community health centers. Here is a list; which is closest to you? I can schedule you for _____.

(If Unable to Get to a Community Health Center):
Can I help you with transportation? I will give your name to the volunteer specialist to help arrange a ride for you.

If High:
A nurse case manager will be calling you to set up a home visit.

Evidence-Based Guidelines

Evidence-based guidelines are a must in any DM program. They are an important and fundamental tool for establishing continuity and quality of care. Guidelines provide a map for care delivery that has been proven through acceptable research techniques. Guidelines are available through associations such as the American Diabetes Association, the American Heart Association, or the Agency for Health Care Policy and Research (AHCPR). An example of a guideline for community-acquired pneumonia is illustrated in Figure 24-2.

   Locating guidelines is not the issue, however. The greatest barrier to guideline implementation is adapting guidelines into multidisciplinary practices and measuring them, which is further complicated by multiple provider settings. For example, following a DM guideline in a hospital setting can be accomplished by establishing protocols and following

Clinical Practice Guideline **ADULT INPATIENT MANAGEMENT OF** **COMMUNITY-ACQUIRED PNEUMONIA**	
Purpose	• Initial selection of antibiotics • Conversion of intravenous to oral antibiotics • Appropriate use of chest radiography
Treatment/ management This guideline reflects expert opinion nationally (ATS) and locally regarding the *initial* management of patients hospitalized for community-acquired pneumonia (CAP). It may not be applicable for all patients with CAP, particularly those with certain risk factors, such as HIV, aspiration, and substance/alcohol abuse. See reverse side for additional references.	**Less severe pneumonia** • Initial intravenous antibiotics choices: 　- Cefuroxime (and erythromycin if *Mycoplasma*, *Legionella*, or *Chlamydia* suspected) 　- Alternative for penicillin-allergic patients: trimethoprin/sulfamethoxazole (Bactrim) +/− erythromycin. **Severe pneumonia** Define as one or more of the following: 1. Respiratory rate >30/min 2. Pao$_2$ (room air) <60 or Sao$_2$ (room air) <91% 3. Mechanical ventilation required 4. Bilateral/multiple lobe involvement 5. Increasing infiltrate by >50% in 48 hours 6. Presence of shock • Initial intravenous antibiotic choices: 　- Ceftazidime or ticarcillin/clavulanate **AND** erythromycin 　- Alternative for penicillin-allergic patients: aztreonam (Azactam) may be substituted for ceftazidime or tacarcillin/clavulanate ***Convert from intravenous to oral antibiotics when:*** 1. Two consecutive oral temperature readings of <100 °F are obtained at least 8 hours apart in the absence of antipyretics 2. Decrease in leukocytosis to <12,000 3. Improved pulmonary signs/symptoms 4. Able to tolerate oral medications *Note: This usually occurs in first 24 to 72 hours of hospitalization in less severe pneumonia* *Note: Chest radiography within the first week on an improving patient is not necessary because the radiography findings typically lag behind the clinical picture.*

Oral Conversion Alternatives		
Intravenous		**Oral**
Erythromycin	**To**	Erythromycin or doxycycline Alternative for erythromycin/doxycycline intolerant patients: Clarithromycin (Biaxin) or Azithromycin (Zithromax)
Cefuroxime or timentin		Cefuroxime (Ceftin) or trimethoprim/ sulfamethoxazole (Bactrim)
Ceftazidime		Cefuroxime (Ceftin) or ciprofloxacin (Cipro)
Ciprofloxacin		Ciprofloxacin (Cipro)
Indications for discharge	Discharge may occur simultaneously or up to 24 hours of switch to oral antibiotics providing no deterioration or other reason for continued hospitalization.	

Figure 24-2　Sample clinical practice guidelines. (From Toni G. Cesta, Case Manager Solutions, LLC, Tucson, Arizona, 1999.)

the patient's progress through a critical pathway or by a multidisciplinary action plan (MAP). In this situation, hospital case managers can track variances and report accordingly.

On the other hand, in provider offices or community clinics, guidelines are turned into flowcharts that are many times used as checklists only. These do not reflect clinical outcomes; rather, they just illustrate clinical practice patterns. Unless the offices and clinics set up clinical protocol flow charts that require recording of real data and DM tracking systems, evidence-based guidelines will only offer limited demonstration of best practice. The key to success is simplicity. An example of a single, easy-to-use guideline is illustrated in Figure 24-3. This guideline was developed for use in a clinic setting to manage uninsured diabetics.

Documentation Methods

Documentation systems for DM offer challenges for individual and multidisciplinary provider settings. Flow charts for clinical protocols and patient education can be included in a patient's chart and operate under the documentation by exception rule (Cesta, Tahan, and Fink, 1997).

Another documentation need is to capture change in individual and group knowledge, behavior, and health status. The Omaha Documentation System (Martin, Leak, and Aden, 1992) offers an excellent vehicle to reflect changes on an interval-determined basis and has been shown to have interrater reliability and validity. Many home health and community nursing practices have adopted this system as their documentation system, and most nursing schools teach this system in their community health nursing courses.

Unfortunately, this system has remained limited to these nursing settings and has not become a common language within other disciplines or clinical settings. Therefore obtaining information on knowledge, behavior, and health status requires separate measurements.

Behavior Modification

Another element of a DM program is helping patients and staff members use specific methods to modify behavior and facilitate changes that will reduce complications or prevent further deterioration. Although many providers offer patient education, it is important to understand what helps people want to change their risky behaviors. These complexities entwine concepts such as culture, perceptions, knowledge, readiness, and value.

These concepts require an in-depth analysis of several theoretical models and how to best apply them to certain DM behaviors. The Health Belief Model (Becker, 1974) offers a theoretical framework to better understand individual behaviors and motivations for change. In this model, the health educator identifies the individual's perceptions through their perceptions of susceptibility and seriousness of the illness. For example, if the health educator wants to teach an individual to perform monthly breast self-examinations, then it is important to know if the individual identifies a strong desire to practice this behavior. In other words, if the participant has had a mother with breast cancer (high susceptibility) and had a mastectomy (high seriousness), then the individual may be more likely to see the importance of the practice of monthly breast self-examinations.

Cues to action are related to socioeconomic status, education level, family influence, and media influence. These cues will vary in importance, depending on culture and beliefs.

Diabetes Quality Indicators: Clinical

St. Elizabeth of Hungary Clinic
140 W. Speedway Blvd
Tucson, AZ 85705-7698
(520) 628-7871

Patient: _____ DOB: _____

MR# _____ Provider: _____

Date/Initials		Frequency	Baseline	3 mo	6 mo	9 mo	1 year
Assessment FS blood glucose	R or F	q visit					
Hb A_{1c}		quarterly					
Blood pressure ≤130/80		q visit					
Urine protein dip		Annual					
Height		Annual					
Weight		q visit					
Body mass index (BMI)		q visit					
Lab Chol/TG <200/200		Annual					
HDL/LDL >45/<100		Annual					
Micro protein (If protein dip negative)		Annual					
BUN/creatinine		Annual					
Interventions Oral agents	Y or N	q visit					
Insulin	Y or N	q visit					
ACE inhibitor if hypertensive	Y or N	q visit					
ACE inhibitor if proteinuric	Y or N	q visit					
Statin	Y or N	q visit					
ASA	Y or N	q visit					
Vaccines Specify (flu, pneumonia, etc.)		Annual					
PE Full physical exam	Y or N	Annual					
Eye exam	Re or C	Annual					
Foot exam	Re or C	q visit					
Self Care SMBG and records	S or SME	q visit					
Meal plan	S or SME	q visit					
Physical activity	S or SME	q visit					
Medication instruction	S or SME	q visit					
Tobacco cessation	S or SME	q visit					

Legend: C = Completed; Re = Referred; F = Fasting; R = Random; SME = Self-Management Education Referral; S = Satisfactory

This flow sheet indicates recommended services to be provided in the continuing care of persons with diabetes. The frequency of each service is a recommendation from the American Diabetes Association. Document values where indicated. Any discussions with patients or significant others should be documented in the "notes" section in date order.

Signature	initials	Signature	initials

Figure 24-3 Diabetes provider clinical protocol. (From Donna Zazworsky, Director of Home Health and Outreach, and Pat Hiller, Consultant, St. Elizabeth of Hungary Clinic, Tucson, Arizona, 2000.)

After evaluating these two components, the final component must not be overlooked—likelihood to action. This component has to do with the benefits and barriers to the desired behavior change. If cost, transportation, or time is not addressed, then the likelihood of behavior change will be jeopardized.

Another model that helps to direct behavior change is Prochaska's Stages of Change Model (1992). In this model, the health educator identifies the behavioral stage of the individual. These stages are dynamic and will vary with individuals in regard to different health behaviors. In the Precontemplation stage, an individual may not know that there is a health problem. It is in this stage that an individual may attend a health fair and have a blood pressure check done only to find out that he or she may have high blood pressure.

In the Contemplation stage, an individual acknowledges that there is a problem and is thinking (contemplating) what actions to take—or if he or she wants to take actions. This is the stage where the health educator can provide more information (brochures, Website information) to help the individual move toward taking action.

In the Action stage, the individual sees a physician or nurse practitioner to verify and treat his or her blood pressure problem. This person may also start on a diet to lose weight. It is critical at this stage that providers be supportive and offer regular feedback on success or relapses.

The Maintenance stage is the most difficult, because this is the commitment to lifestyle change. Eating healthy foods, regular exercise, or not smoking are easy to start but hard to maintain. A provider may suggest a support group, such as Weight Watchers, to help the individual with a long-term strategy.

Finally, the provider cannot overlook the Relapse stage. Many providers will help the individual develop a relapse prevention plan to identify triggers for relapse (e.g., emotional, physical) and strategies to derail the relapse. The key is the ability for the provider to recognize where the individual is in their stages of change and how to guide the individual through the stages.

In addition to these models, providers must have an appreciation for, and appropriate application of, adult learning modalities. They must understand the following:

- When is it best to provide individual education or encourage the person to participate in a group?
- Simply telling a patient about their disease and self-care management is not as effective as having that person perform a return demonstration.

Information Management

An information management system must provide the feedback that is needed to track and demonstrate outcomes identified by the DM team. The organization will need to assess its data sources and establish whether these sources will be able to do the following:

- Query the databases in a number of different ways for problem identification (e.g., ICD-9 code, DRG)
- Turn around reports quickly to provide the needed information for continuous quality improvement

- Provide triggers for high-cost users
- Track outcomes related to clinical, financial, and quality
- Track associated costs related to service utilization
- Mail merge for postcard reminders and targeted information

One pitfall of many administrators is the misconception that tracking service utilization and quality is an adequate DM program. On the contrary, unless the information systems can also accommodate clinical outcomes, such as changes in Hb A_{1c}, or reduction in CHF levels, the program is in essence a utilization management program only.

Outcomes Management

Managing outcomes in a DM program requires the following three categories of measurement indicators: (1) clinical, (2) financial, and (3) quality.

All three must be identified within a comprehensive program to determine structure and process improvements, as well as short- and long-term program success.

Clinical Outcomes

The keystone of a successful DM program is the emphasis placed on clinical outcomes. In other words, is the program really producing the changes in the disease process according to the individual's risk level in the defined disease? For example, when addressing a diabetes disease management program, the bottom line is to decrease and stabilize an individual's Hb A_{1c} within targeted ranges so that a reduction in complications will be realized. All patients would be managed according to the standard diabetes guidelines, which recommend quarterly provider visits. Nevertheless, the higher-risk–stratified individuals would receive the greatest intensity of support services to more aggressively manage their disease.

Setting specific clinical outcomes will better direct service delivery (costs) and quality measurements. Following through on the diabetic example, case management activities and other services (such as individual nutrition counseling) can be focused on those individuals with high Hb A_{1c}s. The intent is to target more intervention strategies (e.g., case management) according to the individuals with higher-risk needs. The lower- and moderate-risk–stratified individuals would still be monitored according to the quarterly clinical protocols but would receive less costly interventions, such as group education and support. The assumption here is that the low- or moderate-risk individuals are managing adequately but still need regular motivation through individual and group activities.

Other clinical outcomes examples include improved respiratory status as measured by lung function testing; improved functional status, mobility, and strength as measured by a manual muscle test and a range of motion test; or improved hemoglobin levels in patients undergoing dialysis.

Financial Outcomes

Financial outcomes are associated with service utilization and complications. For example, CHF is commonly targeted for DM programs because the return on investment is quickly realized through reduced hospital readmission rates. This means that the investment that an organization makes initially to implement a CHF identification process and intervention strategy such as telephonic case management and patient education pays off through avoidance of unnecessary hospital admissions (Venner and Seelbinder, 1996).

Other financial outcomes include reduced length of stay, reduced pharmacy expenses, reduced physician/clinic visits, and reduced surgeries.

Quality Outcomes

Quality outcomes relate to the quality indicators of the program itself. How satisfied are the patients, providers, and health services? Has quality of life improved? All of these indicators have standardized tools for measurement and must be incorporated into the DM program as the third element of outcomes.

An outcomes grid illustrates the areas of measurement that are proposed to be evaluated within each DM program (Table 24-1). Once the grid is completed, a more in-depth process of identification of targets and benchmarks will be established. This is sometimes referred to as a *balance sheet* or a *report card*.

Balance Sheet

The balance sheet is a monthly worksheet that contributes to the continuous quality improvement (CQI) program. This sheet records the following elements:

- The outcome indicators identified for the disease
- The targets to be achieved based on local or national benchmarks
- The "numbers" and "percentages" of individuals meeting the targets
- The "numbers" and "percentages" falling outside the targets, called *variances*
- The reasons for the variances

Table 24-2 presents an example of a balance sheet for diabetes in a clinical setting.

TABLE 24-1
Sample Outcomes Grid

Disease	Clinical Indicator	Financial Indicator	Quality Indicator
CHF	CHF status	Reduced no. of readmission costs	Provider satisfaction
Diabetes	Hb A_{1c}	Reduced no. of amputations	Quality of life: depression
Hip fractures	Improved strength	Reduced no. of hip fracture hospitalizations	Patient satisfaction

CHF, Congestive heart failure.

TABLE 24-2
Balance Sheet for Diabetes in a Clinic Setting: High and Moderate-High Risk

Outcome Indicator	Target/ Benchmark	Number Met Target (%)	Number Variances (%)	Variance Reasons
Hb A$_{1c}$	<8	13 out of 26 (50%) High risk	13 (50%)	Not taking diabetic medications as prescribed because unable to pay for them ($n = 10$) Not following diet ($n = 3$)
Hospitalizations for amputations	<5% of population	0 out of 26	0	
Quality of life: depression	Some, little, or none of the time	20 out of 26	6 (23%)	Poor financial resources to support medication and diet regimen

From Case Manager Solutions, LLC, Tucson, Arizona, 2001.

Continuous Quality Improvement

The CQI process is a well-established vehicle to improve program effectiveness and efficiency. The simple steps of plan-do-check-act (PDCA) (Deming, 1986) are easy to implement but often are overlooked because of the need to closely and carefully track data. Therefore the critical issue of establishing a reliable and easy to access information system methodology must be reiterated.

THE FAST APPROACH TO DISEASE MANAGEMENT

The FAST Approach (Lamb and Zazworsky, 2000) to DM is action oriented and based on the assumption that to effectively care for at-risk populations, there must be a system in place for rapid identification, triage, monitoring, and communication. The FAST components are as follows:

- *Find:* Identify high-risk/high-volume populations using multiple sources, including service use data, pharmacy data, and easy-access referral forms in physician offices.
- *Assess:* Conduct a brief assessment to determine risk for hospitalization, severe complications of chronic illness, and skilled facility placement. Assessments are repeated at key transition points.
- *Stratify:* Match individuals to clinical interventions according to risk level.
- *Treat, Train, and Track:* Follow at-risk individuals across interventions.

The FAST Approach to DM can be applied to any disease entity. It is basically a guideline for an organized DM program, allowing for a logical structure, process, and outcomes framework to be put in place.

Step 1: The Pilot

In 1997, CHF was identified as a major concern for the Carondelet Health Network (CHN), an integrated delivery network in Tucson, Arizona. A multidisciplinary team of physicians, administrators, and nurse case managers were assembled to take an in-depth look at this problem. A closer look at the data revealed that CHF readmission rate was 18% within 30 days and, more alarming, 41% readmission within 1 week posthospitalization.

A 6-month pilot was implemented using community nurse case managers. The results of the study demonstrated a dramatic reduction in readmission rates. The 30-day readmissions went from 18% to 8%, and the 1-week readmissions went from 41% to 0%. These significant findings, along with evidence-based guidelines for community nurse case managers, demonstrated the value of targeted approaches for chronically ill populations.

Step 2: Implementing FAST

Because the organization recognized the impact of a targeted approach, the next step was to focus on the managed care contracts that CHN had global capitated risk. An analysis of these two contracts demonstrated CHF was the number-one and number-three cause of admissions related to volume and costs, respectively. An immediate process was needed to demonstrate a return on investment within 6 months. Therefore the FAST Approach was implemented.

Find

A data management team was able to identify patients who were discharged from the hospital with a CHF diagnosis within the past 18 months. After cross-referencing this list with current case management and home health lists, as well as plan disenrollment lists, a final list of 586 patients was identified.

Assess

A team of five nurses and two health professionals were trained to perform telephone risk assessments to identify potential for hospitalizations using the PRA Plus tool (Boult, Pacala, and Boult, 1995) and a second questionnaire specific to CHF to assess disease self-management. In less than 6 weeks, over 400 individuals were contacted and risk assessed by telephone.

Stratify

Over 400 individuals assessed were then assigned to community nursing interventions depending on their low-, moderate-, or high-risk status. Risk status was primarily dependent on the PRA Plus score; however, the telephone assessor would also take into consideration the CHF Disease Self-Management score to determine if the individual should be placed in a higher- or lower-risk category. The low-risk patients were referred to group education classes either provided by the health plan or the CHN community health centers. The moderate-risk patients were given appointments to meet individually with the nurse practitioner (NP) at one of the community health centers. The high-risk patients were assigned a community nurse case manager who would visit them in their homes.

Track

Daily hospital and ED admissions were tracked through the Carondelet Community Referral Service—a hub for DM and community referrals from the CHN hospitals and physicians. Monthly RUN charts were provided by the data management team to demonstrate inpatient admissions/1000, ED visits/1000, and patient days/1000 based on DRG 127 and the ICD-9 428.

Step 3: Findings

With the ability to track the data closely, the CHF DM team was able to identify problems early and make adjustments accordingly. For example, after the first month of tracking, the team identified that only a small number of low- and moderate-risk patients were willing to attend classes or see the NP for an individual appointment (Table 24-3). Most patients only wanted a telephone follow-up (49%). Conversely, the low- and moderate-risk patients were showing up in the ED for CHF-related problems. Therefore the team quickly revamped the interventions to a telephonic model for all patients using the two community nurse case managers. The result was a decrease in low- and moderate-risk patients showing up in the ED the next month.

Although the RUN charts demonstrated a consistent decrease in all measurements for a consecutive 3-month period, the organization continued to experience negative results overall with their global capitation managed care contracts. In March 1999, CHN renegotiated these contracts back to a fee-for-service model and no longer had the incentive structure to maintain the DM program. Thus the CHF program was discontinued.

TABLE 24-3
Health Plan Comparison of Congestive Heart Failure Data

Plan	Plan A	Plan B
Nursing case management	17% (43)	28% (33)
Telephone follow-up	52% (107)	45% (52)
Referred to CHN classes	12% (26)	2% (2)*
Referred to community health centers for individual NP visit	5% (12)	7% (6)
One-time home visit†	12% (24)	9% (8)
Referred to community nursing case management after one-time home visit	20% (5)	13% (1)

CHN, Carondelet Health Network; NP, nurse practitioner.
*Only indicates referrals to Carondelet congestive heart failure (CHF) classes and not the health plan CHF classes.
†Refers to recommended home visit based on CHF Disease Self-Management Questionnaire but low- or moderate-risk PRA Plus score.

   This change in cost management strategy is the reality of today's volatile healthcare markets. No longer is there the luxury to take 6 to 12 months to demonstrate cost savings. Healthcare organizations must be able to respond more quickly, which is reason enough to try the FAST Approach.

NURSING CASE MANAGEMENT IMPLICATIONS

Nurse case managers provide a vital role in DM programs. It is within a DM framework that nurse case managers demonstrate their greatest impact in clinical, financial, and quality outcomes through management of high-risk subgroups. Therefore it is critical for the case management system to establish a system of structure and process that tracks interventions and delivers outcomes.

Establish a Well-Rounded Documentation System

A good documentation system for case management must capture interventions and changes in knowledge, behavior, and health status. The Omaha System (Martin, Leak, and Aden, 1992) is a popular documentation system for community case management. Developed by the Visiting Nurses Association of Omaha, Nebraska, this tool provides a common language and Likert scale measurement for knowledge, behavior, and health status (KBS).

   Many hospital-based case managers use some type of clinical pathway system to document and track variances and outcomes. Other hospital and community-based case management programs only track resource and utilization management information.

Identify Visit Strategies and Rationale

Nurse case managers are most recognized in a hospital- or insurance-based setting. These settings dictate the type of visits; hospital-based case managers see patients in the hospital only while they are hospitalized, whereas insurance-based case managers tend to practice telephonically due to their regional or national territories (Mahn and Zazworsky, 2000).

   Community-based case managers, whether in independent practice or with an MCO or hospital, usually provide a combination of visits—hospital, home, community, and telephonic. These visits are more costly and time-consuming but can yield the best results when targeting a high-risk subpopulation through a DM program.

Track Interventions, Activities, and Outcomes

Tracking case management interventions, activities, and outcomes follows the same course as any other tracking system. There must be accountability for case management time spent in the following areas:

- Direct care, such as visits and telephone calls
- Indirect care, such as documentation, data entry, and patient conferences
- Administrative, such as CQI meetings and data collection
- Professional education

In addition, tracking patient outcomes becomes another important case management function with the analysis of documentation reports and other reports, such as the balance sheet, which is generated to track the disease and provide valuable input into the CQI process.

SUMMARY

DM is in the forefront of most healthcare organizations and employer groups. It is a critical component to cost control and quality. Nurses are in a key position within DM programs, but they must not be complacent and assume their position is steadfast.

Nurses must demonstrate their value. Documenting clinical, financial, and quality outcomes will strengthen their position within an organization or may even provide a new avenue for independent practice. Either way, nurses have an opportunity to offer a valuable expertise in any DM program.

REFERENCES

Agency for Health Care Policy and Research: *Clinical practice guideline no. 11, heart failure: evaluation and care of patients with left-ventricular systolic dysfunction,* Pub No 94-0612, Rockville, Md, 1994, US Department of Health and Human Services.

Becker MH: *The health belief model and personal health behavior,* Thorofare, NJ, 1974, Charles B Slack.

Boult C, Pacala JT, Boult LB: Targeting elders for geriatric evaluation and management: reliability, validity, and practicality of a questionnaire, *Aging (Milano)* 7(3):159-164, 1995.

Cesta TG, Tahan H, Fink L: *The case manager's survival guide: winning strategies for clinical practice,* St Louis, 1997, Mosby.

Deming WE: *Out of crisis,* Cambridge, Mass, 1986, Center for Advanced Engineering Study, Massachusetts Institute of Technology.

Eichert JH, Patterson RB: Factors affecting the success of disease management, *J Oncol Manag* 7(1):15-18, 1998.

Goldman L, Hashimoto B, Cook EF, et al: Comparative reproducibility and validity of systems for assessing cardiovascular functional class: advantages of a new specific activity scale, *Circulation* 64(6):1227-1234, 1981.

Harrison MB, Toman C, Logan J: Hospital to home: evidence-based education for CHF, *Can Nurse* 94(2):36-42, 1998.

Lamb GS, Zazworsky D: Improving outcomes fast: The FAST approach to disease management, *Advance for Providers of Post-Acute Care* 3(11):28-29, 2000.

Lamb GS, Mahn V, Dahl R: Using data to design systems of care adults with chronic illness, *Manag Care Q* 4(3):46-53, 1996.

Mahn V, Zazworsky D: The advanced practice nurse case manager. In Hamric AB, Spross JA, Hanson CM, editors: *Advanced nursing practice: an integrative approach,* Philadelphia, 2000, WB Saunders.

Martin K, Leak G, Aden C: The Omaha system: a research-based model for decision making, *J Nurs Admin* 22(11):47-52, 1992.

National Multiple Sclerosis Society: *Minimal record of disability for multiple sclerosis,* New York, 1985, The Society.

Parsons K: Personal communication, October 12, 2000.

Peterson KW, Kane DP: Beyond disease management: population-based health management. In Todd WE, Nash D: *Disease management: a systems approach to improving patient outcomes,* Chicago, 1998, American Hospital Association Publications.

Plocher DW: Disease management. In Kongstvedt PR, editor: *The managed care handbook,* ed 3, Gaithersburg, Md, 1996, Aspen.

Prochaska JO, DiClemente CC, Norcross JC: In search of how people change: applications to addictive behaviors, *Am Psychol* 47(9):1102-1114, 1992.

Shelton P, Sager MA, Schraeder C: The community assessment risk screen (CARS): identifying elderly persons at risk for hospitalization or emergency department visit, *Am J Manag Care* 6(8):925-933, 2000.

Todd WE, Nash D: *Disease management: a systems approach to improving patient outcomes,* Chicago, 1998, American Hospital Association.

Venner GH, Seelbinder JS: Team management of congestive heart failure across the continuum, *J Cardiovasc Nurs* 10(2):71-84, 1996.

Ware JE, Snow KK, Dosinski M, et al: *SF-36 health survey manual and interpretation guide,* Boston, 1993, The Health Institute, New England Medical Center.

Wedsicha JA, Bestall JC, Garrod R, et al: Randomized controlled trial of pulmonary rehabilitation in severe chronic obstructive pulmonary disease patients, stratified with the MRC dyspnoea scale, *Eur Respir J* 12:363-369, 1998.

Zander K: Classic nursing management skills and disease management: something old, something new, *Semin Nurse Manag* 5(2):85-90, 1997.

25

Workers' Compensation in Managed Care

Deborah V. DiBenedetto

KEY LESSONS IN THIS CHAPTER

- Although workers' compensation has a small effect on the overall healthcare dollars spent today, its impact is great in terms of its cost to employers.
- Workers' compensation managed care manages costs and lost work time and helps employees return to work.
- Because workers' compensation pays for both medical care and lost wages, it is important that medical providers recognize the financial impact of keeping a person off the job or disabled from work.
- Employers should refer to the disability duration guidelines when determining when employees can return to work.
- Nurses play many important roles in managing the return-to-work process, including direct care, case management, health education, and facilitation.

Workers' compensation (WC) is a no-fault system of benefits provided to employees who sustain injuries and illnesses in the course of their employment. Injuries sustained on the job or in the course of employment are considered occupational. WC laws, first enacted in 1911, provide coverage for occupational injuries and illness and are no-fault or an "exclusive remedy." Before 1911, injured workers had to sue their employers for the cost of medical care and monetary damages. Under WC, injured workers give up some or all of their right to sue for an occupational injury or sustained illness in exchange for medical care, payment of lost wages (indemnity payments), and vocational rehabilitation. To qualify for WC benefits, a person must have incurred an injury or illness that arises out of and in the course of employment, and he or she must incur medical costs, rehabilitation costs, lost wages, or disfigurement. WC is a state-mandated program that covers all employees; each state determines the scope and payment of WC benefits under the respective state's WC law (DiBenedetto et al, 1990-1998).

FINANCIAL IMPACT OF WORKERS' COMPENSATION

Many employers see the cost of dealing with occupational injures as a cost of doing business. Today WC constitutes only about 3% of total medical expenditures; however, 11 million employees suffer work-related injuries, resulting in $111 billion in payments for medical care, wage replacement, and disability payments. More than 50% of the $111 billion is associated with the payment of lost wages (Stefanchek, 1998), and more than 40% to 60% equals the cost of WC medical care (Benda et al, 1998). Studies show that medical care delivered in an unmanaged environment can be as much as 2½ times more costly than caring for the same injury (sustained off the job) under a group health plan or non-WC plan (Stefanchek, 1998; Parry, 1999). On average, 24% of work-related injuries result in lost work time, with an average cost of $19,000 per claim; in a managed care environment, the same claim costs an average of $13,500. Of employers who channel employees to a managed care environment or preferred providers, significant cost savings are further realized (Walter, 1998).

INTEGRATED BENEFIT INITIATIVES AND IMPACT ON WORKERS' COMPENSATION PROGRAMS

Managed Care for Occupational Injuries and Illnesses

In an effort to better manage the double-digit inflation of WC medical care in the late 1980s and 1990s, states began allowing the use of managed care arrangements to lower the cost of occupational injuries and illnesses. WC managed care differs significantly from group health managed care in several ways (Table 25-1). WC managed care requires the management of not only the medical care but the person's disability or lost time from work as well. Because WC pays for both medical care and lost wages (i.e., lost workdays), it is important that medical providers recognize the impact of keeping a person off the job or disabled from work as a result of the occupational injury.

The general objectives for WC managed medical care are as follows (Olin, 1998):
- Controlling the cost of WC claims by achieving the fastest maximum medical improvement
- Securing the earliest return to work (RTW) feasible, given the nature of the workers' injury
- Ensuring the delivery of cost-effective, quality medical care

Managed care techniques have long been part of the WC system, although they may not have been identified as *managed care*. Another term often used is *managed comp*, which indicates that some components of management have been put in place to manage the cost of the WC claim, resultant medical care, lost work time, and other associated costs of the claim (Parry, 1999; DiBenedetto et al, 1996-2002).

TABLE 25-1
Essential Differences Between Group Health and Workers' Compensation Managed Care Models

Element	Group Health	Workers' Compensation
Incidence of injury and illness	Predictable in aggregate for large populations Minimal employer role for incidence Occurs "off-the-job" (nonoccupational) Reflects demographics of workforce and their dependents	Unpredictable Finite relationship to work environment—arises out of and in course of employment Employer accountability for incurred injuries and illnesses Injuries can be prevented through safe work practices and limiting hazard exposures
Medical management or gatekeeper role	PCP; may be generalist, internist, or specialist With females, PCP may be ob/gyn	Requires knowledge of occupational health and medicine On-site employer, occupational health nurse, or physician may be primary contact or gatekeeper Needs appropriately staffed, knowledgeable providers with ready access to medical facility
Medical care	Progressive Often conservative, delays for non-emergency care No emphasis on RTW or disability management	Aggressive, sports medicine approach Emphasis on returning employee to normal functioning and work in timely manner State may have specific treatment guidelines or protocols that must be followed by physician
System financing	Employer-funded, some movement toward "self-insurance" with larger employers Funding may be community rated vs. employer-based Downstream risk sharing Not linked to wage replacement or disability costs Medical care payments limited to coverage in plan or per plan design and employment May preclude payment for motor vehicle (no-fault) injuries	Protracted treatment and lost work days add to cost of WC program Generally funded on fee-for-service, discounted fee schedules Limited use of capitation Medical coverage may last to age 65 or lifetime Reimbursement only if injury/illness is occupational

From DV DiBenedetto & Associates LTD, 1999. (Modified from The Vincam Group, Coral Gables, Florida.)
PCP, Primary care physician; *RTW,* return to work; *WC,* workers' compensation.

Characteristics of WC managed care include the use of the following (DiBenedetto et al, 1996-2002):

- Preferred providers or WC networks
- Negotiated fee schedules or capitated rates
- Treatment protocols
- Disability duration guidelines
- Case management
- Aggressive, facilitated, and early RTW
- Utilization review (UR) and quality assurance

Preferred Providers/Networks

In many states, employers have been able to direct their insured workers to a panel of preferred physicians who are familiar with the WC system and the management of occupational injuries and illnesses. Most often, these medical providers are specialists in occupational health and medicine. The control of the physician panel is a powerful cost-control technique (Stefanchek, 1998). In more recent years, states have allowed the development of formal WC provider networks and preferred provider arrangements. The establishment of these managed comp medical arrangements is a movement that recognizes the need to have an integrated approach to managing both the medical and disability aspects of the case, that is, controlling both healthcare and wage replacement costs.

Because WC pays for both medical care and lost wages (i.e., lost workdays), it is important that medical providers recognize the financial impact of keeping a person off the job or disabled from work. WC managed care differs from group health managed care, in which delivery of medical care and services may be more conservative. In WC, the provider is expected to aggressively assess the injured workers' current condition, provide diagnostic procedures, and plan care, which returns the injured workers to health and normal functioning, including timely RTW.

Providers who care for injured workers must know and understand the employee's work environment and the essential functions of that person's job and work responsibilities to effectively plan care and help the worker return to work as soon as medically possible. It is recommended that treating physicians or provider representatives visit the various workplaces and have a keen understanding of the specific employer workplace issues, exposures, and RTW policies. WC managed care providers must be knowledgeable about the following:

- Occupational health and medicine
- Plant or workplace safety, ergonomics, and preventive work procedures
- The myriad regulations, including WC laws, that affect the delivery of medical care and effective case management

Negotiated Fee Schedules/Capitated Rates

Each state has a different payment or reimbursement methodology for medical care delivered under its WC program. Some states have a standard fee schedule that provides a set dollar amount for care rendered, whereas others use the prevailing "reasonable and customary" fee-for-service methodology. In the WC managed care arena, several payment options have been identified, including the following (Olin, 1998; DiBenedetto et al, 1996-2002):

- Unit-based pricing
- Use of discounted state fee schedules
- Medical services delivered as a fixed percentage of the WC premium
- Capitated arrangements

In states that have established fee schedules, many WC managed care providers or networks will discount the fee schedule by a certain percentage. In some cases, the fee schedule remains at 100%, but the network administrator may discount reimbursement to the providers, keeping the differential to "pay" for administration of the plan or program.

A survey by the American College of Occupational and Environmental Medicine (ACOEM) in 1996 queried its members about their involvement in managed care. Approximately 8% of the 600 respondents indicated that they received over half of their income from managed care arrangements but generally not from a case rate or capitated basis (Harris, 1998).

Treatment Protocols

The ACOEM has developed clinical practice guidelines for potentially work-related health problems in worker populations, which are based on the following (Harris, 1998):

- Presenting complaints
- Emphasis on prevention
- Proper clinical evaluation
- Provision of guidance for medical and disability management

The guidelines are relatively unique in that they address the entire spectrum of management of a presenting problem rather than focusing on a specific diagnosis or procedure, assuming that the diagnosis is correct or that the procedure is warranted.

The guidelines emphasize and advocate using a medical approach of activity limitation and functional recovery, rather than having workers assume a "sick role." The goals of the guidelines include the following (Harris, 1998):

- Providing uniform information to a diverse group of practitioners who care for or manage potentially work-related health concerns
- Providing guidance for case management
- Speeding functional recovery
- Improving the quality of care for potentially work-related health problems, including the following:
  - Improvements in appropriateness
  - Efficiency
  - Effectiveness
  - Reduction of variation in practice

The scope of present complaints include neck, upper back, shoulder, elbow, forearm, wrist, hand, lower back, knee, ankle, foot, and acute eye. The occupational health practitioner should know the scope of treatment, which will ultimately help the worker return to normal functioning as soon as possible. Over 21 states have established treatment guidelines for WC injuries, which may be mandated by the municipality. (Massachusetts has 26 mandatory treatment guidelines.) Although no one specific national treatment plan exists for the myriad of health issues and complaints, the ACOEM guidelines provide a means to evaluate and manage medical care of workers using an occupational medicine approach (DiBenedetto et al, 1996-2002).

Disability Duration Guidelines

When can a person return to work? At what point along the healthcare continuum should RTW be expected? What tools are available for employers, providers, and payers to determine reasonable time frames for return to normal functioning and work? The answer lies in the use of *disability duration guidelines*. Specified recovery guidelines establish a benchmark, or an expected time frame during which a worker recovers from his or her disability. Persons with the same diagnosis or medical condition will recover at different rates and be able to return to work within a general time frame; however, recovery is as variable as a person's individuality. Disability and ability to return to work also depend on the worker's healing or adaptation to illness or injury and the scope of his or her job functions. A variety of disability duration guidelines are available to determine the potential length of a worker's absence due to injury or illness, including *The Medical Disability Advisor*, Workloss Data Institute's *Occupational Disability Guidelines*, and Milliman & Robertson's *Healthcare Management Guidelines*. These guidelines provide both theoretical and evidence-based lengths of disability (DiBenedetto et al, 1996-2002).

Case Management

Case management is a dynamic and cost-effective tool for managing both occupational and nonoccupational disability. In the managed WC arena, it is most often provided by registered professional nurses with an occupational health or insurance background. The focus of WC case management is to help the ill or injured person achieve the highest level of medical improvement and to facilitate his or her successful RTW in the most cost-effective manner (DiBenedetto et al, 1996-2002). The case manager may work for the employer, insurance carrier, managed care organization, or private third-party company. The case manager's primary role is that of advocate to ensure that the injured worker navigates the medical environment, complies with treatment, and works to facilitate his or her timely return to productivity and work as soon as medically possible. The case manager may also function as a benefits administrator for the employer, thus providing a higher level of case coordination with the physician, employee, and supervisor. The case manager may assist with access to or help create the employee's job task analysis, supervisor education, RTW, and follow-up (Harris, 1998). As more employers manage both occupational and nonoccupational lost-time cases consistently, the case manager will generally be more knowledgeable about the employee's medical history, prior claim activities, and periods of disability. The case manager acts as an advocate for the employee and ultimately the employer to facilitate the employee's effective RTW. The physician will find the case manager a highly knowledgeable colleague and a member of the disability management team whose knowledge will augment the medical plan of care and ultimately assist with positive case outcomes, specifically decreased periods of disability through effective RTW.

Aggressive, Facilitated, and Early Return to Work

Over 50% of the cost of WC is associated with the payment of lost wages (DiBenedetto et al, 1996-2002). Injured workers generally receive some percentage of their full pay, often receiving more than they usually receive, since WC benefits are not taxed. Each day the physician keeps a worker off-the-job or disabled, costs are incurred, even though the cost of medical care is capped, or managed. To return an employee to work, the provider must know what work the employee is required to do and what the essential functions of the job entail. Many times, what the employee tells the provider is vastly different from actuality. In addition, job title alone does not necessarily dictate actual job responsibilities. Effective RTW planning requires knowledge of the person's job functions, physical demands, and required physical abilities. The use of functional capacity examinations is an objective measurement process to determine a worker's physical ability to execute certain physical tasks and actions. Both insurers and employers may request independent medical examinations to confirm a person's medical status and ability to return to work or need for job accommodation (DiBenedetto et al, 1996-2002).

Many employers have modified duty or alternate work arrangements available for workers. In fact, it is often easier to get a WC claimant back to work than a person who is disabled from a nonoccupational injury or illness because employers and supervisors recognize the relationship between lost work time and its impact on the cost of the WC program. Barriers to effective RTW include the following:

- Unavailability of modified work
- Supervisor and/or employee discord
- Lack of communication between the provider, employer, and employee
- Medical issues that preclude safe RTW and psychosocial issues that impede or prevent the worker from reentering the workforce
- Transportation issues

Many employees return to a level of normal functioning but are unable to tolerate their commute to work. This problem is a significant barrier to effective RTW, but neither the employer nor the doctor is responsible for the employee getting to work. Once a person is medically capable of meeting his or her job task responsibilities and there is work available at the employer's work site, the employee should be released to work. Often the employer, insurer, or case manager can help investigate alternative means of transportation that are appropriate, given the situation.

Work hardening is a form of physical therapy that mimics actual work demands or job tasks and functions. Actual exercises and work-simulated activities are monitored by a professional healthcare worker, generally a registered physical therapist, who helps the employee gradually build up job task tolerance (DiBenedetto et al, 1996-2002).

Injured workers with permanent disabilities are protected under the Americans with Disabilities Act (ADA). The provider needs to let the insurer and employer know as soon as possible if an employee's injury will result in permanent disability and loss of functioning. If a resultant medical condition limits the person's ability to perform the essential functions of his or her job, the employer is obligated to consider reasonable accommodations that would allow the employee to return to work.

If injured workers are unable to return to work or if they have a permanent disability that precludes them from executing the work for which they were hired and trained, the WC system provides vocational rehabilitation. The injured worker will have assistance from qualified vocational rehabilitation counselors (also considered to be case managers) in assessing their vocational and RTW options. Vocational rehabilitation may be provided by the respective state's Office of Vocational Rehabilitation or through the private sector (insurers or independent third parties).

UTILIZATION REVIEW AND QUALITY ASSURANCE

UR is performed on a retrospective, concurrent, and prospective basis in managed WC programs. In managed care arrangements, routine medical care is usually provided under the purview of the treating physician or gatekeeper. UR is required in most states and forms the basis for reimbursement, especially in a fee-for-service, or fee-schedule WC system. It is important to provide all relevant medical information to the carrier or adjuster for approval of medical procedures. In true managed care arrangements, the cost of the care is part of the managed care contract, and the provider or network assumes the actual cost of care. Most managed WC programs operate on a noncapitated basis, however, and thus UR is an important tool in managing access and cost of care, especially in nonemergency situations. The longer the wait for approval, many times the carrier requires independent medical opinions to confirm the need for specialized care or treatment, and the impact on indemnity payments is heightened. Thus the longer the wait for care, the more lost workdays ensue.

Many states require that WC managed care organizations demonstrate appropriate delivery of care through establishing UR and quality assurance programs with distinct lines of accountability to the state. To respond to the public need, the American Accreditation Healthcare Commission/Utilization Review Accreditation Commission (URAC),* has established the only national standards for accrediting WC/UR programs and provider networks. Because each state defines the components of its WC managed care program and there is considerable variation in the scope of programs and delivery of care, national accreditation by a recognized quality assurance body is imperative to protect public interests regarding care delivery.

URAC is a not-for-profit entity founded in 1990 to establish accreditation standards for managed healthcare organizations. Generally, states recognize URAC accreditation for management of both WC networks and UR programs in one of the following two ways: (1) *deemed status,* in which the accredited programs are exempt from some or all of the respective state's licensure requirements, or (2) *mandated status,* in which accreditation by URAC is required as a condition of state licensure.

---

*For more information, see the URAC Website: http://www.urac.org.

SUMMARY

The delivery of WC managed care has been evolving to more than just "discounted health care for occupational injuries and illnesses" (Nikolaj, 1998, p 380). WC managed care has a broader focus that includes prevention of work-related injuries, including environmental scanning and assessment for safety and health hazards; injury-prevention programs that are workplace-specific; and employee training, education, and information on safe and healthy work practices (DiBenedetto et al, 1996-2002). The WC managed care market is moving toward integrated benefits and is of ultimate value when part of an employer's overall disability management strategy, which is a concerted effort to manage both occupational and nonoccupational injuries and illnesses and resultant lost work time in a consistent manner.

In WC, there is a direct connection between the person's medical status, the providers' findings, and the employee's eligibility for wage replacement. Although the employee is eligible for a percentage of lost wages, it is imperative that treatment is rendered within the context of a sports medicine approach, meaning that treatment is provided immediately with a focus on returning the individual to his or her preinjury state, and that the individual returns to work as soon as medically possible. Providers should release the injured worker to modified duty or alternate work as soon as it is practical. Most employers have alternate work arrangements available. The sooner an employee returns to work, the greater the cost savings. The combination of managed care and aggressive RTW efforts saves both the cost of medical care and indemnity (wage replacement) payments. As states continue to move toward a managed approach to WC medical care, the medical and business communities must be proactive in ensuring that all workers have timely and appropriate medical care with an eye on the end goals: facilitated return to normal functioning and return to productivity, or return to work.

REFERENCES

Benda CG et al: *Liability and risk management in managed care*, Gaithersburg, Md, 1998, Aspen.

DiBenedetto DV et al: *The OEM occupational health and safety manual*, Beverly Farms, Mass, 1990-1998, OEM Press.

DiBenedetto DV et al: *Principles of workers' compensation and disability case management course*, Yonkers, NY, 1996-2002, DV DiBenedetto & Associates, Ltd.

Harris J: *Managed care: occupational medicine state of the art reviews*, Philadelphia, 1998, Hanley & Belfus.

Nikolaj S: *Healthcare management in workers' compensation: occupational medicine state of the art reviews*, Philadelphia, 1998, Hanley & Belfus.

Olin M: *The Standard guide to workers' compensation*, ed 4, Boston, 1998, Standard.

Parry T: *Occupational versus nonoccupational benefits: looking beyond system aggregate experience*, San Francisco, 1999, Integrated Benefits Institute.

Stefanchek MG: *WC managed care sourcebook: new strategies for success in a growing marketplace*, New York, 1998, Faulkner & Gray.

Walter JM: *Managed care can help reduce your workers' comp costs: occupational hazards*, Waco, Tex, 1998, Stevens.

ADDITIONAL READINGS

American College of Occupational and Environmental Medicine Position Statement: *Eight best ideas for workers' compensation reform*, Chicago, 1997, ACOEM.

DiBenedetto DV: *Workers' compensation and disability management: OEM report,* OEM Health Information, Beverly Farms, Mass, 1995, OEM Press.

DiBenedetto DV: *Total health and productivity management: foundation for integrated benefit programs, OEM report,* Beverly Farms, Mass, 1999, OEM Press.

Leopold RS: *OEM internet companion: summer update,* Beverly Farms, Mass, 1997, OEM Press.

Workers' compensation third-party claim management information sourcebook and survey results, Stamford, Conn, 1999, Tillinghast-Towers Perrin Consulting.

1999 Workers' compensation year book, Washington, DC, 1998, LRP.

I·N·D·E·X